ATS-104 ADMISSION TEST SERIES

This is your PASSBOOK for...

U.S. Medical Licensing Examination (USMLE)

Test Preparation Study Guide Questions & Answers

NLC®

NATIONAL LEARNING CORPORATION®

National Learning Corporation

212 Michael Drive, Syosset, NY 11791
(516) 921-8888 • www.passbooks.com
E-mail: info@passbooks.com

PUBLISHED IN THE UNITED STATES OF AMERICA

PASSBOOK® SERIES

THE *PASSBOOK® SERIES* has been created to prepare applicants and candidates for the ultimate academic battlefield – the examination room.

At some time in our lives, each and every one of us may be required to take an examination – for validation, matriculation, admission, qualification, registration, certification, or licensure.

Based on the assumption that every applicant or candidate has met the basic formal educational standards, has taken the required number of courses, and read the necessary texts, the *PASSBOOK® SERIES* furnishes the one special preparation which may assure passing with confidence, instead of failing with insecurity. Examination questions – together with answers – are furnished as the basic vehicle for study so that the mysteries of the examination and its compounding difficulties may be eliminated or diminished by a sure method.

This book is meant to help you pass your examination provided that you qualify and are serious in your objective.

The entire field is reviewed through the huge store of content information which is succinctly presented through a provocative and challenging approach – the question-and-answer method.

A climate of success is established by furnishing the correct answers at the end of each test.

You soon learn to recognize types of questions, forms of questions, and patterns of questioning. You may even begin to anticipate expected outcomes.

You perceive that many questions are repeated or adapted so that you can gain acute insights, which may enable you to score many sure points.

You learn how to confront new questions, or types of questions, and to attack them confidently and work out the correct answers.

You note objectives and emphases, and recognize pitfalls and dangers, so that you may make positive educational adjustments.

Moreover, you are kept fully informed in relation to new concepts, methods, practices, and directions in the field.

You discover that you are actually taking the examination all the time: you are preparing for the examination by "taking" an examination, not by reading extraneous and/or supererogatory textbooks.

In short, this PASSBOOK®, used directedly, should be an important factor in helping you to pass your test.

UNITED STATES MEDICAL LICENSING EXAMINATION®
(USMLE®)

INTRODUCTION

The United States Medical Licensing Examination® (USMLE®) is a three-step examination for medical licensure in the United States and is sponsored by the Federation of State Medical Boards (FSMB) and the National Board of Medical Examiners® (NBME®). The Composite Committee, appointed by the FSMB and NBME, establishes policies for the USMLE program. Membership includes representatives from the FSMB, NBME, Educational Commission for Foreign Medical Graduates (ECFMG®), and the American public.

The USMLE assesses a physician's ability to apply knowledge, concepts, and principles, and to demonstrate fundamental patient-centered skills, that are important in health and disease and that constitute the basis of safe and effective patient care. Each of the three Steps complements the others; no Step can stand alone in the assessment of readiness for medical licensure. Because individual medical licensing authorities make decisions regarding use of USMLE results, you should contact the jurisdiction where you intend to apply for licensure to obtain complete information. Also, the FSMB can provide general information on medical licensure.

THE THREE STEPS OF THE USMLE

Step 1 assesses whether you understand and can apply important concepts of the sciences basic to the practice of medicine, with special emphasis on principles and mechanisms underlying health, disease, and modes of therapy. Step 1 ensures mastery of not only the sciences that provide a foundation for the safe and competent practice of medicine in the present, but also the scientific principles required for the maintenance of competence through lifelong learning.

Step 2 assesses whether you can apply medical knowledge, skills, and understanding of clinical science essential for the provision of patient care under supervision and includes emphasis on health promotion and disease prevention. Step 2 ensures that due attention is devoted to principles of clinical sciences and basic patient-centered skills that provide the foundation for the safe and competent practice of medicine.

Step 3 assesses whether you can apply medical knowledge and understanding of biomedical and clinical science essential for the unsupervised practice of medicine, with emphasis on patient management in ambulatory settings. Step 3 provides a final assessment of physicians assuming independent responsibility for delivering general medical care.

STEP 1

Step 1 includes test items in the following content areas:

- anatomy
- behavioral sciences
- biochemistry
- microbiology
- pathology
- pharmacology
- physiology
- interdisciplinary topics, such as nutrition, genetics and aging.

Step 1 is a broadly based, integrated examination. Test items commonly require you to perform one or more of the following tasks:

- interpret graphic and tabular material;
- identify gross and microscopic pathologic and normal specimens;
- apply basic science knowledge to clinical problems.

Step 1 classifies test items along two dimensions: system and process, as shown in the following table:

System**

25%–35% General principles

65%–75% Individual organ systems

- hematopoietic/lymphoreticular
- nervous/special senses
- skin/connective tissue
- musculoskeletal
- respiratory
- cardiovascular
- gastrointestinal
- renal/urinary
- reproductive
- endocrine
- immune

Process

20%–30% Normal structure and function

40%–50% Abnormal processes

15%–25% Principles of therapeutics

10%–20% Psychosocial, cultural, occupational and environmental considerations

* Percentages are subject to change at any time. See the USMLE website for the most up-to-date information.

** The general principles category includes test items concerning those normal and abnormal processes that are not limited to specific organ systems. Categories for individual organ systems include test items concerning those normal and abnormal processes that are system specific.

STEP 2 – Clinical Knowledge (CK)

Step 2 CK includes test items in the following content areas:

- internal medicine
- obstetrics and gynecology
- pediatrics
- preventive medicine
- psychiatry
- surgery
- other areas relevant to provision of care under supervision

Most Step 2 CK test items describe clinical situations and require that you provide one or more of the following:

- diagnosis
- prognosis
- indication of underlying mechanisms of disease
- the next step in medical care, including preventive measures

Step 2 CK is a broadly based, integrated examination. It frequently requires interpretation of tables and laboratory data, imaging studies, photographs of gross and microscopic pathologic specimens, and results of other diagnostic studies. Step 2 CK classifies test items along two dimensions: disease category and physician task, as shown in the following table:

Normal Conditions and Disease Categories

- Normal growth and development and general principles of care
- Individual organ systems or types of disorders
    - immunologic disorders
    - diseases of the blood and blood-forming organs
    - mental disorders
    - diseases of the nervous system and special senses
    - cardiovascular disorders
    - diseases of the respiratory system
    - nutritional and digestive disorders
    - gynecologic disorders
    - renal, urinary, and male reproductive systems
    - disorders of pregnancy, childbirth, and the puerperium
    - disorders of the skin and subcutaneous tissue
    - diseases of the musculoskeletal system and connective tissue
    - endocrine and metabolic disorders

Physician Task

15%–20% Promoting preventive medicine and health maintenance
20%–35% Understanding mechanisms of disease
25%–40% Establishing a diagnosis
15%–25% Applying principles of management

* Percentages are subject to change at any time. See the USMLE website for the most up-to-date information.

STEP 2 – CLINICAL SKILLS (CS)

Step 2 CS assesses whether you can demonstrate the fundamental clinical skills essential for safe and effective patient care under supervision. There are three subcomponents of Step 2 CS (see Table 3): Integrated Clinical Encounter (ICE), Communication and Interpersonal Skills (CIS), and Spoken English Proficiency (SEP).

Step 2 CS uses standardized patients, i.e., people trained to portray real patients. You are expected to establish rapport with the patients, elicit pertinent historical information from them, perform focused physical examinations, answer questions, and provide counseling when appropriate. After each interaction with a patient, you will record pertinent history and physical examination findings, list diagnostic impressions, and outline plans for further evaluation, if necessary. The cases cover common and important situations that a physician is likely to encounter in common medical practice in clinics, doctors' offices, emergency departments, and hospital settings in the United States.

The cases that make up each administration of the Step 2 CS examination are based upon an examination blueprint. An examination blueprint defines the requirements for each examination, regardless of where and when it is administered. The sample of cases selected for each examination reflects a balance of cases that is fair and equitable across all examinees. While the set of cases administered on a given day will differ from the set of cases administered on another day, each set of cases is comparable.

The intent is to ensure that examinees encounter a broad spectrum of cases reflecting common and important symptoms and diagnoses. The criteria that are used to define the blueprint and create individual examinations focus primarily on presenting complaints and conditions. Presentation categories include, but are not limited to, cardiovascular, constitutional, gastrointestinal, genitourinary, musculoskeletal, neurological, psychiatric, respiratory, and women's health. Examinees will see cases from some, but not all, of these categories. The selection of cases is also guided by specifications relating to acuity, age, gender, and type of physical findings presented in each case.

The Subcomponents of Step 2 CS

Integrated Clinical Encounter (ICE)

- Data gathering – patient information collected by history taking and physical examination
- Documentation – completion of a patient note summarizing the findings of the patient encounter, diagnostic impression, and initial patient workup

Communication and Interpersonal Skills (CIS)

- Questioning skills
- Information-sharing skills
- Professional manner and rapport

Spoken English Proficiency (SEP)

- Clarity of spoken English communication within the context of the doctor-patient encounter

STEP 3

Step 3 is organized along two principal dimensions: clinical encounter frame and physician task. Step 3 content reflects a data-based model of generalist medical practice in the United States.

Encounter frames capture the essential features of circumstances surrounding physicians' clinical activity with patients. They range from encounters with patients seen for the first time for non-emergency problems, to encounters with regular patients seen in the context of continued care, to patient encounters in (life-threatening) emergency situations. Encounters occur in clinics, offices, skilled nursing care facilities, hospitals, emergency departments, and on the telephone. Each test item in an encounter frame also represents one of the six physician tasks. For example, initial care encounters emphasize taking a history and performing a physical examination. In contrast, continued care encounters emphasize decisions regarding prognosis and management.

High-frequency, high-impact diseases also have an effect on how the content of Step 3 is organized. Clinician experts assign clinical problems related to these diseases to individual clinical encounter frames to represent their occurrence in generalist practice.

USMLE Step 3 Specifications*

Clinical Encounter Frame

20%–30% Initial care
50%–60% Continued care
15%–25% Emergency care

Physician Task

8%–12% Obtaining history and performing physical examination
8%–12% Using laboratory and diagnostic studies
8%–12% Formulating most likely diagnosis
8%–12% Evaluating severity of patient's problems
8%–12% Applying scientific concepts and mechanisms of disease
45%–55% Managing the patient

- health maintenance
- clinical intervention
- clinical therapeutics
- legal and ethical issues

Primum® Computer-Based Case Simulations (CCS)

Step 3 examinees test using two formats: multiple-choice questions and *Primum* computer-based case simulations (CCS), a testing format that allows you to provide care for a simulated patient. You decide which diagnostic information to obtain and how to treat and monitor the patient's progress. The computer records each step you take in caring for the patient and scores your overall performance. This format permits assessment of clinical decision-making skills in a more realistic and integrated manner than other available formats.

In *Primum* CCS, you may request information from the history and physical examination; order laboratory studies, procedures, and consultants; and start medications and other therapies. Any of the thousands of possible entries that you type on the "order sheet" are processed and verified by the "clerk." When you have confirmed that there is nothing further you wish to do, you decide when to reevaluate the patient by advancing simulated time. As time passes, the patient's condition changes based on the underlying problem and your interventions; results of tests are reported, and results of interventions must be monitored. You suspend the movement of simulated time as you consider next steps. While you cannot go back in time, you can change your orders to reflect your updated management plan.

The patient's chart contains, in addition to the order sheet, the reports resulting from your orders. By selecting the appropriate chart tabs, you can review vital signs, progress notes, patient updates, and test results. You may care for and move the patient among the office, home, emergency department, intensive care unit, and hospital ward.

The cases used in the CCS portion of the Step 3 examination are based upon a CCS examination blueprint. The blueprint defines the requirements for CCS examination forms. The CCS blueprint is used to construct CCS examination forms focusing primarily on presenting symptoms and presenting locations. Presenting symptoms relate to the Step 3 Problem/Disease List and are associated with the central nervous system, eye/ear/nose/mouth/throat, respiratory system, circulatory system, digestive system, behavioral/emotional disorders, musculoskeletal system, skin/subcutaneous tissue, endocrine/nutrition/metabolic disorders, kidneys/urinary tract, reproductive system, pregnancy/childbirth, neonate/childhood illnesses, blood and blood-forming organs, infectious/parasitic diseases, injuries/wound/toxic effects/burns, and health maintenance issues. Presenting locations include the outpatient office, emergency department, inpatient unit, intensive care unit, and the patient's home.

You will see cases related to some, but not all, of these problem/disease and location categories. The intent is to ensure that all examinees encounter a broad range of cases reflecting common and important symptoms and diagnoses. The selection of cases is also guided by specifications relating to age and gender. Each CCS examination form is structured to reflect a balance of cases that is fair and equitable for all examinees.

Test Lengths and Formats

Step 1 has approximately 322 multiple-choice test items, divided into seven 60-minute blocks, administered in one eight-hour testing session.

Step 2 CK has approximately 352 multiple-choice test items, divided into eight 60-minute blocks, administered in one nine-hour testing session.

Step 2 CS has 12 patient cases. You will have 15 minutes for each patient encounter and 10 minutes to record each patient note. If you do not use the entire 15 minutes for the patient encounter, the remaining time will be added to the time you have to record the patient note. The testing session is approximately eight hours.

Step 3 has approximately 480 multiple-choice test items, divided into blocks of 35 to 50 items. You will have 45 to 60 minutes to complete each of these blocks. There are approximately nine computer-based case simulations, with one case in each block. You will have a maximum of 25 minutes to complete each of these blocks. Step 3 is administered in two eight-hour testing sessions.

HOW TO TAKE A TEST

You have studied long, hard and conscientiously.

With your official admission card in hand, and your heart pounding, you have been admitted to the examination room.

You note that there are several hundred other applicants in the examination room waiting to take the same test.

They all appear to be equally well prepared.

You know that nothing but your best effort will suffice. The "moment of truth" is at hand: you now have to demonstrate objectively, in writing, your knowledge of content and your understanding of subject matter.

You are fighting the most important battle of your life—to pass and/or score high on an examination which will determine your career and provide the economic basis for your livelihood.

What extra, special things should you know and should you do in taking the examination?

I. YOU MUST PASS AN EXAMINATION

A. WHAT EVERY CANDIDATE SHOULD KNOW

Examination applicants often ask us for help in preparing for the written test. What can I study in advance? What kinds of questions will be asked? How will the test be given? How will the papers be graded?

B. HOW ARE EXAMS DEVELOPED?

Examinations are carefully written by trained technicians who are specialists in the field known as "psychological measurement," in consultation with recognized authorities in the field of work that the test will cover. These experts recommend the subject matter areas or skills to be tested; only those knowledges or skills important to your success on the job are included. The most reliable books and source materials available are used as references. Together, the experts and technicians judge the difficulty level of the questions.

Test technicians know how to phrase questions so that the problem is clearly stated. Their ethics do not permit "trick" or "catch" questions. Questions may have been tried out on sample groups, or subjected to statistical analysis, to determine their usefulness.

Written tests are often used in combination with performance tests, ratings of training and experience, and oral interviews. All of these measures combine to form the best-known means of finding the right person for the right job.

II. HOW TO PASS THE WRITTEN TEST

A. BASIC STEPS

1) Study the announcement

How, then, can you know what subjects to study? Our best answer is: "Learn as much as possible about the class of positions for which you've applied." The exam will test the knowledge, skills and abilities needed to do the work.

Your most valuable source of information about the position you want is the official exam announcement. This announcement lists the training and experience qualifications. Check these standards and apply only if you come reasonably close to meeting them. Many jurisdictions preview the written test in the exam announcement by including a section called "Knowledge and Abilities Required," "Scope of the Examination," or some similar heading. Here you will find out specifically what fields will be tested.

2) Choose appropriate study materials

If the position for which you are applying is technical or advanced, you will read more advanced, specialized material. If you are already familiar with the basic principles of your field, elementary textbooks would waste your time. Concentrate on advanced textbooks and technical periodicals. Think through the concepts and review difficult problems in your field.

These are all general sources. You can get more ideas on your own initiative, following these leads. For example, training manuals and publications of the government agency which employs workers in your field can be useful, particularly for technical and professional positions. A letter or visit to the government department involved may result in more specific study suggestions, and certainly will provide you with a more definite idea of the exact nature of the position you are seeking.

3) Study this book!

III. KINDS OF TESTS

Tests are used for purposes other than measuring knowledge and ability to perform specified duties. For some positions, it is equally important to test ability to make adjustments to new situations or to profit from training. In others, basic mental abilities not dependent on information are essential. Questions which test these things may not appear as pertinent to the duties of the position as those which test for knowledge and information. Yet they are often highly important parts of a fair examination. For very general questions, it is almost impossible to help you direct your study efforts. What we can do is to point out some of the more common of these general abilities needed in public service positions and describe some typical questions.

1) General information

Broad, general information has been found useful for predicting job success in some kinds of work. This is tested in a variety of ways, from vocabulary lists to questions about current events. Basic background in some field of work, such as sociology or economics, may be sampled in a group of questions. Often these are principles which have become familiar to most persons through exposure rather than through formal training. It is difficult to advise you how to study for these questions; being alert to the world around you is our best suggestion.

2) Verbal ability

An example of an ability needed in many positions is verbal or language ability. Verbal ability is, in brief, the ability to use and understand words. Vocabulary and grammar tests are typical measures of this ability. Reading comprehension or paragraph interpretation questions are common in many kinds of civil service tests. You are given a paragraph of written material and asked to find its central meaning.

IV. KINDS OF QUESTIONS

1. Multiple-choice Questions

Most popular of the short-answer questions is the "multiple choice" or "best answer" question. It can be used, for example, to test for factual knowledge, ability to solve problems or judgment in meeting situations found at work.

A multiple-choice question is normally one of three types:

- It can begin with an incomplete statement followed by several possible endings. You are to find the one ending which best completes the statement, although some of the others may not be entirely wrong.
- It can also be a complete statement in the form of a question which is answered by choosing one of the statements listed.
- It can be in the form of a problem – again you select the best answer.

Here is an example of a multiple-choice question with a discussion which should give you some clues as to the method for choosing the right answer:

When an employee has a complaint about his assignment, the action which will best help him overcome his difficulty is to

A. discuss his difficulty with his coworkers
B. take the problem to the head of the organization
C. take the problem to the person who gave him the assignment
D. say nothing to anyone about his complaint

In answering this question, you should study each of the choices to find which is best. Consider choice "A" – Certainly an employee may discuss his complaint with fellow employees, but no change or improvement can result, and the complaint remains unresolved. Choice "B" is a poor choice since the head of the organization probably does not know what assignment you have been given, and taking your problem to him is known as "going over the head" of the supervisor. The supervisor, or person who made the assignment, is the person who can clarify it or correct any injustice. Choice "C" is, therefore, correct. To say nothing, as in choice "D," is unwise. Supervisors have and interest in knowing the problems employees are facing, and the employee is seeking a solution to his problem.

2. True/False

3. Matching Questions

Matching an answer from a column of choices within another column.

V. RECORDING YOUR ANSWERS

Computer terminals are used more and more today for many different kinds of exams.

For an examination with very few applicants, you may be told to record your answers in the test booklet itself. Separate answer sheets are much more common. If this separate answer sheet is to be scored by machine – and this is often the case – it is highly important that you mark your answers correctly in order to get credit.

VI. BEFORE THE TEST

YOUR PHYSICAL CONDITION IS IMPORTANT

If you are not well, you can't do your best work on tests. If you are half asleep, you can't do your best either. Here are some tips:

1) Get about the same amount of sleep you usually get. Don't stay up all night before the test, either partying or worrying—DON'T DO IT!
2) If you wear glasses, be sure to wear them when you go to take the test. This goes for hearing aids, too.
3) If you have any physical problems that may keep you from doing your best, be sure to tell the person giving the test. If you are sick or in poor health, you relay cannot do your best on any test. You can always come back and take the test some other time.

Common sense will help you find procedures to follow to get ready for an examination. Too many of us, however, overlook these sensible measures. Indeed, nervousness and fatigue have been found to be the most serious reasons why applicants fail to do their best on civil service tests. Here is a list of reminders:

- Begin your preparation early – Don't wait until the last minute to go scurrying around for books and materials or to find out what the position is all about.
- Prepare continuously – An hour a night for a week is better than an all-night cram session. This has been definitely established. What is more, a night a week for a month will return better dividends than crowding your study into a shorter period of time.
- Locate the place of the exam – You have been sent a notice telling you when and where to report for the examination. If the location is in a different town or otherwise unfamiliar to you, it would be well to inquire the best route and learn something about the building.
- Relax the night before the test – Allow your mind to rest. Do not study at all that night. Plan some mild recreation or diversion; then go to bed early and get a good night's sleep.
- Get up early enough to make a leisurely trip to the place for the test – This way unforeseen events, traffic snarls, unfamiliar buildings, etc. will not upset you.
- Dress comfortably – A written test is not a fashion show. You will be known by number and not by name, so wear something comfortable.
- Leave excess paraphernalia at home – Shopping bags and odd bundles will get in your way. You need bring only the items mentioned in the official notice you received; usually everything you need is provided. Do not bring reference books to the exam. They will only confuse those last minutes and be taken away from you when in the test room.

- Arrive somewhat ahead of time – If because of transportation schedules you must get there very early, bring a newspaper or magazine to take your mind off yourself while waiting.
- Locate the examination room – When you have found the proper room, you will be directed to the seat or part of the room where you will sit. Sometimes you are given a sheet of instructions to read while you are waiting. Do not fill out any forms until you are told to do so; just read them and be prepared.
- Relax and prepare to listen to the instructions
- If you have any physical problem that may keep you from doing your best, be sure to tell the test administrator. If you are sick or in poor health, you really cannot do your best on the exam. You can come back and take the test some other time.

VII. AT THE TEST

The day of the test is here and you have the test booklet in your hand. The temptation to get going is very strong. Caution! There is more to success than knowing the right answers. You must know how to identify your papers and understand variations in the type of short-answer question used in this particular examination. Follow these suggestions for maximum results from your efforts:

1) Cooperate with the monitor

The test administrator has a duty to create a situation in which you can be as much at ease as possible. He will give instructions, tell you when to begin, check to see that you are marking your answer sheet correctly, and so on. He is not there to guard you, although he will see that your competitors do not take unfair advantage. He wants to help you do your best.

2) Listen to all instructions

Don't jump the gun! Wait until you understand all directions. In most civil service tests you get more time than you need to answer the questions. So don't be in a hurry. Read each word of instructions until you clearly understand the meaning. Study the examples, listen to all announcements and follow directions. Ask questions if you do not understand what to do.

3) Identify your papers

Civil service exams are usually identified by number only. You will be assigned a number; you must not put your name on your test papers. Be sure to copy your number correctly. Since more than one exam may be given, copy your exact examination title.

4) Plan your time

Unless you are told that a test is a "speed" or "rate of work" test, speed itself is usually not important. Time enough to answer all the questions will be provided, but this does not mean that you have all day. An overall time limit has been set. Divide the total time (in minutes) by the number of questions to determine the approximate time you have for each question.

5) Do not linger over difficult questions

If you come across a difficult question, mark it with a paper clip (useful to have along) and come back to it when you have been through the booklet. One caution if you do this – be sure to skip a number on your answer sheet as well. Check often to be sure that you have not lost your place and that you are marking in the row numbered the same as the question you are answering.

6) Read the questions

Be sure you know what the question asks! Many capable people are unsuccessful because they failed to read the questions correctly.

7) Answer all questions

Unless you have been instructed that a penalty will be deducted for incorrect answers, it is better to guess than to omit a question.

8) Speed tests

It is often better NOT to guess on speed tests. It has been found that on timed tests people are tempted to spend the last few seconds before time is called in marking answers at random – without even reading them – in the hope of picking up a few extra points. To discourage this practice, the instructions may warn you that your score will be "corrected" for guessing. That is, a penalty will be applied. The incorrect answers will be deducted from the correct ones, or some other penalty formula will be used.

9) Review your answers

If you finish before time is called, go back to the questions you guessed or omitted to give them further thought. Review other answers if you have time.

10) Return your test materials

If you are ready to leave before others have finished or time is called, take ALL your materials to the monitor and leave quietly. Never take any test material with you. The monitor can discover whose papers are not complete, and taking a test booklet may be grounds for disqualification.

VIII. EXAMINATION TECHNIQUES

1) Read the general instructions carefully. These are usually printed on the first page of the exam booklet. As a rule, these instructions refer to the timing of the examination; the fact that you should not start work until the signal and must stop work at a signal, etc. If there are any special instructions, such as a choice of questions to be answered, make sure that you note this instruction carefully.

2) When you are ready to start work on the examination, that is as soon as the signal has been given, read the instructions to each question booklet, underline any key words or phrases, such as least, best, outline, describe and the like. In this way you will tend to answer as requested rather than discover on reviewing your paper that you listed without describing, that you selected the worst choice rather than the best choice, etc.

3) If the examination is of the objective or multiple-choice type – that is, each question will also give a series of possible answers: A, B, C or D, and you are called upon to select the best answer and write the letter next to that answer on your answer paper – it is advisable to start answering each question in turn. There may be anywhere from 50 to 100 such questions in the three or four hours allotted and you can see how much time would be taken if you read through all the questions before beginning to answer any. Furthermore, if you

come across a question or group of questions which you know would be difficult to answer, it would undoubtedly affect your handling of all the other questions.

4) If the examination is of the essay type and contains but a few questions, it is a moot point as to whether you should read all the questions before starting to answer any one. Of course, if you are given a choice – say five out of seven and the like – then it is essential to read all the questions so you can eliminate the two that are most difficult. If, however, you are asked to answer all the questions, there may be danger in trying to answer the easiest one first because you may find that you will spend too much time on it. The best technique is to answer the first question, then proceed to the second, etc.

5) Time your answers. Before the exam begins, write down the time it started, then add the time allowed for the examination and write down the time it must be completed, then divide the time available somewhat as follows:
   - If 3-1/2 hours are allowed, that would be 210 minutes. If you have 80 objective-type questions, that would be an average of 2-1/2 minutes per question. Allow yourself no more than 2 minutes per question, or a total of 160 minutes, which will permit about 50 minutes to review.
   - If for the time allotment of 210 minutes there are 7 essay questions to answer, that would average about 30 minutes a question. Give yourself only 25 minutes per question so that you have about 35 minutes to review.

6) The most important instruction is to read each question and make sure you know what is wanted. The second most important instruction is to time yourself properly so that you answer every question. The third most important instruction is to answer every question. Guess if you have to but include something for each question. Remember that you will receive no credit for a blank and will probably receive some credit if you write something in answer to an essay question. If you guess a letter – say "B" for a multiple-choice question – you may have guessed right. If you leave a blank as an answer to a multiple-choice question, the examiners may respect your feelings but it will not add a point to your score. Some exams may penalize you for wrong answers, so in such cases only, you may not want to guess unless you have some basis for your answer.

7) Suggestions
   a. Objective-type questions
      1. Examine the question booklet for proper sequence of pages and questions
      2. Read all instructions carefully
      3. Skip any question which seems too difficult; return to it after all other questions have been answered
      4. Apportion your time properly; do not spend too much time on any single question or group of questions
      5. Note and underline key words – all, most, fewest, least, best, worst, same, opposite, etc.
      6. Pay particular attention to negatives
      7. Note unusual option, e.g., unduly long, short, complex, different or similar in content to the body of the question
      8. Observe the use of "hedging" words – probably, may, most likely, etc.

9. Make sure that your answer is put next to the same number as the question
10. Do not second-guess unless you have good reason to believe the second answer is definitely more correct
11. Cross out original answer if you decide another answer is more accurate; do not erase until you are ready to hand your paper in
12. Answer all questions; guess unless instructed otherwise
13. Leave time for review

b. Essay questions
1. Read each question carefully
2. Determine exactly what is wanted. Underline key words or phrases.
3. Decide on outline or paragraph answer
4. Include many different points and elements unless asked to develop any one or two points or elements
5. Show impartiality by giving pros and cons unless directed to select one side only
6. Make and write down any assumptions you find necessary to answer the questions
7. Watch your English, grammar, punctuation and choice of words
8. Time your answers; don't crowd material

8) Answering the essay question

Most essay questions can be answered by framing the specific response around several key words or ideas. Here are a few such key words or ideas:

M's: manpower, materials, methods, money, management
P's: purpose, program, policy, plan, procedure, practice, problems, pitfalls, personnel, public relations

a. Six basic steps in handling problems:
1. Preliminary plan and background development
2. Collect information, data and facts
3. Analyze and interpret information, data and facts
4. Analyze and develop solutions as well as make recommendations
5. Prepare report and sell recommendations
6. Install recommendations and follow up effectiveness

b. Pitfalls to avoid
1. Taking things for granted – A statement of the situation does not necessarily imply that each of the elements is necessarily true; for example, a complaint may be invalid and biased so that all that can be taken for granted is that a complaint has been registered
2. Considering only one side of a situation – Wherever possible, indicate several alternatives and then point out the reasons you selected the best one
3. Failing to indicate follow up – Whenever your answer indicates action on your part, make certain that you will take proper follow-up action to see how successful your recommendations, procedures or actions turn out to be
4. Taking too long in answering any single question – Remember to time your answers properly

EXAMINATION SECTION

EXAMINATION SECTION
TEST 1

DIRECTIONS: Each question or incomplete statement is followed by several suggested answers or completions. Select the one that BEST answers the question or completes the statement. *PRINT THE LETTER OF THE CORRECT ANSWER IN THE SPACE AT THE RIGHT.*

1. The pain, fever, and headache of acute maxillary sinusitis may be BEST relieved by 1.____

   A. penicillin
   B. adequate drainage
   C. aureomycin
   D. autogenous vaccine

2. The course of *virus* tracheobronchitis will be shortened by treatment with 2.____

   A. aerosol penicillin
   B. aureomycin
   C. erythromycin
   D. none of the above

3. The treatment of choice for infectious hepatitis is 3.____

   A. bed rest and diet
   B. methionine
   C. aureomycin
   D. intraheptol

4. A comatose patient has a clearcut history and clinical findings indicating a brain tumor in the posterior fossa of the skull. 4.____
   Of the following, the MOST dangerous diagnostic procedure is

   A. lumbar puncture
   B. vertebral artery angiogram
   C. electroencephalogram
   D. ventroculogram

5. The PRIMARY objective of the procedure known as debride-ment of an accidental wound is to 5.____

   A. remove contaminating bacteria
   B. excise skin and thus promote open drainage of the wound
   C. remove non-viable tissue
   D. permit the immediate closure of the skin wound

6. A patient complains of low back pain after a fall. There is anaesthesia about the external malleolus and an absent ankle jerk. 6.____
   The MOST likely diagnosis is

   A. spinal cord tumor
   B. herniated intervertebral disk
   C. sciatica
   D. sacroiliac sprain

7. A 40-year-old man presents with a spontaneous fracture of the femur, severe anemia, marked weight loss, enlarged liver, mild clinical icterus, multiple vitamin deficiencies, and a history of moderate diarrhea for several months. 7.____
   The one of the following diagnoses which is MOST likely, presuming all the above findings relate to a single disorder, is

   A. sprue syndrome
   B. cirrhosis of the liver
   C. pernicious anemia
   D. pellagra

8. Patients with chronic tophaceous gout 8.____

A. rarely die as a result of their disease
B. rarely have severe arteriosclerosis
C. seldom have articular destruction
D. seldom have related renal disease

9. The combination of low back pain and urinary retention in a 55-year-old man should warrant, in addition to other examinations, the determination of the 9.____

A. alkaline phosphatase
B. plasma protease
C. serum amylase
D. acid phosphatase

10. An elevated serum calcium concentration often appears in the course of 10.____

A. sarcoidosis
B. myxedema
C. hypoparathyroidism
D. uremia due to chronic diffuse glomerulonephritis

11. Nephrocalcinosis is MOST characteristic of 11.____

A. Paget's disease, hyperparathyroidism, myositis ossificans
B. tuberculosis of the kidneys, vitamin D intoxication, hyperparathyroidism
C. hyperparathyroidism, vitamin C intoxication, renal tubular necrosis
D. Paget's disease, tuberculosis of the kidneys, renal tubular necrosis

12. A patient with chronic sinusitis and associated recurrent respiratory tract infections develops intractable productive coughing with occasional small hemoptysis. 12.____
The one of the following diagnostic procedures which would be MOST significant in establishing a diagnosis of bronchiectasis is

A. an x-ray of the chest
B. a bronchogram
C. laryngoscopy
D. examination of sputum for 3 layer formation

13. The one of the following disease in which examination of the bone marrow is LEAST likely to be helpful in establishing the diagnosis is 13.____

A. aplastic anemia
B. leukemia
C. Hodgkin's disease
D. hypersplenism syndrome

14. Of the following tests, the one which would be MOST diagnostic of rheumatoid arthritis is 14.____

A. antistreptolysin-O determination
B. blood calcium and phosphorus determination
C. erythrocyte sedimentation test
D. hemolytic streptococcus agglutination test

15. The sudden onset of pain radiating down the back of the left leg with the finding of an absent ankle jerk on the left in a previously well 40-year-old patrolman suggests the diagnosis of 15.____

A. sciatic neuritis
B. lumbosacral sprain
C. tabetic crisis
D. herniated vertebral disc

16. The MOST common type of surgical metabolic alkalosis due to an increase in bicarbonate ion results from 16.____

A. vomiting
B. diarrhea
C. sweating
D. high urine output

17. The one of the following laboratory determinations which has the GREATEST value in establishing a diagnosis of prostatic carcinoma is elevated blood serum 17.____

A. acid phosphatase
B. chloride
C. cholesterol
D. potassium

18. A patient has been on gastric suction for five days. It is noted on rounds that there is moderate cyanosis, the pulse rate is 90, the blood pressure reading 86/60 mm. Hg, and there is a positive Chvostek's sign. The MOST likely diagnosis is 18.____

A. perforated ulcer
B. hypochloremic alkalosis
C. acidosis
D. gastrointestinal hemorrhage

19. Coma due to acute alcoholism is associated with 19.____

A. high blood level of alcohol
B. Battle's sign
C. spinal fluid oozing from the nose
D. hemiplegia

20. Silicosis is caused by the dust of 20.____

A. coal
B. silicates
C. iron
D. silica

21. Occupational lead poisoning in the United States is MOST frequently acquired by 21.____

A. absorption through the skin
B. ingestion
C. inhalation
D. implantation from trauma

22. A patient develops nausea, vomiting, and diarrhea a few hours after having eaten a *contaminated* meal.
The MOST probable etiology is acute 22.____

A. trichiniasis
B. bacillary dysentery
C. botulism
D. staphylococcal toxin poisoning

23. Increased severity of infection following cessation of the administration of ACTH or cortisone is MOST likely to occur when either of the drugs has been given to patients with 23.____

A. viral diseases
B. bacterial endocarditis
C. staphylococcal sepsis
D. tuberculosis

24. Published data up to the present time indicate that the one of the following which has an especially effective symbiotic antibacterial action is 24.____

A. bacitracin-sulfadiazine
B. terramycin-aureomycin
C. penicillin-streptomycin
D. penicillin-chloramphenicol

25. The quantity of NaCl in the spinal fluid is characteristically reduced in ______ meningitis. 25.____

A. meningococcus
B. syphilitic
C. tuberculous
D. pneumococcal

26. In the course of typhoid fever, a positive blood culture is MOST frequently obtained during the ______ week. 26.____

A. 1st
B. 2nd
C. 3rd
D. 4th

27. The association of normal urinary concentrating capacity and azotemia is consistent with the diagnosis of uremia in 27.____

A. unilateral atrophic pyelonephritis
B. acute malignant nephrosclerosis
C. polycystic renal disease
D. bilateral atrophic pyelonephritis

28. The normal renal whole blood flow per minute, as measured by the p-aminohippurate clearance, is MOST NEARLY ______ cc. 28.____

A. 300
B. 600
C. 1200
D. 2500

29. The normal renal glomerular filtration rate per minute, as measured by the insulin clearance, is MOST NEARLY ______ cc. 29.____

A. 75
B. 130
C. 600
D. 1200

30. Numerous elliptical calcific shadows about 1/2 inch in length are seen in several x-ray films of the four extremities of a patient.
These are MOST likely due to 30.____

A. buckshot
B. cysticercosis
C. Trichinella spiral is
D. bismuth injections

31. Acute amebic dysentery is MOST readily diagnosed by 31.____

A. proctoscopy
B. stool culture
C. direct smear of stool
D. complement fixation test

32. Brucellosia is an infectious disease of human beings which may be acquired through ingestion or through the skin.
The one of the following which CANNOT be a source of this infection is a 32.____

A. cow
B. goat
C. pig
D. horse

33. The mechanism explaining the clinical picture observed in carbon monoxide poisoning is 33.____

A. hemolysis of red blood cells
B. a chemical union of the carbon monoxide with the hemoglobin of the red blood cells
C. transformation of the carbon monoxide to carbon dioxide in the blood
D. arrest of oxidation in the tissues by enzyme interference

34. The one of the following solvents which is safest, toxi-cologically, for household dry cleaning is 34.____

A. benzine
B. benzene
C. carbon tetrachloride
D. benzol

35. The method of preventing occupational mercury poisoning which is generally considered to be LEAST desirable is 35.____

A. enclosing the hazardous process
B. rotating worker at intervals to less hazardous exposure
C. the use of masks or respirators
D. the use of exhaust ventilation

36. A 25-year-old man develops a unilateral plèural effusion of clear straw-colored fluid of high specific gravity. He complains of easy fatigue; and slight weight loss, a low grade fever, and a tender epididymis are the only positive clinical findings in addition to the foregoing. Of the following,the MOST probable diagnosis is 36.____

A. rheumatic fever
B. lupus erythematosus
C. bronchogenic carcinoma with pleural metastases
D. tuberculosis

37. In a patient with cough, fever, signs of shifting consolidation, and x-ray evidence of patchy consolidation, a cold agglutinin titer of 1:500 is observed on the tenth day of the disease. 37.____
This titer may be interpreted as

A. proof of the diagnosis of atypical virus pneumonia
B. compatible with but not proof of the diagnosis of atypical virus pneumonia
C. probably unrelated to the respiratory tract disease
D. pathognomonic evidence of primary (idiopathic) cryoglobulinemia

38. The MOST usual incubation period of tetanus in patients who have NOT received prophylactic treatment is ______ to ______ days. 38.____

A. 2; 3
B. 5; 10
C. 25; 28
D. 85; 90

39. Of the following, the one which is NOT a good index of the activity of the infection in the follow-up of a patient with known long-standing pulmonary tuberculosis, previously adequately treated, is 39.____

A. presence of post-tussic rales in the affected areas
B. presence of Koch's bacillus in sputum
C. erythrocyte sedimentation rate
D. body weight determined weekly

40. Amyl nitrite is used in the treatment of cyanide poisoning because it 40.____

A. forms methemoglobin which competes successfully with ferricytochrome for cyanide ions
B. improves the coronary circulation
C. combines directly with the cyanide ions
D. stimulates the respiratory center

41. The characteristic electrocardiographic alteration in hyperpotassemia is 41.___

A. elevation of the S-T segments
B. heart block
C. increase in the height of T waves
D. a variety of ectopic rhythms

42. The one of the following which is MOST useful in determining the cause of bronchial asthma in a patient is a(the) 42.___

A. history
B. skin test
C. sputum smear
D. eosinophile test

43. Following the use of a household cleaning compound to remove spots from his uniform, a policeman becomes jaundiced. 43.___
The compound which he used MOST probably c.ontained

A. lauryl sulfate
B. ammonia
C. benzine
D. carbon tetrachloride

44. A patient with inoperable bronchiectasis develops a progressive anemia in association with his chronic infection. 44.___
Of the following, the plan of specific therapy of the anemia which is indicated is administration of

A. repeated transfusions
B. vitamin B_{12} and colloidal iron by mouth
C. saccharated iron oxide intravenously
D. liver extract and Brewer's yeast by mouth

45. A routine x-ray in a 40-year-old man reveals a discrete, *soft,* round nodule less than 1 1/2 cm. in diameter in the periphery of the lower right lung field. 45.___
The one of the following procedures which should be followed is to

A. take no action since nodules of this type are insignificant
B. institute prompt anticoagulation therapy
C. plan prompt thoractomy and excision of nodule if its nature cannot otherwise be positively established
D. give a one month's trial of intensive chemotherapy with one or more antibiotics

46. A 64-year-old male with chronic pulmonary emphysema is admitted with acute pneumonia, is deeply cyanotic, and is immediately placed in an oxygen tent. He is maintained in a high oxygen atmosphere continuously for four days, at which time he is noted to go gradually into coma with a respiratory rate of 6 per minute, and to become increasingly cyanotic. The carbon dioxide content of the arterial blood was found to be 90 volumes percent. CORRECT treatment for this man is 46.___

A. administration of caffeine sodium benzoate
B. immediate removal from the oxygen tent and the use of intermittent oxygen only
C. increase in penicillin dosage
D. administration of aureomycin

47. A 40-year-old comatose male with cold, clammy skin, temperature 97°F., bilateral Babinski reflexes, no nuchal rigidity, and no other abnormal physical findings has a catheterized urine which shows albuminuria +, glucose ++, no acetone or diacetic, rare red blood cell and white blood cell per high power field. Serum area nitrogen is 23 mg./100 cc. Of the following, the BEST diagnosis is 47.____

A. diabetic acidosis
B. insulin shock
C. meningitis
D. uremia

48. Syncope following physical exertion suggests 48.____

A. adrenal cortical adenoma
B. pheochromocytoma
C. islet cell adenoma of pancreas
D. thyroid adenoma

49. Crooke's hyalinization of cells is COMMONLY associated with 49.____

A. diabetes mellitus
B. lupus erythematosus
C. Gushing's syndrome
D. acromegaly

50. Acrocyanosis is a disturbance of the 50.____

A. hemoglobin
B. capillary bed
C. platelets
D. red cells

KEY (CORRECT ANSWERS)

1. B	11. B	21. C	31. C	41. C
2. D	12. B	22. D	32. D	42. A
3. A	13. C	23. B	33. B	43. D
4. A	14. D	24. C	34. A	44. A
5. C	15. A	25. C	35. C	45. C
6. B	16. A	26. A	36. D	46. B
7. A	17. A	27. B	37. B	47. B
8. A	18. B	28. C	38. B	48. C
9. D	19. A	29. B	39. A	49. C
10. A	20. D	30. B	40. A	50. B

TEST 2

DIRECTIONS: Each question or incomplete statement is followed by several suggested answers or completions. Select the one that BEST answers the question or completes the statement. *PRINT THE LETTER OF THE CORRECT ANSWER IN THE SPACE AT THE RIGHT.*

1. The one of the following which is the BEST treatment for causalgia is 1.____

   A. rhizotomy
   B. chordotomy
   C. sympathectomy
   D. lobotomy

2. To sympathectomize the lower extremities successfully, one MUST 2.____

   A. remove lumbar ganglions 1-2-3
   B. remove lumbar ganglions 3-4-5
   C. section sympathetic trunk between dorsal ganglions 8-9
   D. remove ganglion chain from D6 to 15

3. A patient has a hard mass in the thyroid and osseous metastasis which shows moderate uptake of radioactive iodine. 3.____
   The OPTIMUM treatment in this case is

   A. total thyroidectomy and systemic radioactive iodine therapy
   B. total thyroidectomy and irradiation of the metastasis
   C. irradiation of the gland and the metastasis
   D. systemic radioactive iodine therapy alone

4. The one of the following with which Paget's disease of the bone (osteitis deformans) is MOST commonly associated is 4.____

   A. elevated serum calcium and diminished serum phosphorus
   B. elevated alkaline phosphatase
   C. elevated nonprotein nitrogen
   D. reversal of the albumin-globulin ratio

5. A bullet that may have grazed or perforated the ascending colon before lodging within the spinal canal has caused paraplegia. 5.____
   The one of the following which you would choose as the FIRST measure in treatment is

   A. laminectomy for removal of bullet
   B. observation for 24 hours
   C. exploratory laparotomy
   D. antibiotic therapy for 24 hours

6. A small pupil, ptosis of the upper eyelid, and enophthalmos (Norner's syndrome) indicate a spinal nerve root lesion at a vertebral level of 6.____

   A. cervical 1-2
   B. cervical 4-5
   C. cervical 7-thoracic 1
   D. thoracic 3-4

7. The diagnosis of bladder neck obstruction due to benign or malignant enlargement of the prostate gland is BEST established by 7.____

A. a cystogram
B. urethrocystoscopy
C. a rectal digital examination
D. determination of amount of residual urine

8. The anatomical structure USUALLY involved in the production of a direct inguinal hernia is 8.____

A. Poupart's ligament
B. conjoint tendon
C. external oblique fascia
D. transversalis fascia

9. The popliteal artery can be acutely occluded in the 6th decade and 9.____

A. there is no danger of gangrene
B. gangrene develops in 100 percent of cases
C. gangrene develops in two-thirds of cases
D. gangrene develops in not more than 10% of cases

10. Congenital arteriovenous fistulae of the forearm at times are accompanied by increased growth of the hand. 10.____
This is MOST probably due to the fact that

A. collateral arterial blood supply is stimulated by the fistulae and overnourishes the part
B. increased venous pressure distal to the fistulae influences growth
C. oxygen uptake by tissues distal to the fistulae is increased
D. oxygenated blood is diverted into the venous system and nourishes the part by retrograded flow

11. The age specific death rate for accidental death for males and females in the United States is HIGHEST in the age group 11.____

A. 5 through 14 years
B. 15 through 24 years
C. 25 through 44 years
D. 65 years and older

12. Following a *head cold,* a young man complains of slight dyspnea and a harassing cough productive of 1/2 -1 cup of non-foul, occasionally blood-streaked green mucopurulent sputum daily. Examination of the chest reveals scattered wheezes and rhonchi from apices to bases over both lung fields anteriorly, posteriorly, and in the axillae. The chest x-ray is negative. 12.____
The PROBABLE diagnosis of this illness is

A. viral pneumonia
B. acute tracheobronchitis
C. bronchial asthma
D. disseminated tuberculosis

13. A young policeman complains of low grade fever, malaise, headache, and increasing asthenia for one week. Physical examination shows a temperature of 101F. and hypertrophy of lymphoid tissue in posterior pharynx with generalized lymphadenopathy. The liver edge is palpable and tender and the edge of the spleen is palpable and tender. There is no icterus. 13.____
The diagnosis of this illness is MOST likely to be

A. infectious mononucleosis
B. Hodgkin's disease
C. acute leukemia
D. infectious hepatitis

14. Amebic hepatitis is BEST treated by 14.___

A. needle aspiration of liver and injection of emetine hydrochloride
B. open surgical drainage
C. radiation x-ray therapy
D. chloroquine therapy

15. A 55-year-old man complains of easy fatigue, night sweats, weight loss of two weeks duration. Examination of blood reveals 8,000 white blood cells per cubic millimeter, 3,000,000 red blood cells per cubic millimeter, hemoglobin of 12.5 gm./100 cc., diminished number of platelets, occasional nucleated red cells, and less than 1 percent immature white cells. 15.___
The one of the following diagnoses which is MOST unlikely is

A. pernicious anemia in relapse
B. aleukemic leukemia
C. lupus erythematosus disseminatus
D. multiple myeloma

16. A 55-year-old male, who has worked in the quarries of Barre, Vermont, complains of dyspnea, marked peripheral edema, and palpitations during the past three months. Examination reveals cyanosis, hepatomegaly, sinus tachycardia, fibrosis of the lungs, and an elevated venous pressure. 16.___
Treatment for this patient should include

A. no oxygen
B. quinidine to relieve the tachycardia
C. digitalization
D. a high carbohydrate diet

17. The MOST useful of the following tests in the diagnosis of a suspected case of disseminated lupus erythematosus would be 17.___

A. examination of the urine
B. examination of the bone marrow
C. examination of the blood for cold agglutinins
D. erythrocyte sedimentation test

18. The one of the following which does NOT occur in a patient receiving cortisone or corticotropin is 18.___

A. peptic ulcer
B. psychosis
C. retention of potassium
D. glycosuria

19. Of the following, the one which is NOT a collagen disease is 19.___

A. Hodgkin's disease
B. lupus erythematosus disseminatus
C. dermatomyositis
D. scleroderma

20. Recurrence of acute gout is BEST prevented by regular administration of small doses of 20.____

A. cinchophen
B. colchicine
C. salicylates
D. benemid

21. The one of the following drugs which is useful in the treatment of myasthenia gravis is 21.____

A. curare
B. neostigmine
C. cortisone
D. quinidine

22. The one of the following which is MOST helpful in establishing the diagnosis of polycystic renal disease is 22.____

A. retrograde pyelogram
B. asymptomatic uremia for a period of years
C. family history of polycystic renal disease
D. palpation of masses in both flanks

23. The longest periods of survival with uremia are USUALLY seen in patients with 23.____

A. chronic glomerulonephritis
B. polycystic renal disease
C. intercapillary glomerulosclerosis
D. unilateral atrophic pyelonephritis

24. Systolic hypertension is COMMONLY seen in association with 24.____

A. coarctation of the aorta
B. acute glomerulonephritis
C. sclerosis of the aorta
D. pheochromocytoma

25. A *paradoxical pulse* is USUALLY caused by 25.____

A. cardiac tamponade
B. myocardial infarction
C. cardiac decompensation
D. auricular fibrillation

26. A *paradoxical pulse* is characterized by 26.____

A. a faster rate during inspiration than during expiration
B. a faster rate during expiration than during inspiration
C. diminished force or absence during inspiration
D. inequality of rates at the cardiac apex and radial artery

27. Of the following agents, the one which produces a persistent increase in plasma volume is 27.____

A. dextran
B. norepinephrine
C. dextrose solution
D. saline solution

28. The child born of a mother who has had German measles during the last month of pregnancy is very apt to have 28.____

A. congenital cardiac defects
B. congenital cataract
C. club foot
D. none of the above

29. Of the following, the one which is MOST effective in the treatment of typhoid fever is 29.____

A. chloramphenicol
B. streptomycin
C. sulfaguanidine
D. aureomycin

30. The one of the following which, in association with rheumatic heart disease, is MOST suggestive of subacute bacterial endocarditis is 30.____

A. prolonged fever
B. persistent microscopic hematuria
C. a single blood culture positive for streptococcus viridans
D. splenomegaly

31. The MOST reliable clinical evidence of active rheumatic carditis is 31.____

A. changing P-R interval in the electrocardiogram
B. acute joint inflammation
C. unusual blood sedimentation rate
D. fever

32. A patient who has refractory chronic urethritis, conjunctivitis, and arthritis has a disease which is referred to as 32.____

A. Weber-Osier syndrome
B. Libman-Sacks disease
C. Reiter's syndrome
D. Pick's disease

33. An American businessman returned by Airplane from Mexico on September 30 and registered in a New York hotel with his wife. Five days after arrival, he became very ill with fever and a hemorrhagic skin rash. He shortly became comatose. The hotel physician had to make an immediate differential diagnosis among smallpox, Rocky Mountain spotted fever, typhus, and meningococcus meningitis.
The microscope would be of GREATEST immediate diagnostic assistance in 33.____

A. smallpox
B. Rocky Mountain spotted fever
C. typhus
D. meningococcus meningitis

34. Assume that the hotel physician made a tentative diagnosis of smallpox in the case described in Question 33.
The one of the following colurses of action which is MOST appropriate in handling such a case is 34.____

A. to keep the patient strictly isolated in his hotel room and cared for by the hotel physician
B. for the hotel physician to telephone the epidemio-logical service of the New York City Health Department and request assistance
C. to transfer the patient to a private hospital via private ambulance
D. to transfer the patient immediately to his house in Connecticut and notify the Connecticut State Department of Health

35. In the treatment of simple hypochromic, microcytic anemia of chronic blood loss, such as might occur with hemorrhoids, the antianemic agent of choice is 35.____

A. vitamin B_{12}
B. $FeSO_4$
C. folic acid
D. B_{12} and $FeSO_4$

36. A 60-year-old man complains of progressive dyspnea on exertion and chronic cough for a number of years. He was gassed in Vietnam but was able to do heavy physical work without difficulty after discharge from the Army. Examination reveals a blood pressure reading of 106/60 mm. Hg, diminished breath sounds, rhonchi and rales in both lungs and percussion note which is hyperresonant. By x-ray, the heart is small and lung fields very clear with accentuated hilar markings. The electrocardiogram shows right axis deviation and inverted T waves in lead V_1. Vital capacity is 80 percent of normal, and the oxygen saturation of the arterial blood is 84 percent with a CO_2 content of 80 percent. The cause of these symptoms is MOST likely to be 36.____

A. cardiac insufficiency
B. tuberculosis
C. pulmonary insufficiency due to chronic emphysema
D. chlorine poisoning

37. The one of the following diseases whose etiological agent does NOT belong to the general group of Rickettsia is 37.____

A. Q fever
B. tularemia
C. typhus fever
D. Rocky Mountain spotted fever

38. A disorder of copper metabolism has been found in 38.____

A. Wilson's disease
B. Von Gierke's disease
C. Milkman's syndrome
D. Kimmelstiel-Wilson's disease

39. *Spider angiomata* appearing in patients with cirrhosis of the liver are GENERALLY believed to be caused by 39.____

A. photosensitivity due to a disturbance of porphyrin metabolism
B. failure of the liver to catabolize estrogens
C. deficiency of B-complex vitamins
D. elevated venous pressure

40. Of the following drugs, the one which has been found useful in the detection of pheochromocytoma is 40.____

A. hydrazinophthalazine
B. benzedrine
C. pyribenzamine
D. benzodioxane

41. Paget's disease of bone is characteristically associated with ______ serum calcium, ______ serum inorganic phosphate, ______ serum alkaline phosphatase. 41.____

A. high; normal; high
B. high; high; high
C. normal; normal; high
D. normal; high; high

42. A man thirty-five years of age has a large, firm solitary nodule in the right lobe of the thyroid gland, unassociated with hyperthyroidism. The BEST management is 42.____

   A. no treatment
   B. surgery
   C. administration of radioiodine
   D. radiotherapy

43. Classical subacute bacterial (Strept. viridans) endocarditis usually does NOT occur when 43.____

   A. rheumatic subcutaneous nodules are present
   B. auricular fibrillation is absent
   C. only a single valve has rheumatic involvement
   D. there have not been repeated previous attacks of active rheumatic fever

44. An IMPORTANT factor in the differentiation of infectious hepatitis from serum hepatitis is the 44.____

   A. difference in incubation period
   B. degree of jaundice
   C. presence or absence of gastrointestinal symptoms
   D. characteristic abnormalities in hepatic function tests

45. Streptomycin is MOST disappointing in the treatment of 45.____

   A. colon bacillus pyelitis
   B. Friedlaender's bacillus pneumonia
   C. influenza bacillus meningitis
   D. typhoid fever

46. A man of 30 presents with a classical history and x-ray evidence of gastric ulcer. Symptomatically, he makes an excellent response to diet and antiacid therapy; an x-ray at the end of three months of treatment shows a slight decrease in the size of the lesion. The management should be to 46.____

   A. gastroscope patient and attempt to obtain exfoliated gastric mucosal cells for cytologic study
   B. continue diet and antiacids as long as symptomatic improvement continues and the x-ray lesion does not increase in size
   C. continue diet and antiacids but in addition place patient on restricted activity for 30 days to help speed the rate of healing
   D. discharge patient from close supervision, to return only if he develops disturbing symptoms again

47. Norepinephrine in therapeutic dosage raises the blood pressure in association with 47.____

   A. increased cardiac output, unchanged peripheral vascular resistance, tachycardia
   B. increased cardiac output, reduced peripheral vascular resistance, unchanged pulse rate
   C. unchanged cardiac output, increased peripheral vascular resistance, tachycardia
   D. reduced cardiac output, increased peripheral vascular resistance, bradycardia

48. In view of present-day medical and surgical advances, all asymptomatic patients with the murmur of mitral stenosis should have 48.____

A. regular medical examinations
B. digitalis
C. limited physical activity
D. the operation of mitral commissurotomy as a preventive measure

49. Two hours after a motorcycle accident, the victim lapses into a coma and the right pupil dilates. X-rays show a fracture line that crosses the right middle meningeal artery channel and extends into the right frontal sinus. The MOST likely diagnosis is 49.____

A. cerebral contusion and edema of the right temporal lobe
B. subdural hematoma
C. post-traumatic progressive intracranial aerocele
D. epidural hematoma

50. The one of the following which is the BEST treatment for the condition described in Question 49 is 50.____

A. administration of caffeine sodium benzoate and oxygen
B. trephination
C. intravenous hypertonic glucose
D. lumbar puncture

KEY (CORRECT ANSWERS)

1. C	11. D	21. B	31. A	41. C
2. A	12. B	22. A	32. C	42. B
3. B	13. A	23. B	33. D	43. A
4. B	14. D	24. C	34. B	44. A
5. C	15. A	25. A	35. B	45. D
6. C	16. C	26. C	36. C	46. A
7. B	17. B	27. A	37. B	47. D
8. D	18. C	28. D	38. A	48. A
9. C	19. A	29. A	39. B	49. D
10. A	20. B	30. C	40. D	50. B

EXAMINATION SECTION
TEST 1

DIRECTIONS: Each question or incomplete statement is followed by several suggested answers or completions. Select the one that BEST answers the question or completes the statement. *PRINT THE LETTER OP THE CORRECT ANSWER IN THE SPACE AT THE RIGHT.*

1. In primary atypical (presumably viral) pneumonia, the one of the following blood findings that is COMMON is 1.____

   A. leucocytosis
   B. agglutination of sheep's red cells by the patient's blood serum
   C. cold agglutinins in the serum
   D. secondary anemia

2. In simple acute tuberculous pleurisy with effusion, the one of the following findings which is characteristic upon physical examination is 2.____

   A. bronchophony
   B. increase of vocal fremitus
   C. egophony
   D. succussion splash

3. Sulfadiazine is USUALLY efficacious in the treatment of pneumonia caused by 3.____

   A. tubercle bacillus
   B. Friedlander bacillus (Klebsiella pneumoniae)
   C. Hemophilus influenzae
   D. streptococcus

4. In a patient who has retrosternal pain and is found to have acute swelling with crepitus of the soft tissues above the clavicle, the one of the following which is the PROBABLE diagnosis is 4.____

   A. retropharyngeal abscess
   B. rupture of the pericardium
   C. mediastinal emphysema
   D. ruptured gastric ulcer

5. In acute diaphragmatic pleurisy involving the central part of the diaphragm, the patient is LIKELY to complain of pain in the 5.____

   A. neck and shoulder
   B. lateral part of the chest between the third and sixth ribs
   C. center of the chest between the second and fifth ribs
   D. interscapular region

6. In acute tuberculous lobar pneumonia, the finding which is TYPICAL is blood leucocytes 6.____

   A. below 4,000
   B. between 4,000 and 10,000
   C. between 10,000 and 20,000
   D. above 20,000

7. Colchicine is the drug of choice in 7.______

A. rheumatic fever
B. rheumatoid arthritis
C. gonorrheal arthritis
D. gout

8. The one of the following diseases involving the joints, of which subcutaneous nodules are characteristic, is 8.______

A. gonorrheal arthritis
B. osteoarthritis
C. rheumatic fever
D. tubercular arthriti

9. A 22-year-old male has complained for the past three weeks of epigastric pain two to three hours after meals. He is relieved of pain by food and alkalis but has pain during the night. For the past week, he has been vomiting, chiefly at night. Gastro-intestinal x-ray series reveal a small ulcer niche at the pylorus, with considerable five-hour and some twenty-four hour gastric retention. 9.______
The PREFERRED initial treatment is a

A. transthoracic vagotomy
B. posterior gastro-enterostomy
C. gastric resection and gastro-jejunostomy
D. medical regimen consisting of decompression of stomach at night and a modified form of *stenosis diet*

10. A suspected obstructing lesion of the descending colon is BEST visualized by 10.______

A. plain prone film of the abdomen
B. a gastro-intestinal series
C. signoidoscopy
D. barium enema

11. In a gastro-intestinal x-ray series, an enlargement of the duodenal sweep with displacement downward and to the right is often significant of 11.______

A. anomalous position of the stomach
B. tumor of head of pancreas
C. partial obstruction of jejunum
D. enlargement of the left lobe of the liver

12. Radioactive phosphorus has been found useful in the treatment of certain diseases. The one of the following diseases in which it is of NO use is 12.______

A. acute myelogenous leukemia
B. chronic myelogenous leukemia
C. chronic lymphatic leukemia
D. polycythemia vera

13. A 58-year-old patient presents the following symptoms: for several months he had noticed weakness, sore tongue, acroparesthesia and diarrhea; examination reveals pallor, absence of position and vibration sensation in the feet, and an atrophic tongue; blood count shows a macrocytic anemia. 13.______
The one of the following which will cause the BEST response of reticulocytosis is

A. folic acid 20 mgm daily
B. ferrous sulphate 2 g daily

C. thiamin chloride 100 mgm daily
D. transfusion of whole blood 500 cc daily

14. BAL (British Anti-Lewisite) is used to counteract the toxic effects of 14.____

A. atropine
B. mercury
C. morphine
D. barbiturates

15. Charcot triad consists of 15.____

A. nystagmus, scanning speech, intention tremor
B. dysarthria, dysphagia, acroparesthesias
C. paraplegia, vesical difficulty, amblyopia
D. pain, temperature dissociation, weakness, hyperactive reflexes

16. Untreated syphilis will cause clinical cardiovascular involvement in ______ of the cases. 16.____

A. 100%
B. 75%
C. 50%
D. less than 25%

17. A patient with a history of a chancre fifteen years ago presents himself for medical care. When the chancre was discovered, his blood Wasserman reaction was *four plus.* He received intravenously 26 injections of arsenical preparation at weekly intervals and 26 of bismuth intramuscularly at weekly intervals. He now exhibits a *three plus* Wasserman reaction, a negative spinal fluid examination, and no demonstrable evidence of visceral involvement. The one of the following courses which SHOULD be followed is 17.____

A. quantitative blood Wasserman determinations at intervals of three months, as a guide to further therapy
B. a course of 26 arsenicals intravenously at weekly intervals
C. administering 2,400,000 units of penicillin in seven and one-half days
D. discharging the patient

18. A patient has a history of hay fever beginning each year about August 15th. Skin tests show he is equally sensitive to (1) giant ragweed, (2) oak pollen, (3) timothy. A course of treatment is planned with antigens.
The one of the following courses which is MOST acceptedis a course of 18.____

A. ragweed *alone*
B. oak *alone*
C. timothy *alone*
D. the three in combination

19. The one of the following findings which would MOST likely be associated with chronic alcoholism is 19.____

A. bilateral wrist drop
B. bilateral foot drop
C. a combination of A and B
D. unilateral foot drop

20. The average duration of action of a dose of protamine zinc insulin is 20.____

A. one-half hour to one hour
B. four to six hours
C. twenty to twenty-four hours
D. twelve to sixteen hours

21. A 30-year-old male, about twenty pounds overweight for his age and height, is subjected to a glucose-tolerance test with the following results: 21.____

Fasting blood sugar - 90 mgms per 100 cc
Fasting urine specimen - contains no sugar

100 grams of glucose are fed to him after the specimens have been collected, and subsequent tests show the following:

Blood sugar, one hour after glucose ingestion - 204 mgms per 100 cc
Urine sugar, one hour after glucose ingestion - 0.25%
Blood sugar, two hours after glucose ingestion - 90 mgms per 100 cc
Urine sugar, two hours after glucose ingestion - faint trace

This man has a sugar-tolerance curve which demonstrates

A. normal curve
B. diabetic type (decreased sugar tolerance)
C. increased sugar tolerance
D. alimentary glycosuria

22. A 35-year-old male is forty-five pounds overweight for his age and height. He has no symptoms and is being examined solely in connection with employment. Several of his urine specimens are tested and show from 0.25% glucose to none at different times and are negative for ketone bodies. A fasting blood sugar (venous) is 160 mgms per 100 cc. The CORRECT way to manage this patient at this stage is to 22.____

A. reduce his weight by diet
B. reduce his weight by diet and thyroid medication
C. allow him to follow his usual diet and routine -i.e., no treatment is necessary
D. use insulin and a diet of the same caloric content as he has been eating habitually (securing urine tests that are sugar-free and blood sugars that are normal)

23. In hyperthyroidism, there is 23.____

A. need for increased vitamin B content in the diet given to the patient
B. need for decreased vitamin B content in the diet
C. no need for change in vitamin B content of diet as compared to normal
D. no need for an increase in vitamin B content of diet unless iodine therapy is resorted to

24. Of the following, pellagra is due to deficiency of 24.____

A. thiamine
B. pantothenic acid
C. riboflavin
D. nicotinic acid (niacin)

25. The MAJORITY of cases of obesity in adults are due to 25.____

A. overeating (exogenous) as to total caloric needs
B. thyroid deficiency
C. pituitary deficiency
D. excess carbohydrate ingestion without excessive caloric intake

26. Death of patients with essential hypertension is MOST frequently caused by disease of the 26.____

A. heart B. brain C. kidneys D. lungs

27. The congenital defect with which diastolic hypertension is MOST frequently associated is 27.____

A. persistent ductus arteriosus
B. pulmonary stenosis
C. coarctation of the aorta
D. ventricular septal defect

28. Hematuria is TYPICALLY present in 28.____

A. bichloride of mercury injury to the kidneys
B. acute diffuse glomerulonephritis
C. toxemia of pregnancy
D. acute pyelonephritis

29. Of the following, the BEST agent in the treatment of faucial diphtheria is 29.____

A. streptomycin
B. diphtheria antitoxin
C. penicillin
D. sulfadiazine

Questions 30-35.

DIRECTIONS: Questions 30 through 35, inclusive, are to be answered after a consideration of the facts presented in Case A which is described below.

CASE A:

A 54-year-old police officer presents himself for advice with the following information:

Present History: For one year, he has had vague abdominal symptoms of flatulence, belching, dysphagia, distress after meals, and frequent bowel movements (up to ten daily), normal in consistency and appearance. Appetite has remained good. He has gained fifteen pounds in weight. He has complained of frequent subocci-pital headaches. Rapid palpitations, increased sweating, and momentary sharp pain lateral to the left nipple have been noticed at home. His sleep has been restless. He frequently gets up at night and eats a cracker which, he says, quiets him and permits him to sleep better.

Past History: Usual childhood exanthemata with no residua.

Family History: Father died at 56 years of age of carcinoma of stomach. Mother died at 79 years of age of congestive heart failure. Only brother who had lived with him died of metastatic carcinoma two years ago at the age of 50.

Physical Examination: This shows a rather apprehensive male of 55, obese, in no acute distress.

Positive Findings: Pulse varies 76-110, sinus arrhythmia, blood pressure 160-140 systolic, 80-70 diastolic.

30. The one of the following diagnoses which might explain all of the symptoms in Case A is 30.____

A. hypothyroidism
B. hypertensive heart disease with anginal syndrome
C. carcinoma of the stomach
D. anxiety state

31. If Case A had hyperthyroidism, all symptoms could be explained on that condition alone EXCEPT for 31.____

A. frequent bowel movements
B. gain in weight
C. palpitation
D. restlessness at night

32. If Case A has hypertensive heart disease, the one of the following laboratory findings which would help establish the diagnosis is 32.____

A. protein in urine
B. increase in blood urea
C. fixation of urinary specific gravity
D. cardiac enlargement on x-ray

33. If, in Case A, you suspect carcinoma of the stomach, the one of the following laboratory findings which would be of GREATEST significance is 33.____

A. erythrocyte sedimentation rate increased
B. decrease in white blood count
C. achlorhydria
D. occult blood in stool

34. If Case A were suffering from anxiety state, he would show 34.____

A. equal and overactive knee jerks
B. dorsiflexion of great toe in plantar reflex
C. unequal pupils
D. absent cremasteric reflexes

35. The one of the following courses which would be MOST helpful in determining whether or not the diagnosis in Case A should be anxiety state is 35.____

A. obtaining further history
B. finding a normal stomach on radiographic study
C. finding a normal electrocardiogram
D. finding an absent gag reflex

36. Cardiovascular syphilis is USUALLY syphilis of the 36.____

A. peripheral arteries
B. coronary arteries
C. myocardium
D. aorta

37. The characteristic murmur of aortic insufficiency is 37.____

A. low-pitched and rumbling
B. high-pitched and blowing
C. heard best with the patient supine
D. heard best at the apex

38. In young subjects with rheumatic heart disease, the MOST frequent of the following causes of heart failure is 38.____

A. overexertion
B. active rheumatic carditis
C. emotional trauma
D. pericardial effusion

39. The MOST common cause of right ventricular failure is 39.____

A. tight mitral stenosis
B. advanced cor pulmonale
C. pulmonary stenosis
D. left ventricular failure

40. The diagnosis of mitral insufficiency in a young subject is justified if there is a systolic murmur at the apex which is 40.____

A. loud and harsh
B. transmitted
C. associated with cardiac enlargement
D. accompanied by a loud third sound

41. Clinically, auricular fibrillation must be differentiated from 41.____

A. auricular flutter with complete A-V block
B. auricular flutter with 1-to-4 ventricular response
C. auricular flutter with varying ventricular response
D. normal sinus rhythm with alternating left bundle branch block

42. Generalized arteriolar vasoconstriction causes an increase PRINCIPALLY in ______ pressure. 42.____

A. systolic blood
B. diastolic blood
C. pulse
D. capillary blood

43. Radiographically, the characteristic shape of the cardiac silhouette in well-established hypertensive heart disease is 43.____

A. boot-shape
B. water-bottle shape
C. straightened left border due to obliteration of the cardiovascular angle
D. caused by prominence of the pulmonary conus .

44. Of the following diseases, the one MOST likely to be followed by glomerular nephritis is 44.____

A. mumps
B. diphtheria
C. chicken pox
D. scarlet fever

45. Of the following diseases, the one in which increased titre of heterophile antibodies is an IMPORTANT diagnostic aid is 45.____

A. typhus fever
B. infectious mononucleosis
C. lymphocytic choriomeningitis
D. influenza

46. Of the following diseases, the one in which perforation of the bowel is MOST likely to occur is 46.____

A. amebiasis
B. bacillary dysentery
C. typhoid fever
D. typhus fever

47. Of the following diseases, the one in which a marked leucocytosis is MOST likely to be found is 47.____

A. lobar pneumonia
B. primary atypical pneumonia
C. pulmonary tuberculosis
D. influenza

48. Of the following diseases, the one in which a moderate leucopenia is MOST characteristic is 48.____

A. Weil's disease
B. brucellosis
C. actinomycosis
D. scarlet fever

49. Of the following, the one in which fever with recurring skin lesion simulating erythema-nodosum is MOST commonly seen is 49.____

A. paratyphoid infections
B. chronic meningococcus sepsis
C. malaria
D. lymphogranuloma venereum

50. Erysipelas is COMMONLY associated with infection by 50.____

A. staphylococcus aureus
B. H. influenzae
C. escherichia coli
D. streptococcus hemolyticus

KEY (CORRECT ANSWERS)

1. C	11. B	21. D	31. B	41. C
2. C	12. A	22. A	32. D	42. A
3. D	13. A	23. A	33. D	43. B
4. C	14. B	24. D	34. A	44. D
5. A	15. A	25. A	35. A	45. B
6. C	16. D	26. A	36. D	46. C
7. D	17. A	27. C	37. B	47. A
8. C	18. A	28. B	38. B	48. B
9. D	19. B	29. B	39. D	49. B
10. D	20. C	30. D	40. C	50. D

TEST 2

DIRECTIONS: Each question or incomplete statement is followed by several suggested answers or completions. Select the one that BEST answers the question or completes the statement. *PRINT THE LETTER OF THE CORRECT ANSWER IN THE SPACE AT THE RIGHT.*

1. The one of the following conditions in which the basal metabolic rate is NOT likely to be elevated is 1.____

   A. metastatic carcinoma of the cervical lymph glands
   B. Hodgkin's disease
   C. lymphosarcoma
   D. acute lymphatic leukemia

2. Of the following results, the one which is obtained after a section of the vagus nerves for peptic ulcer is that it 2.____

   A. increases nocturnal secretion in the stomach
   B. increases the motility of the stomach
   C. diminishes the nocturnal secretion from the stomach
   D. has no effect on the nocturnal secretion of the stomach

3. In an indirect inguinal hernia, the relation of the sac at the neck to the deep epigastric artery is that the sac lies _______ to the artery. 3.____

   A. lateral
   B. medial
   C. posterior
   D. anterior

4. The effect of prolonged ascorbic acid depletion in a healing wound is 4.____

   A. an increase of collagen and reticulum
   B. no increase on collagen formation
   C. lack of collagen and reticulum
   D. no change in reticulum

5. The one of the following conditions with which osteitis fibrosa cystica is USUALLY associated is 5.____

   A. hyperthyroidism
   B. hyperparathyroidism
   C. Addison's disease
   D. hypothyroidism

6. The one of the following effects which the pre-operative preparation of the hyperthyroid patient with thiouracil ALONE produces is that it 6.____

   A. increases the vascularity of the thyroid gland
   B. increases the basal metabolic rate
   C. diminishes the vascularity of the thyroid gland
   D. has no effect on the vascularity of the thyroid gland

7. Certain effects follow the establishment of an arterio-venous fistula between the femoral vessels. 7.____
   The one of the following which is NOT such an effect is

A. acceleration of the heart
B. a marked elevation of the diastolic pressure
C. a continuous vibratory thrill
D. dilatation and hypertrophy of the heart

8. In performing a saphenous ligation for varicose veins, the one of the following veins which you would NOT ligate is the _______ , vein. 8.____

A. lateral superficial femoral
B. inferior epigastric
C. superficial circumflex
D. superficial external pudendal

9. The one of the following conditions in which splenectomy would be INADVISABLE is 9.____

A. acute lymphatic leukemia
B. sarcoma of the spleen
C. congenital hemolytic icterus
D. essential thrombocytopenic purpura

10. The one of the following methods which you would NOT use to estimate the amount of fluid to replace in a thermal burn is 10.____

A. hematocrit estimation
B. estimation of plasma protein
C. estimation of surface area of body involved
D. estimation of the degree of the burn

11. The muscles which act as flexors at the metacarpophalangeal joints and extensors of the fingers at both interphalangeal joints are the 11.____

A. flexor digitorum profundus
B. lumbricals
C. brachalis
D. pronator quadratus

12. The position of the posterior tibial nerve at the ankle is 12.____

A. behind the lateral malleolus
B. in front of the ankle between the two malleoli
C. between the medial malleolus and the tendo Achillis
D. in back of the ankle halfway between the two malleoli

13. Of the following, the one which is NOT a liver function test is the 13.____

A. glucose tolerance test
B. determination of alkaline phosphatase
C. determination of albumin-globulin ratio
D. determination of acid phosphatase in the blood

14. The condition associated with shock in which hemoconcen-tration is MOST apt to occur is 14.____

A. burns
B. compound fracture of the femur
C. hemorrhage
D. coronary thrombosis

15. The condition in which disruption of a post-operative abdominal wound is LIKELY to occur is 15.____

A. when sutured with alloy steel wire
B. hypoproteinemia
C. vitamin A deficiency
D. vitamin D deficiency

16. In intravascular clotting or thrombosis, the one factor which is NOT important is 16.____

A. injury to vessel wall
B. slowing of the bloodstream
C. lack of vitamin C
D. increased viscosity of the blood

17. A man jumps from a height of 10 feet and lands on his feet but does not fall to the ground. Ten hours later, he is admitted to the hospital with the clinical signs and symptoms of an acute abdomen. 17.____
Of the following, the measure MOST likely to indicate the correct diagnosis is

A. three-position x-ray of the abdomen
B. intravenous pyelogram
C. x-ray of the spine
D. laboratory study of blood volume and content

18. A patient is admitted with a pathological fracture of the femur. The laboratory findings include: calcium normal, phosphorus normal, alkaline phosphatase slightly elevated, acid phosphatase elevated, serum N.P.N. normal, albumin globulin ratio normal. 18.____
In addition to management of the fracture, the procedure MOST likely to be indicated is

A. parathyroidectomy
B. orchidectomy
C. local radiotherapy to the fracture
D. thyroidectomy; oral administration of irradiated iodine

19. The BEST treatment for an incised wound which divides all flexor tendons at the level of the proximal interphalangeal joint of a finger is 19.____

A. careful repair of all divided structures, including the tendon sheath
B. repair of profundus tendon and suture of the sub-limis to it
C. repair of profundus tendon and excision of the sub-limis
D. repair of the sublimis and excision of profundus tendon

20. Of the following, the mechanism LEAST likely to injure the right brachial plexus is violent 20.____

A. flexion and abduction of the head to the right
B. extension and abduction of the head to the left

C. depression of the right shoulder
D. drawing backward of the right shoulder

21. Following prolonged treatment of a severely infected tendon sheath in the hand, an adult patient develops a clinical fibrous ankylosis of the shoulder on the same side. This is MOST commonly the result of 21.____

A. metastatic infection
B. errors of omission in the treatment of the finger
C. subdeltoid bursitis
D. Sudeck's atrophy

22. The cause of traumatic subdural hematoma is ALWAYS a(n) 22.____

A. fracture of the skull
B. extensive head injury
C. severe or mild head injury
D. tear in the middle meningeal artery

23. An alcoholic patient with a three-inch laceration of the scalp is found on the street. In treating the laceration, it is MOST important to 23.____

A. cleanse the wound, sprinkle sulfa powder in it, suture it and drain it
B. thoroughly cleanse and debride and suture the wound
C. palpate for skull fracture before closing the wound
D. debride the scalp edges

24. A patient falls down the subway stairs. He is a little dazed but gets up and rides home. Two hours later, he becomes drowsy and develops a left hemiplegia. You see him three hours after the accident. He is then comatose and has a contusion of the scalp. The method of treatment should be 24.____

A. immediate operation
B. immediate air studies to see if an expanding blood clot is present and localizing it
C. complete bed rest, dehydration, and lumbar puncture
D. observation for localizing signs; x-ray of the skull

25. Immediate loss of all motor and sensory power below the level of a spinal cord lesion resulting from a fracture dislocation of a cervical vertebra would indicate the presence of 25.____

A. permanent complete cord injury
B. hematomyelia
C. doubtful permanent complete cord injury
D. partial cord injury

26. Treatment of acute fracture dislocation of the cervical vertebrae with cord compression should be treated by 26.____

A. plaster jacket
B. traction and possible later laminectomy
C. extension in bed with careful nursing and observation
D. immediate laminectomy

27. A patient received a gunshot wound of the upper third of the arm, and has since suffered with intense burning pain over the posterior aspect of the thumb and first dorsal interosseus space. The pain was relieved temporarily by novocaine block of the stellate ganglion. He is MOST likely suffering from a 27.____

A. causalgia of the median nerve
B. causalgia of the radial nerve
C. severance of a nerve
D. vacular injury

28. Epileptic seizures of the Jacksonian type beginning in a man of thirty years would MOST likely be of _______ origin. 28.____

A. idiopathic
B. hereditary
C. functional
D. organic

29. A 60-year-old male severely contused his right hand. The skin and soft parts were not split open. X-ray revealed a simple oblique fracture of the shaft of the second meta carpal with no displacement.
The one of the following which is the PREFERRED treatment is 29.____

A. immobilization in extension in plaster cast
B. partial mobilization over a roller bandage
C. complete mobility of hand and fingers
D. immobilization with finger traction

30. A simple fracture through the mid-part of the left carpal scaphoid, without displacement of fragments, in a 20-year-old male showed no x-ray evidence of healing following adequate plastic immobilization for a two-month period. The IMMEDIATE subsequent treatment of choice would be 30.____

A. to remove cast and institute motion
B. continued adequate immobilization in plaster
C. drilling across fracture site
D. insertion of bone peg

31. A policeman injured his right hand. X-ray revealed a simple fracture through the neck of the fifth metacarpal. Of the following, the PREFERRED treatment would be immobilization with 31.____

A. the fifth finger held in semi-flexion
B. straight finger traction
C. digit in hyper-extension
D. the metacarpal phalangeal joint flexed to a ninety degree (90°) angle

32. A forty-five caliber bullet passing through several layers of heavy wool clothing causes a through-and-through wound of the knee joint. X-ray revealed no fracture.
Of the following, the PREFERRED treatment would be 32.____

A. immobilization with local use of penicillin
B. debridement of external wounds and immobilization
C. adequate debridement of external wounds and exploration of knee joint
D. adequate debridement of external wounds with saline irrigation of joint through one of the openings

33. A policeman was stabbed in the abdomen several times with an ice pick. Examination twenty minutes later revealed a soft non-tender abdomen with several oblique puncture tracts through the recti sheaths and anterior abdominal wall. A probe could be passed through the tracts with slight difficulty.
Of the following, the SUBSEQUENT treatment should be 33.____

A. observation in a hospital
B. debridement of the abdominal wall wounds
C. exploratory laparotomy
D. surface dressings; patient discharged to home

34. The diagnosis of a severe ankle sprain has been made clinically. X-ray reveals no fracture. With intravenous anesthesia, the affected ankle was manipulated under the fluoroscope. A moderate subluxation of the talus, as compared to the other ankle, was found.
The BEST results in such a case are obtained by 34.____

A. adhesive strapping
B. novocaine injection with active mobility
C. ethyl chloride spray
D. immobilization in a plaster walking cast

35. A fireman fell across an iron railing sustaining multiple fractures of the left ninth, tenth, and eleventh ribs in the mid-axillary line. Physical examination revealed no other apparent injuries.
The patient would BEST be treated by 35.____

A. adhesive strapping of affected side
B. novocaine block of affected ribs
C. circular adhesive dressings
D. novocaine block of affected ribs with hospitalization for observation

36. In the city, a reportable communicable disease MUST be reported in writing to the Department of Health 36.____

A. in a regular weekly summary of communicable disease patients attended during preceding seven days
B. only if the patient is admitted to a special hospital for communicable diseases
C. when patient refuses to cooperate in the protection of the health of other persons
D. within twenty-four hours after the case is diagnosed

37. The one of the following diseases which, when diagnosed in an adult, may have the MOST serious public health implications and hence should be brought immediately to the attention of the public health authorities is 37.____

A. scarlet fever
B. mumps
C. chicken pox
D. measles

38. Some observers question the wisdom of using penicillin in the immediate treatment of early gonorrhea because 38.____

A. many common strains of the gonococcus have been found to be penicillin resistant
B. it may mask a simultaneous primary syphilitic infection
C. streptomycin has been found to be a cheaper, more effective, and less toxic therapeutic agent

D. to be effective against the gonococcus, penicillin blood levels must reach concentrations attainable only by parenteral administration; thus, penicillin treatment is too cumbersome and inconvenient

39. An American child of Italian parentage is severely burned and receives a transfusion from his father. Three weeks later, he develops progressive fever and chills, anemia, and slight jaundice. 39.____
The MOST likely diagnosis is

A. homologous serum jaundice
B. quartan malaria
C. syphilis
D. yellow fever

40. Serological tests for syphilis are 40.____

A. non-specific and provide only presumptive evidence of infection which must be confirmed by careful history and physical examination
B. specific and definite diagnosis of syphilis may be made on obtaining a positive result. Syphilitic infection can be excluded when a negative test is obtained
C. specific, and definite diagnosis of syphilis may be made on obtaining a positive reaction. The tests are not sufficiently sensitive to give a positive reaction in all syphilitic individuals
D. non-specific, and a positive test may be obtained occasionally in non-syphilitic patients. They are sufficiently sensitive so that a negative test excludes the possibility of syphilis.

41. In an attempt to control endemic typhus, the one of the following measures which should be instituted is eradication of 41.____

A. rats, mice, and fleas
B. body lice
C. dogs and ticks
D. bedbugs

42. A 27-year-old male was seen with a severe febrile illness of twelve days' duration. Onset has been gradual with increasing malaise, headache, prostration, and with a rash extending over almost the entire body, but more pronounced on the extremities. At first, the rash was light red and tended to blanch on pressure; with passage of time, the rash became petechial and lesions could be found on the palms of the hands and the soles of the feet. The patient, who had lived in or around New York City all his life, gave a history of having been on a three-day camping tripon eastern Long Island about ten days before onset. On examination, temperature was found to be 104,2 Fahrenheit, pulse 130 per minute, respiration 20 per minute. The major physical findings were a slightly enlarged spleen and diffuse muscle tenderness on pressure. Laboratory tests showed: hemoglobin 12.5 gms per 100 cc blood; R.B.C. 4,960,000 per cram; W.B.C. 14,500 per cmm; blood culture - negative; lumbar puncture - negative; agglutination tests: P. tularensis - negative; B. abortus -negative; E. typhosa - (0) 1:40, (H) 1:80; B. proteus -(OX 19) 1:320, (OX-2) 1:180. The PRESUMPTIVE diagnosis is 42.____

A. typhoid fever
B. endemic typhus fever
C. Rocky Mountain spotted fever
D. rickettsial pox

43. A veteran without a history of prior malaria is seen with intermittent fever of several days' duration. Thin blood smears on each of two different days are negative for malaria parasites. 43.____
The veteran SHOULD

A. receive a therapeutic trial with an anti-malarial drug, as quinine, atabrine, or chloroquine
B. receive therapy with penicillin or sulfonamides
C. be injected with adrenalin in an attempt to mobilize parasites into the blood
D. have thick blood films examined to exclude malaria before any therapy is given

44. A patient who had amebiasis has recurrent severe attacks of diarrhea. The stools are consistently negative for amebae and shigellae. The mucous membrane of the colon is normal, and x-rays of the colon negative. No pus or blood in the stool. 44.____
The patient should receive

A. amebicidal drugs
B. sulfonamides
C. both amebicidal and sulfonamide drugs
D. only symptomatic therapy

45. An OUTSTANDING clinical finding in persons suffering from chronic industrial mercury poisoning is 45.____

A. hematuria
B. severe anemia
C. jaundice
D. tremor of the hand

46. The MOST important route of absorption of industrial poisons is the 46.____

A. gastro-intestinal tract
B. skin
C. respiratory tract
D. direct implantation in tissues

47. Early signs of excessive exposure to x-ray or radium can BEST be detected by periodic 47.____

A. chest x-rays
B. urinalysis
C. liver function tests
D. blood counts

48. The one of the following which is pathogenic for man is ______ coli. 48.____

A. Endamoeba
B. Balantidium
C. Eimeria
D. Scobicia

49. The LEADING cause of loss of time from work among industrial workers is 49.____

A. occupational diseases
B. non-occupational diseases
C. occupational injuries
D. non-occupational injuries

50. The effectiveness of BAL (2, 3 dimercapto-propanol) in arsenic poisoning is due to the affinity of arsenic for 50.____

A. hemoglobin
B. sulfhydryl groups
C. cholesterol
D. cephalin

KEY (CORRECT ANSWERS)

1. A	11. B	21. B	31. D	41. A
2. C	12. C	22. C	32. C	42. C
3. A	13. D	23. C	33. C	43. D
4. C	14. A	24. A	34. D	44. D
5. B	15. B	25. C	35. D	45. D
6. A	16. C	26. B	36. D	46. C
7. B	17. C	27. B	37. C	47. D
8. B	18. B	28. D	38. B	48. B
9. A	19. C	29. C	39. B	49. B
10. D	20. A	30. B	40. A	50. B

EXAMINATION SECTION

TEST 1

DIRECTIONS: Each question or incomplete statement is followed by several suggested answers or completions. Select the one that BEST answers the question or completes the statement. *PRINT THE LETTER OF THE CORRECT ANSWER IN THE SPACE AT THE RIGHT.*

1. Following the inhalation of irritating gas, such as chloride or phosgene, the physician should watch for the development of 1.____
   A. heart failure with peripheral edema
   B. bronchopneumonia
   C. reactivation of old tuberculosis
   D. pneumonoconiosis

2. The only one of the following neoplasms of the chest which commonly gives rise to hemoptysis is 2.____
   A. dermoid cyst B. chondroma of the bronchus
   C. neurofibroma D. bronchial adenoma

3. A man, aged 22, healthy six months ago, is now discovered to have a soft cottony shadow 2 centimeters in diameter in the upper part of one lung. He has been gaining weight. Physical examination reveals no abnormalities. Patient feels entirely well. The resumptive diagnosis is tuberculosis. PROPER management is 3.____
   A. collapse of the lung by artificial pneumothorax and permit patient to continue working
   B. sanatorium treatment
   C. no treatment because the disease is inactive
   D. allowing the man to work, but with re-examination once a month

4. A veteran who was healthy except for attacks of malaria, dysentery and scrub typhus in the South Pacific develops general malaise and loses weight several months after returning home. He starts to expectorate 4 to 8 ounces of reddish-brown sputum which is liquid and odorless. Dullness is found at the base of the right lung. The diagnosis suggested is 4.____
   A. pulmonary infarct
   B. abscess of the lung due to dysentery bacillus
   C. amebic abscess of the liver
   D. rickettsial pneumonia

5. A 60-year-old man who has been a marble cutter develops dyspnea, becomes weak, and loses weight, but has no fever. X-ray of the chest shows widely scattered stringy and nodular lesions in both lungs. The PROBABLE diagnosis is 5.____
   A. hematogenous tuberculosis B. pneumoconiosis
   C. primary cancer of the lung D. metastatic carcinoma

6. A putrid lung abscess is USUALLY due to 6.____
   A. infected embolus
   B. infarct which becomes secondarily infected
   C. aspiration of infectious material from the mouth
   D. secondary infection of pneumococcal pneumonia

7. A 45-year-old patient coughs up blood and then develops dyspnea, persistent wheezing in one lung, and fever over a period of six months. 7.____
He MOST probably has
   A. tuberculosis
   B. bronchiectasis
   C. primary cancer of the lung
   D. metastatic cancer of the lung

8. Chronic cor pulmonale may be related to 8.____
   A. pneumonoconiosis
   B. diaphragmatic adhesions
   C. chronic tuberculosis at the apex
   D. systemic arteriosclerosis

9. Acute spontaneous pneumothorax without pleural effusion in a young man who does not become dyspneic is BEST treated by 9.____
   A. withdrawal of gas from the chest
   B. artificial pneumothorax
   C. bed rest
   D. oxygen inhalation

10. The cause of edema in the nephrotic stage of chronic diffuse glomerulonephritis is 10.____
   A. increased venous pressure
   B. decreased osmotic pressure of the blood
   C. increased capillary permeability
   D. inability of the kidney to excrete sodium

11. The elevation of mean blood pressure in patients with essential hypertension is due CHIEFLY to 11.____
   A. increased cardiac output
   B. increased blood volume
   C. increased peripheral resistance
   D. decreased elasticity of the arteries

12. In a patient with an abnormally elevated blood urea, the BEST evidence that intrinsic renal disease is the basis for the elevation is 12.____
   A. presence of abnormal amounts of protein in the urine
   B. marked reduction of urine volume
   C. generalized edema
   D. fixation of the specific gravity 1.010 of the urine

13. The occurrence of bilateral papilledema indicates progress from 13.____
   A. benign to malignant nephrosclerosis
   B. acute to chronic diffuse glomerulonephritis
   C. normal sized to contracted kidneys
   D. acute to chronic pyelonephritis

14. In the normal kidney, urea undergoes 14.____
    A. tubular reabsorption
    B. tubular secretion
    C. glomerular filtration
    D. glomerular filtration and tubular resorption

15. Patients manifest the nephrotic syndrome and hypertension with 15.____
    A. intercapillary glomerular sclerosis
    B. atrophic pyelonephritis
    C. acute diffuse glomerulonephritis
    D. polycystic renal disease

16. Subjectively, uncomplicated syphilitic aortitis is characterized by 16.____
    A. retrosternal pain of anginal type
    B. paroxysmal dyspnea
    C. no symptoms
    D. aortalgia

17. Of the following, the POOREST average prognosis is observed in cardio-vascular syphilis with 17.____
    A. coronary osteal stenosis
    B. uncomplicated aortitis
    C. aortic insufficiency
    D. aneurysm of aorta

18. An electrocardiogram displaying a depressed S-T segment and an inverted T-wave in Leads I, V_L, and V_5 in a patient with cardiovascular syphilis would make one suspect 18.____
    A. gumma of the myocardium
    B. left ventricular hypertrophy with or without coronary osteal stenosis
    C. diffuse syphilitic myocarditis
    D. aneurysm of the ascending aorta

19. In congestive heart failure, the circulating plasma volume is 19.____
    A. decreased
    B. variable, usually decreased
    C. unchanged
    D. decreased

20. Radiographically, left auricular enlargement is seen BEST in the ____ view. 20.____
    A. right anterior oblique
    B. left anterior oblique
    C. postero-anterior
    D. left lateral

21. Radiographically, right ventricular hypertrophy is seen BEST in the _____ view. 21.____
    A. left anterior oblique
    B. right anterior oblique
    C. left lateral
    D. postero-anterior

22. In rheumatic heart disease with mitral stenosis, a high-pitched valvular sound in early diastole, heard best in the pulmonic area, is MOST likely 22.____
    A. the opening snap of mitral stenosis
    B. a loud third heart sound
    C. a split second sound
    D. a protodiastolic gallop rhythm

23. Because digitaline nativelle (digitoxin) is a glucoside which comes in crystalline form which can be measured precisely, the daily maintenance dose 23.____
   A. is 0.002 mg
   B. is 0.2 mg
   C. is 2.0 mg
   D. must nevertheless be determined by trial and error

24. Arterial vascular insufficiency of an extremity may manifest itself by 24.____
   A. red, warm skin
   B. pale, warm skin
   C. rubor on elevation, pallor on dependency
   D. red, cool skin

25. By *vasomotor gradient* is meant the difference in vaso-meter activity and hence in temperature between the 25.____
   A. head and feet
   B. thorax and abdomen
   C. proximal and distal parts of an extremity
   D. hands and feet

26. The term *claudication* means 26.____
   A. arthralgia   B. limping   C. pain   D. cramp

27. The characteristic electrocardiographic pattern which results from myocardial infarction secondary to closure of the ramus descendens posterior of the right coronary artery is similar to the electrocardiographic pattern seen in 27.____
   A. Ayerza's disease   B. pulmonary embolization
   C. advance mitral stenosis   D. Chagas' disease

28. When subacute bacterial endocarditis due to streptococcus viridens is encountered during the so-called *bacteria-free* stage, an associated impairment of renal function with azotemia is MOST frequently caused by 28.____
   A. focal embolic glomerulonephritis
   B. subacute or chronic diffuse glomerulonephritis
   C. renal infarction
   D. bilateral pyelonephritis

29. The MOST constant of the clinical features of chronic cor pulmonale is 29.____
   A. edema   B. clubbed fingers
   C. enlarged liver   D. cyanosis

30. For four or five days prior to having a glucose tolerance test, a patient omits all foods containing sugar from his diet and eats little of any foods containing carbohydrates. Such a procedure will 30.____
   A. in no way alter the result of his glucose tolerance test
   B. increase his glucose tolerance
   C. decrease his glucose tolerance
   D. still yield a high fasting blood-sugar but give a normal blood-sugar at the end of two hours following the taking of glucose involved in the test

31. In the majority of cases of hyperthyroidism, 31.____
   A. the blood iodine concentration is normal
   B. the blood iodine concentration is decreased
   C. the blood iodine concentration is increased
   D. there is increased excretion of iodine in urine, feces, etc., but the blood concentration of iodine is normal because thyroid iodine is increased

32. In hypothyroidism, when desiccated thyroid medication is resorted to, the 32.____
   A. lower the basal metabolism, the larger the initial dose of desiccated thyroid should be
   B. lower the basal metabolism, the smaller the initial dose of desiccated thyroid should be
   C. dose should be related to the weight of the patient
   D. dose should be related to the amount of myxedematous swelling (edema) of the patient

33. Of the following, the MOST accurate description of what occurs in well-defined hyperpituitarism is 33.____
   A. fasting hyperglycemia and diminished glucose tolerance
   B. fasting hyperglycemia but increased glucose tolerance
   C. normal blood-sugar and sugar tolerance
   D. hypoglycemia

34. Of the following, the MOST accurate description of findings in hypoparathyroidism is _____ blood serum calcium, _____. 34.____
   A. low; spontaneous fractures
   B. low; high blood serum phosphorus, tetany
   C. high; tetany
   D. high; low blood serum phosphorus

35. A freshly voided urine specimen which contains glucose is being tested for the presence or absence of glucose (copper-reducing substance). To 2½ cc of Benedict's Qualitative Solution, in good condition and correctly prepared, five drops of urine have been added. The mixture has been boiled over a Bunsen burner, but the reagent does not change in color nor in clarity when the test tube is removed. The patient reports the specimen as containing *no sugar.* The erroneous report of *no sugar* is due to the fact that 35.____
   A. too much Benedict's Solution was used in proportion to the amount of urine used in the test
   B. too little Benedict's Solution was used
   C. the contents of the test tube were not allowed to cool before the reading of the results
   D. too little urine was used

36. Hedberden's nodes are characteristic of 36.____
   A. rheumatoid arthritis
   B. gout
   C. osteoarthritis
   D. rheumatic fever

37. Tuberculous arthritis is characteristically 37.____
   A. monarticular in distribution and usually evidences very little inflammation, i.e., heat and redness
   B. polyarticular in distribution and usually involves the smaller joints
   C. associated with high fever and involvement of the temporomandibular joints
   D. associated with an involvement of the great toe

38. Of the following skin diseases, the one with which rheumatoid arthritis is frequently enough associated to be recognized as a clinical syndrome is 38.____
   A. herpes B. psoriasis C. seborrhea D. scabies

39. Of the following, the CORRECT statement is: 39.____
   A. Rheumatoid arthritis is predominantly a disease of the female sex, the incidence being roughly three-to-one greater among females.
   B. Patients with rheumatoid arthritis are generally about evenly distributed between male and female. The disease shows no sex predominance.
   C. Marie Struempell spondylosis (rheumatoid spondylosis) shows a marked difference in sex distribution, the disease affecting females in a ratio to males of about ten to one.
   D. The disease gout does not occur more frequently in males than in females, the sex distribution being about equal.

40. It is GENERALLY agreed that the cause of osteoarthritis is 40.____
   A. the series of physiological and pathological changes which occur in a joint when it is subjected to prolonged and often repeated injury and wear and tear
   B. intestinal toxicity
   C. a chronic infectious process
   D. a prolonged allergy which involves the joints

41. The one of the following diseases involving the joints of which subcutaneous nodules are characteristic is 41.____
   A. serum sickness involving the joints
   B. pneumococcal arthritis
   C. rheumatoid arthritis
   D. Charcot's joint

42. Lipping and osteophyte formation of the spine by x-ray examination is characteristic and diagnostic of 42.____
   A. Marie Struempell spondylosis or rheumatoid arthritis of the spine
   B. gonorrheal arthritis of the spine
   C. metastatic invasion of the spine
   D. osteoarthritis of the spine

Questions 43-45.

DIRECTIONS: Questions 43 through 45 are to be answered after a consideration of the facts presented in Case B, which is described below.

CASE B

A patient is brought to a hospital after he has been knocked down by a truck. He has extensive contusions, abrasions, and lacerations.

43. Case B would be given tetanus toxoid if he had 43.____
   A. dirt in his wounds
   B. a history of serum sickness
   C. been a discharged soldier with the Purple Heart
   D. a history of previous injections of tetanus antitoxin

44. Case B would be given tetanus antitoxin because he 44.____
   A. was under 25 years of age
   B. had a history of previous injection of antitoxin
   C. had a history of previous injections of tetanus toxoid
   D. had no history of previous injection of tetanus toxoid

45. If Case B were treated with tetanus antitoxin and developed serum sickness, *lumphadenopathy* would be expected to develop 45.____
   A. regional to site of injection
   B. in a particularized fashion
   C. regional to site of infection
   D. regional to site of wounds

Questions 46-50.

DIRECTIONS: Questions 46 through 50 are to be answered after consideration of the facts presented in Case C, which is described below.

CASE C

A 39-year-old policeman was admitted to a hospital for observation. He was brought in following a verbal altercation with his desk sergeant. He had reported late for duty; and when he tried to explain his tardiness, he claimed the sergeant became abusive. He was held at the precinct for examination by the police psychiatrist who had been seeing this policeman at weekly intervals for several months. After examination at the precinct, the psychiatrist recommended that the policeman be hospitalized. In the psychiatric hospital, the patient claimed on further questioning that his promotion on the force was being blocked because of his religious affiliations. He also felt that the police psychiatrist, who had been following him, wanted him hospitalized to *get him out of the way*. He was suspicious of his co-workers. Past history revealed that he had finished school in his late teens and joined the Navy. After several years of service in the Navy, he had joined the police force. His record on the police force had shown only two minor infractions of the rules for which he had been fined. When the war began, he rejoined the Navy and had four years of creditable service. While in the Navy, he was hospitalized for four months and given a medical discharge because of *emotional trouble*.

He was reinstated on the police force and had *easy duty* since. His mental examination showed him to be oriented. His intellectual resources were normal. He showed a tendency to unwarranted suspicion, and this extended even to his domestic life in which he accused his wife of infidelity. Actually, his wife was a devoted, sincere person. No discussion could dissuade him of his erroneous ideas.

46. The one of the following which would help MOST in making a diagnosis of Case C is 46.____
    A. electroencephalographic test
    B. examination of the spinal fluid
    C. Binet-Simon intelligence test
    D. Rorschach test

47. The one of the following which would help MOST in making a diagnosis in Case C is 47.____
    A. a high sedimentation rate
    B. additional history from patient that his fellow officers were jealous of his good record and that in order to prevent him from being promoted had engineered his hospitalization
    C. loss of vibration sensation in feet
    D. history of poor school record

48. The one of the following diagnoses which would be the MOST probable from the data given in Case C is 48.____
    A. paranoid psychosis
    B. anxiety state
    C. psychopathic personality
    D. alcoholic hallucinations

49. In Case C, if the diagnosis were alcoholic hallucinations, the one of the following which you would NOT expect to find is 49.____
    A. tenderness of the calf
    B. tenderness of the sole
    C. positive Babinski sign
    D. loss of position sensation in the feet

50. If the diagnosis in Case C were psychopathic personality, the course MOST frequently to occur would be 50.____
    A. episodes of severe depression with intermittent elation
    B. development of gross paralysis
    C. progressive deterioration of intellectual ability
    D. continuing asocial and amoral behavior

KEY (CORRECT ANSWERS)

1.	B	11.	C	21.	B	31.	C	41.	C
2.	D	12.	D	22.	C	32.	B	42.	D
3.	B	13.	A	23.	D	33.	A	43.	C
4.	C	14.	D	24.	D	34.	B	44.	D
5.	D	15.	A	25.	C	35.	C	45.	A
6.	C	16.	C	26.	B	36.	C	46.	D
7.	C	17.	A	27.	B	37.	A	47.	B
8.	A	18.	B	28.	B	38.	B	48.	A
9.	C	19.	D	29.	D	39.	A	49.	C
10.	B	20.	A	30.	C	40.	A	50.	D

TEST 2

DIRECTIONS: Each question or incomplete statement is followed by several suggested answers or completions. Select the one that BEST answers the question or completes the statement. *PRINT THE LETTER OF THE CORRECT ANSWER IN THE SPACE AT THE RIGHT.*

1. If the diagnosis in a case were paranoid psychosis, the MOST frequent trait to be watched for is 1.____
   A. assaultive behavior
   B. burglary
   C. convulsions
   D. hemiplegia

2. In acute infectious hepatitis with jaundice, an increasing urobilinogenuria is evidence of 2.____
   A. complicating extra-hepatic obstruction
   B. progressive liver necrosis
   C. diminishing intra-hepatic obstruction
   D. marked intra-hepatic obstruction

3. In a patient with evidence of obstructive jaundice, a palpable enlargement of the gallbladder suggests 3.____
   A. an obstruction of the common duct due to extrinsic pressure
   B. carcinoma of the gallbladder
   C. calculus in the common duct
   D. suppurative cholangitis

4. Sigmoidoscopic examination of a patient complaining of chronic diarrhea with mucus and blood reveals ulcerations varying in size from a pinhead to an inch in diameter. The larger ulcers have rolled hyperemic margins and undermined edges, so-called flask-shaped ulcers, which extend to the submucosa. They are usually covered with a yellowish or greenish black slough. These ulcers are insensitive to pain when scraped. There are intervening patches of mucous membrane, quite normal in appearance. 4.____
   Of the following, this picture is USUALLY seen in
   A. bacillary dysentery
   B. non-specific ulcerative colitis
   C. tuberculous colitis
   D. amebic dysentery

5. Blumer's shelf is 5.____
   A. a stricture of the rectum due to lymphogranuloma venereum
   B. an abnormal dilation of the rectal ampulla
   C. carcinoma of the anterior rectal wall
   D. a malignant infiltration of the pelvic floor between the anterior rectal wall and the bladder or uterus

6. Carcinoid or Argentaffin tumors are MOST commonly found in the 6.____
   A. stomach
   B. small intestine
   C. colon
   D. rectum

7. A 32-year-old male with an eight-year history of peptic ulcer is seen in the hospital three hours after a copious hematemesis. This is his first bleeding episode. His skin and mucous membranes are pale; extremities are warm. Pulse rate is 90 per minute, regular and good quality. His blood pressure is 116 over 70. The hematocrit is 43#, hemoglobin is 12.6 grams, the RBC is 3,800,000. The PREFERRED initial treatment would be 7.____
   A. blood transfusion 500 cc
   B. plasma transfusion 500 cc
   C. either A or B, and 1000 cc of 5% glucose in saline by clysis
   D. sedation and the initiation of a modified feeding regimen

8. An obese woman of forty with a history of recurrent dyspepsia is suddenly seized with severe epigastric pain, radiating to chest and back, and severe vomiting. She goes into a shock-like state, with grayish cyanosis. The major physical finding is a board-like rigidity of the upper abdomen. Blood examination shows a polymorphonuclear leukocytosis, hemoconcentration, and an amylase (Sornogyi method) of 860. 8.____
   The LOGICAL diagnosis is
   A. acute coronary occlusion
   B. acute pancreatitis
   C. ruptured peptic ulcer
   D. acute cholecystitis with cholelithiasis

9. John Brown has been in a traffic accident. He is in shock and needs a blood transfusion. His blood type if RH positive. 9.____
   The one of the following statements which applies BEFORE transfusion is given is that
   A. ordinary typing would be sufficient
   B. the history of previous transfusion is necessary
   C. he needs donor with RH positive blood
   D. he needs donor with RH negative blood

10. The one of the following rays which radioactive phosphorus emits is 10.____
    A. alpha B. beta C. gamma D. others

11. The BEST single index to the severity of H. influenza meningitis is 11.____
    A. spinal fluid cell count B. spinal fluid sugar
    C. spinal fluid protein D. stained smear of spinal fluid

12. Of the following, the cause of San Joaquin Valley fever is 12.____
    A. rickettsia B. filterable virus
    C. fungus D. gram-positive cocci

13. Of the following infections, the one in which blackwater fever is MOST likely to occur is 13.____
    A. leishmaniasis B. vivax malaria
    C. quartan malaria D. falciparura malaria

14. The insect vector of Rocky Mountain spotted fever is the 14.____
    A. tick B. louse C. mite D. flea

15. Of the following, the test which is MOST valuable in the diagnosis of typhus fever is 15.____
    A. Paul B. Frei C. Widal D. Weil-Felix

16. A patient weighing 70 kilograms is severely burned (25% of the body). The amount of daily nitrogen which would be required to maintain a positive nitrogen balance in such a patient is _____ grams a day. 16.____
    A. 5 B. 12 C. 20 D. 60

17. The one of the following conditions in which uribilinogen is likely to be ABSENT in the urine is 17.____
    A. carcinoma of the head of the pancreas
    B. stones in the gallbladder
    C. cirrhosis of the liver
    D. acute yellow atrophy of the liver

18. The one of the following organs which NORMALLY elaborates acid phosphatase is the 18.____
    A. liver B. prostate gland
    C. bone marrow D. spleen

19. The percentage which MOST NEARLY represents the five-year survival rate in Hodgkin's disease is 19.____
    A. 1% B. 20% C. 50% D. 90%

20. The percentage of cases of carcinoma of the rectum in which a downward or retrograde spread occurs is MOST NEARLY 20.____
    A. 5% B. 50% C. 80% D. 90%

21. The APPROXIMATE amount of fluid excreted normally per day in the gastrointestinal tract is _____ cc. 21.____
    A. 520 B. 3200 C. 5200 D. 8200

22. To determine the degree of vasospasms in a case of thrombo-angiitis obliterans, you should 22.____
    A. take oscillometric readings
    B. perform an intradermal salt test
    C. immerse both forearms in water at a temperature of 50°F for 20 minutes
    D. inject the posterior tibial nerve with 5 cc of 2% novocaine solution

23. After ligating the inferior vena cava, the one of the following veins or systems of veins which does NOT take part in establishing collateral circulation is the 23.____
    A. ascending lumbar veins B. azygos veins
    C. inferior mesenteric veins D. internal vertebral plexus

24. The one of the following substances which inhibits the production of prothrombin in the liver is 24.____
A. heparin B. dicoumarol C. vitamin K D. glucose

25. On entering the abdominal cavity from the chest, the relationship of the two vagi nerves USUALLY is 25.____
A. right vagus enters behind the esophagus and is distributed to the posterior surface of the stomach while the left vagus is on the anterior aspect
B. right vagus lies on the anterior surface and the left vagus on the posterior surface
C. both vagi lie on the posterior aspect of the stomach
D. both vagi lie on the anterior surface of the stomach

26. In the case of complete portal vein block, MOST of the portal blood is then conveyed to the parenchyma of the liver by the 26.____
A. hepatic vein B. hepatic artery
C. esophageal veins D. middle hemorrhoidal veins

27. A patient with gastro-jejuno-colic-fistula suffers rapid weight loss and diarrhea. These symptoms can MOST likely be attributed to 27.____
A. loss of food from the stomach into the colon
B. loss of hydrochloric acid from the stomach into the colon
C. improper diet
D. the irritation set up by the entrance of colonic gases and contents into the stomach

28. Of the following micro-organisms, the one which is resistant or slightly susceptible to penicillin activity in vitro is 28.____
A. gonococcus B. bacillus coli
C. staphylococcus aureus D. clostridium welchii

29. Following a severe convulsion, as in electric shock therapy, the patient complains of persistent mediastinal pain.
This is MOST likely to be a result of injury to 29.____
A. pleuropulmonary mechanism B. cardiac mechanism
C. bony skeleton D. peripheral nerves

30. The one of the following which is MOST likely to be encountered as evidence of a lesion complicating a fracture of the olecranon is weak or absent power to 30.____
A. extend wrist B. abduct the thumb
C. spread the fingers D. flex the interphalangeal joints

31. The one of the following lesions in which dyspnea accompanied by cyanosis of the face and neck is MOST likely to be present several hours after injury is 31.____
A. tear of the ligamentum nuchae
B. crushing injury of chest
C. fracture of the fifth cervical vertebra
D. dislocation of the jaw

32. The MOST efficient of the following measures to bring about early relief of circulatory embarrassment accompanying a grossly displaced supracondylar fracture is 32.____
    A. reduction of the displaced fracture fragments
    B. flexion of the elbow
    C. extension of the elbow
    D. immobilization and elevation of the arm without reduction

33. A patient is admitted with a severely crushed pelvis. He is in profound shock. The one of the following procedures which is MOST likely to be of little or no help in evaluating the intactness of his genito-urinary tract is 33.____
    A. injection and attempted withdrawal of sterile saline from the bladder
    B. retrograde cystography
    C. catherization
    D. intravenous pyelography

34. The one of the following in which atrophy of the deltoid is NOT a characteristic concomitant is 34.____
    A. long standing rupture of the stipraspinatus tendon
    B. chronic subdeltoid bursitis due to calcium deposit
    C. long standing painful acromioclavicular arthritis
    D. chronic suppuration in the shoulder joint

35. The one of the following to which hip pathology MOST frequently produces referred pain is the 35.____
    A. buttock
    B. groin
    C. knee
    D. lateral side of the thigh

36. The one of the following muscle groups which is of LEAST importance in producing the characteristic displacement of a subtrochanteric fracture of the femur is the 36.____
    A. lesser glutei
    B. ilio-psoas
    C. external rotators
    D. gluteus maximus

37. The one of the following lesions MOST commonly characterized by the sudden onset of complete inability to actively extend the interphalangeal joint of the thumb as a late complication is 37.____
    A. Colles' fracture
    B. carpal scaphoid fracture
    C. fracture through base of first metacarpal
    D. complex dislocation of first metacarpophalangeal joint

38. An injured ankle shows the following fractures by x-ray: a transverse fracture of the medial malleolus and a fracture through the junction of the middle and lower one-third of the fibular shaft. Neither fracture is displaced sufficiently to require reduction. Of the following, the lesion MOST likely to result in persistent pain and disability is 38.____
    A. fracture of the medial malleolus
    B. fracture of the fibula
    C. associated ligamentous damage
    D. aseptic necrosis of the talus

39. Of the following, the MOST common cause for continued elevation of temperature, pulse, respiration, white blood count, and erythrocyte sedimentation rate during the first two weeks following a simple comminuted fracture of the femoral shaft treated by traction is 39.____
   A. local tissue damage
   B. venous complications
   C. pulmonary complications
   D. the effect of traction upon the extremity

40. In a fracture of the femoral neck, the one of the following MOST likely to predispose to bony union is 40.____
   A. a varus deformity of the head fragment
   B. a valgus deformity of the head fragment
   C. a normal relationship between head and neck
   D. external rotation of the neck on the head

41. Of the following nerves, the one MOST commonly injured in a dislocation of the shoulder is 41.____
   A. median B. axillary C. radial D. ulnar

42. Persistent wrist pain on forcing the extremes of pronation and supination following a Colles' fracture can MOST frequently be relieved by an operative procedure on the 42.____
   A. radius B. ulna
   C. radiocarpal ligaments D. pronator quadratus

43. During the first six months following a fractured elbow and after the primary injury has healed, the therapeutic program of choice for the management of progressive stiffening of the joint accompanied by the roentgenological appearance of calcification in the region of the brachialis muscle is 43.____
   A. normal use within pain limits
   B. restriction of use
   C. physiotherapy and passive stretching of the joint
   D. complete rest of the joint by use of a splint

44. A patient is admitted with an incomplete transverse fissure fracture through the shaft of the femur. X-rays demonstrate the bone to be somewhat bowed with coarse trabeculations and a thickened cortex. He also complains of deafness and tinnitus. 44.____
   The condition MOST likely to be found responsible for the latter complaints is
   A. Paget's disease B. Addison's disease
   C. hyperthyroidism D. rickets

45. Following a penetrating wound at the base of the neck in the posterior cervical triangle, it is noted that there is a drooping of the shoulder with a wing scapula rotated downwards and outwards, and there is an abnormal contour of the base of the neck. 45.____
The MOST likely lesion is damage to the
   A. long thoracic nerve of Bell
   B. dorsal scapula nerve
   C. spinal accessory nerve
   D. supra scapula nerve

46. In a postero-lateral herniation of a lumbar intervertebral disk, the nucleus pulposus MOST often ruptures the 46.____
   A. ligamentum flavum
   B. annulus fibrosus
   C. dentate ligament
   D. interspinous ligament

47. Symptoms indicating operation for traumatic subdural hematoma MOST frequently occur 47.____
   A. at any time from hours to months after injury
   B. a few hours after a head injury
   C. a few months after injury
   D. within the first few hours or a few months after injury

48. The one of the following traumatic lesions in which a fracture of the skull is NEARLY ALWAYS present is 48.____
   A. contusion of the brain
   B. subarachnoid hemorrhage
   C. laceration of the brain
   D. hemorrhage from the middle meningeal artery

49. A patient is very ill with pneumonia, despite large doses of sulfadiazine. Suddenly, he develops weakness of the left arm and leg and becomes s4emi-stuporous. The stupor gradually clears, and the weakness of the left side improves a little, but after three weeks a papilledema of four diopters appears. 49.____
The patient is PROBABLY suffering from
   A. meningitis
   B. brain abscess
   C. cerebral thrombosis with softening
   D. cerebral hemorrhage

50. An adult develops over a period of months weakness and numbness of the entire left side of his face. He has been almost totally deaf in the left ear for five years. 50.____
The MOST likely diagnosis is a
   A. tumor of the eighth nerve
   B. neuritis
   C. chronic otitis media or petrositis
   D. cerebral tumor

KEY (CORRECT ANSWERS)

1.	A	11.	B	21.	D	31.	B	41.	B
2.	C	12.	C	22.	D	32.	A	42.	B
3.	A	13.	D	23.	C	33.	D	43.	A
4.	D	14.	A	24.	B	34.	A	44.	A
5.	D	15.	D	25.	A	35.	C	45.	C
6.	B	16.	D	26.	B	36.	D	46.	B
7.	D	17.	A	27.	D	37.	A	47.	A
8.	B	18.	B	28.	B	38.	C	48.	D
9.	A	19.	B	29.	C	39.	A	49.	B
10.	B	20.	A	30.	C	40.	B	50.	A

TEST 3

DIRECTIONS: Each question or incomplete statement is followed by several suggested answers or completions. Select the one that BEST answers the question or completes the statement. *PRINT THE LETTER OF THE CORRECT ANSWER IN THE SPACE AT THE RIGHT.*

1. Following a bullet wound of the upper third of the arm, a patient shows, in addition to other signs, atrophy of the thenar eminence and inability to flex the distal phalanx of the index finger. 1.____
   He MOST likely sustained an injury of the
   A. brachial artery B. ulnar nerve
   C. median nerve D. radial nerve

2. A male, 50 years of age, experienced a severe pain the left inguinal region while lifting a heavy object. Examination revealed a direct inguinal hernia. 2.____
   Of the following, the anatomical structure which was PRIMARILY involved is the
   A. external oblique fascia B. transversal is fascia
   C. transversus abdomenus muscle D. conjoined tendon

3. A normal knee joint in ten degrees of flexion shows some lateral instability. 3.____
   Of the following, this instability is due to injury of _____ ligament(s).
   A. cruciate
   B. fibular collateral
   C. tibial collateral
   D. tibial and fibular collateral ligaments and cruciate

4. All structures of the anterior aspect of the left wrist, 3 inch proximal to the flexor crease, are severed by a knife. Preparations for surgical repair have been completed. The wrist is viewed in the anatomical position. The structures are identified prior to repair. The flexor carpi radialis muscle lies _____ to the tendons of the flexor digitorum sublimis. 4.____
   A. anterior B. posterior C. perpendiclar D. medial

5. In the normal anatomical relationship of the bones of the wrist joint, the greater multangular (trapezium) articulates with 5.____
   A. lunate and third metacarpal B. lunate and second metacarpal
   C. navicular and first metacarpal D. triquetrum and lunate

6. A patient with a third degree burn of the dorsum of the hand and fingers has the greatest assurance of a good functional result if the treatment followed is 6.____
   A. pressure dressings with skin grafting in 4 to 6 weeks
   B. daily dressings with sulfa ointment
   C. daily active in motion in warm saline with skin grating in 3 to 4 weeks
   D. daily active motion in warm saline with skin grafting in 10 to 14 days

7. A simple complete fracture of the upper third of radius is sustained by a young adult. Closed reduction is attempted. To obtain an adequate reduction, the arm and hand should be held in 7.____
   A. pronation B. supination C. mid-position D. extension

8. Of the following places of work, cases of byssinosis are MOST likely to be found in 8.____
   A. mines
   B. foundries
   C. woodworking shops
   D. cotton mills

9. At the present time, a number of substances are used in place of lead in the manufacture of paints. Of the following, the one which is NOT used for this purpose is 9.____
   A. litharge B. zinc oxide C. lithopone D. titanium oxide

10. Orthotolidine is commonly used in testing for 10.____
    A. bacteria in milk
    B. bacteria in water
    C. arsenic in food
    D. chlorine in water

11. In determining the source of an outbreak of food poisoning traced to a particular meal, the MOST important step is to 11.____
    A. examine bacteriologically every item of food served at the meal
    B. determine the attack rates for each food served for those who partook of the food and those who did not partake of the food
    C. examine the stools of all who became ill
    D. examine the stools of all food handlers who prepared the meal

12. Gram for gram, the one of the following foods which is the RICHEST source of nicotinic acid is 12.____
    A. banana B. corn meal C. calf liver D. spinach

13. In a trichinosis lawsuit, the item of food which was MOST likely the cause of trichinosis was 13.____
    A. raw ground beef
    B. pork processed under federal inspection for consumption without additional cooking
    C. federally inspected fresh ham eaten raw
    D. homemade thoroughly cooked sausage

14. A veteran with known and treated schistosomiasis acquired on Leyte develops two years later, convulsions, and signs of an expanding intracranial lesion. This is PROBABLY 14.____
    A. a malignant brain tumor
    B. a hydatid cyst
    C. schistosomiasis of the brain
    D. an amebic abscess

15. A food handler is found to have cysts of Endamoeba histolytica in the stool but is asymptomatic. This food handler should 15.____
    A. never be employed as a food handler
    B. be treated with emetine and then re-employed
    C. be observed and treated only if symptoms develop
    D. be treated with amebicidal drugs by mouth and then re-employed if the stools are negative

16. A patient consumed a mixture of raw ground beef and pork. A year later, he had convulsions. X-ray showed calcified shadows (1-2 cm long) in the muscles. The patient MOST likely had 16.____
    A. multiple hydatid cysts
    B. trichinosis
    C. cysticercosis (Taenia solium)
    D. the larval stage of the beef tapeworm

17. One of the following worms which is endemic in the United States is 17.____
    A. Hymenolepis nana
    B. Schistosoma mansoni
    C. Ancylostoma duodenale
    D. Clonorchis sinensis

18. The metabolism of lead in the body CLOSELY resembles that of 18.____
    A. sodium
    B. potassium
    C. calcium
    D. iron

19. Measles occurs only occasionally in the adult population because 19.____
    A. the control of measles has become so effective that it is a rapidly disappearing disease in all age groups
    B. one attack of measles produces a life-long immunity and the disease is sufficiently prevalent to result in almost universal infection during childhood
    C. hormonal changes associated with adolescence produce a high degree of non-specific immunity effective against measles, as well as the other so-called communicable diseases of childhood
    D. exposure to measles rarely occurs after school days

20. The HIGHEST yield of tuberculosis cases will be found by the routine x-ray examination of 20.____
    A. admissions to general hospitals
    B. school children
    C. adult familial contacts of known cases
    D. industrial workers

21. The PROPER interpretation of a positive reaction to a tuberculin test is that the person is 21.____
    A. suffering from active tuberculosis
    B. immune to invasion by the tubercle bacillus
    C. susceptible to invasion by the tubercle bacillus
    D. sensitive to tuberculo-protein by virtue of previous or present infection with tubercle bacillus

22. A typhoid fever patient CANNOT be released from isolation in the city until 22.____
    A. ten days after temperature reaches and remains normal and thereafter until two stools, taken not less than forty-eight hours apart, are negative
    B. the Widal test becomes negative
    C. one week after recovery
    D. the patient signs a pledge not to work as a food handler

23. Syphilis may be communicable 23.____
    A. up to four years after acquiring the disease (except that females during the childbearing period may transmit infection in uterine life to their children for longer periods of time)
    B. only while the primary lesion is visible
    C. from the appearance of the primary lesion until the disappearance of the secondary lesion
    D. only while one or another of the serological tests for syphilis is positive

24. Of the following procedures, the one which would be MOST important in producing a safe drinking water is 24.____
    A. treating the reservoir with copper sulphate
    B. chlorination
    C. aeration
    D. screening

25. The drug of choice for the termination of an acute attack of vivax malaria is 25.____
    A. quinine
    B. quinacrine (atabrine)
    C. totaquine
    D. plasmochin

KEY (CORRECT ANSWERS)

1. C
2. B
3. B
4. A
5. C

6. D
7. B
8. D
9. A
10. D

11. B
12. C
13. C
14. C
15. D

16. C
17. A
18. C
19. B
20. C

21. D
22. A
23. A
24. B
25. B

EXAMINATION SECTION
TEST 1

DIRECTIONS: Each question or incomplete statement is followed by several suggested answers or completions. Select the one that *BEST* answers the question or completes the statement. *PRINT THE LETTER OF THE CORRECT ANSWER IN THE SPACE AT THE RIGHT.*

1. Prenatal care begins 1.____

   A. before conception
   B. early in the prenatal period
   C. with a positive Ascheim Zondek test
   D. the fourth month of the prenatal period

2. *One* of the *BEST* methods to use to teach home nursing and child care is 2.____

   A. programmed instruction
   B. student-centered activity instruction
   C. teacher-centered developmental instruction
   D. the use of work books

3. The *PRINCIPAL* objective of the home nursing course is to teach 3.____

   A. the practice of simple nursing techniques
   B. the deviations from normal health
   C. how to interpret the doctor's reports
   D. how to maintain, protect, and improve personal and family health

4. The Emerson Birtheez machine is used in obstetrics to 4.____

   A. *accelerate* action of abdominal muscles
   B. *decompress* diaphragm and overcome nausea
   C. *accelerate* breathing and aid 2nd stage of labor
   D. *decompress* abdominal muscles and accelerate labor

5. Sex of a baby is determined by 5.____

   A. the "x" chromosomes in the ovum
   B. the "x and Y' chromosomes in the sperm cell
   C. pre-natal influences
   D. following a definite known pattern of selection

6. Although there is no nerve connection between the mother and the fetus, it has been established that the fetus has been influenced by 6.____

   A. emotional immaturity of the mother-to-be
   B. excessive fatigue
   C. narcotic addiction of the mother-to-be
   D. undesirable environmental contacts

7. Blood specimens must be collected from all newborn infants 7.____

A. at birth
B. within 24 hours after birth
C. on the day of discharge from the hospital
D. at one month of age

8. Testing of newborn infants for phenylketonuria is 8.____

A. voluntary
B. required by state law
C. required by federal law
D. is *not* required

9. At each regular visit for routine examination of the pregnant woman, the following procedures are carried out: 9.____

A. Blood pressure, weight, urinalysis
B. Ascheim-Zondek test, R.E. factor
C. Wasserman, hemoglobin, weight
D. Basal metabolism, hemoglobin, chest x-ray

10. In the young, 10.____

A. untreated diabetes mellitus runs a relatively more rapid and more uniformly fatal course than in older patients
B. diabetes is easily detected and is simple to manage
C. diabetes may be corrected by simple surgery
D. early diagnosis and treatment of diabetes does not arrest its fatal course

11. When pregnancy occurs, the corpus luteum reaches full development 11.____

A. in about seven months and retrogresses after the delivery of the baby
B. and produces progesterone during the full term of pregnancy
C. at about the fourth month and produces progesterone
D. in about eight days and then deteriorates quickly

12. Nutritional studies show that 12.____

A. babies of mothers on poor diets are in excellent condition at birth
B. newborn babies are not affected by the mother's diet
C. the pregnant woman, following natural instincts, will select a wellbalanced diet
D. some complications of pregnancy may result from an inadequate diet

13. The *MOST* common presentation at birth is 13.____

A. frank breech
B. head or cephalic
C. shoulder
D. full breech

14. Toxemia of pregnancy characterized by a sudden elevation in blood pressure, albuminuria, and edema in a previously normal gravida is known as 14.____

A. eclampsia
B. hypertensive vascular disease without superimposed acute toxemia
C. unclassified toxemia
D. pre-eclampsia

15. Physical care in pediatric nursing *includes* 15.____

   A. understanding the health problems, their treatment and means of prevention
   B. maintaining quiet, cleanliness, and freedom from distraction
   C. limiting parental visits to the hospital
   D. stress on feeding

16. Tetanic contractions on the pregnant uterus usually indicate 16.____

   A. fetal distress
   B. accelerated descent and rotation
   C. that a ruptured uterus is imminent
   D. occurrence of perineal lacerations

17. The *FIRST* indication that the baby is gaining control of his muscles is when he 17.____

   A. lifts his chin while lying on his abdomen
   B. really smiles
   C. turns his head in response to sound
   D. lifts his chest while lying on his abdomen

18. The mouth of the infant should be 18.____

   A. washed gently dally with tap water
   B. washed gently each day with sterile water
   C. inspected after each feeding
   D. inspected as part of the bath routine

19. A study comparing the desirability of giving an infant a formula warmed to body temperature and one direct from the refrigerator has shown that there is 19.____

   A. frequent regurgitat ion from the cold formula
   B. a disturbed sleep pattern from the cold formula
   C. a more stable weight gain with the warmed formula
   D. no significant difference

20. In the care of newborn infants, the intramuscular injection of vitamin K is *MOST* valuable in 20.____

   A. preventing intracranial hemorrhage
   B. preventing cord hemorrhage
   C. stimulating the assimilation of calcium
   D. treating circumcision hemorrhage

21. For the purposes of treatment of a baby, the definition of prematurity is *BEST* expressed by the phrase *birth after viability AND* 21.____

   A. before the 8th month
   B. before the 20th week
   C. before the 9th month
   D. weight under 2500 grams

22. Congenital defects in the fetus often result if, in early pregnancy, a woman contracts 22.____

   A. scarlet fever
   B. German measles
   C. whooping cough
   D. pneumonia

23. During pregnancy, the mother should gain *about* 23.____

A. 15 pounds B. 10 pounds C. 20 pounds D. 25 pounds

24. A "demand" schedule means feeding the baby 24.____

A. every four hours
B. every three hours
C. when he's hungry
D. when he awakens

25. The leading cause of death of children between 1-5 years of age is 25.____

A. home accidents
B. rheumatic fever
C. pneumonia
D. cancer

KEY (CORRECT ANSWERS)

1. A
2. B
3. D
4. D
5. B

6. C
7. C
8. B
9. A
10. A

11. C
12. D
13. B
14. D
15. A

16. C
17. A
18. D
19. A
20. B

21. D
22. B
23. C
24. C
25. A

TEST 2

DIRECTIONS: Each question or incomplete statement is followed by several suggested answers or completions. Select the one that *BEST* answers the question or completes the statement. *PRINT THE LETTER OF THE CORRECT ANSWER IN THE SPACE AT THE RIGHT.*

1. When the pediatrician adds egg yolk to the infant's diet, on the first day add 1.____

   A. one drop B. five drops
   C. half a yoke D. one teaspoonful

2. During the first year of life, the infant should be in-noculated to prevent 2.____

   A. smallpox, diphtheria, whooping cough
   B. diphtheria, measles, tetanus
   C. scarlet fever, smallpox, whooping cough
   D. diphtheria, measles, smallpox

3. First-aid treatment of nosebleed in a young child calls for 3.____

   A. permitting child to lie flat on back
   B. sitting child in chair; tipping head back
   C. allowing child to sit up, head bent forward, applying cold compress at back of neck and nostrils
   D. assisting child to blow nose, then pressing nostrils shut

4. Thumb-sucking usually indicates that the baby 4.____

   A. is insecure and discontented
   B. is hungry and likes the sensation of sucking
   C. needs something to handle and play with
   D. has been poorly trained

5. The protein requirement for infants is 5.____

   A. the *same* per kilogram or pound of body weight as for adults
   B. *less* per kilogram or pound of body weight than for adults
   C. is *slightly higher* per kilogram or pound of body weight than for adults
   D. *much higher* per kilogram or pound of body weight than for adults

6. Boiling milk for the baby's formula 6.____

   A. reduces the size of the fat globules
   B. makes a smaller curd to aid digestion
   C. makes a more perfect emulsion
   D. reduces the water content

7. It is considered safer from the standpoint of the mother's health to have the first child between the ages of 7.____

   A. 18 and 19 B. 20 and 24 C. 25 and 28 D. 29 and 30

8. To meet the need for iron, a baby under four months of age is furnished 8.____

   A. egg yolk given 2 or 3 times a week
   B. whole grain cereals
   C. an entire egg yolk each day
   D. green vegetables

9. The constant temperature to be maintained for a premature infant is 9.____

   A. 68-72° F   B. 80-89° F   C. 90-99° F   D. 100-105° F

10. It is *important* to advise the mother of a new baby to protect it by 10.____

   A. impressing upon her the fact that the baby's mind is like a clean slate; everything he hears will be deeply engraved
   B. explaining that personality cannot be improved, but health can be improved
   C. helping her to interpret the baby's physical needs
   D. encouraging her to fondle the baby often, to develop a sense of security

11. There are certain symptoms of illness in children that a mother must learn to observe and heed early. One of these is: 11.____

   A. Brow feels hot to the touch
   B. Lack of appetite for a day
   C. Dry skin, hot and flushed
   D. Rapid pulse after exertion or play

12. The ossification of children's bones ends 12.____

   A. during infancy
   B. during the later pre-school years
   C. during the early pre-school years
   D. just before puberty

13. The child's bones have an area of growth 13.____

   A. at the upper end only
   B. at the lower end only
   C. at both ends
   D. from the center upward and downward

14. During the prepubertal growth acceleration period and during adolescence, 14.____

   A. there is no need for vitamin D
   B. the need for vitamin D is more universal
   C. the need for vitamin D is the same as for the younger child
   D. vitamin E may replace vitamin D

15. Diphtheria innoculations should be given at the age of 15.____

   A. 2 years   B. 6 weeks
   C. 9 months   D. admission to school

16. When brown sugar is used in the infant's formula (in place of refined sugar), the mineral content is 16.____

A. reduced
B. slightly increased
C. not affected
D. greatly increased

17. The infantile stomach is completely emptied of a feeding in 17.____

A. less than 1 hour
B. 5 to 6 hours
C. 1 to 4 hours
D. none of these

18. The protein content of mother's breast milk compared with that of cow's milk is 18.____

A. the same
B. greater
C. less
D. more granular

19. The average amount of sleep required by an infant at the age of six months is 19.____

A. 20 hours B. 17 hours C. 15 hours D. 14 hours

20. A baby should be immunized against diphtheria 20.____

A. *before* the sixth month
B. *between* the sixth month and the first year
C. *during* the second year
D. *between* the second and third year

21. The prenatal transmission of syphilis can usually be prevented by the institution of effective treatment before the 21.____

A. second month
B. third month
C. fifth month
D. sixth month

22. The *HIGHEST* degree of motor control which an average child of 13 months would be expected to reach is the ability to 22.____

A. pull himself into a sitting position and to sit unsupported
B. creep about the playpen and to pull himself into a standing position
C. stand alone and walk with some assistance
D. walk alone with no support

23. The use of x-ray for determining pregnancy, missed abortion, disproportion, etc., is thought to impose the risk of 23.____

A. affecting the mental development of the child
B. affecting the tonicity of uterine musculature
C. producing malformation in subsequent offspring
D. sterilizing the woman

24. The daily use of mineral oil for prevention of constipation in pregnancy is considered *unwise* because 24.____

A. it centers attention on the use of drugs, rather than diet, to stimulate elimination
B. it increases the tendency to nausea
C. the fatty substance slows the digestion of protein foods
D. the oily coating over the intestinal mucosa interferes with the absorption of vitamins

25. The feeding interval for normal young infants should be based upon 25.____

A. early training in habits of regularity
B. four-hour rest periods between feedings
C. individual digestive capacities
D. the 24-hour nutritional requirements

KEY (CORRECT ANSWERS)

1. A
2. A
3. C
4. B
5. D

6. B
7. B
8. A
9. B
10. A

11. C
12. D
13. C
14. B
15. C

16. B
17. C
18. C
19. C
20. B

21. C
22. D
23. C
24. A
25. C

ANATOMIC SCIENCES
EXAMINATION SECTION
TEST 1

DIRECTIONS: Each question or incomplete statement is followed by several suggested answers or completions. Select the one that BEST answers the question or completes the statement. *PRINT THE LETTER OF THE CORRECT ANSWER IN THE SPACE AT THE RIGHT.*

1. When stratified squamous epithelium thickens, the 1.____

   A. rete pegs increase in size and the intercellular bridges become more evident
   B. basement membrane becomes more irregular and the dermis acquires an increased lymphatic supply
   C. stratum spinosum becomes less evident and the basement membrane thickens
   D. number of vascular capillaries in the dermis increases and more sweat glands develop

2. In growth of the neuron, there is an essential synthesis of axoplasm to accommodate for increasing axonal length. This material is synthesized 2.____

   A. within the cell body
   B. in connective tissue
   C. within Schwann cells
   D. within the axon itself

3. The cells in the adrenal gland that secrete epinephrine are the ______ cells. 3.____

   A. medullary
   B. zona fasciculata
   C. zona glomerulosa
   D. zona reticularis

4. The blood vessels which empty into the right atrium are the 4.____

   A. pulmonary and bronchial veins
   B. superior vena cava, coronary sinus and hemiazygos vein
   C. superior and inferior venae cavae and coronary sinus
   D. coronary sinus and pulmonary veins

5. Surgical excision of the parotid gland endangers the facial nerve as well as the 5.____

   A. hypoglossal nerve
   B. motor nerves to the muscles of mastication
   C. external carotid artery and auriculotemporal nerve
   D. lesser occipital nerve and spinal accessory nerve

6. The elements that are present during development and growth of the alveolar process are the 6.____

   A. osteoblasts, osteoclasts, osteoid
   B. perichondrium, osteoblasts, periosteal bud
   C. osteoblasts, osteoid, megakaryocytes
   D. periosteum, epiphyseal ossification centers, osteoblasts

7. An efferent lymphatic channel and an afferent lymphatic channel in lymph nodes *differ* in that the efferent vessel 7.____

   A. is located in the hilus region of the gland, whereas the afferent vessel enters the gland elsewhere
   B. contains numerous myeloid white blood cells, whereas the afferent vessel contains few, if any, white blood cells
   C. has no valve structure, whereas the afferent vessel has a valve component
   D. is lined partially with reticuloendothelial cells, whereas the afferent vessel is lined totally with endothelial cells

8. The function of the posterior lobe of the hypophysis involves the storage and release of 8.____

   A. thyrotropic hormone and gonadotropic hormone
   B. thyrotropic hormone and vasopressin (ADH)
   C. oxytocin and gonadotropic hormone
   D. vasopressin (ADH) and oxytocin

9. The adult parotid gland can be distinguished by 9.____
   I. mucous acini *only*
   II. relatively long secretory ducts
   III. mucous acini with serous demilunes
   IV. serous acini *only*
   V. long intercalated ducts

   The CORRECT answer is:

   A. I, II, III
   B. II, III, IV
   C. II, IV, V
   D. III, IV, V

10. The inguinal ligament runs between the 10.____

    A. pubic tubercle and the iliac tubercle
    B. symphysis pubis and the inferior iliac spine
    C. anterior superior iliac spine and the pubic tubercle
    D. anterior and posterior superior iliac spines

11. The ligamentum arteriosum is 11.____

    A. a ligament connecting the liver to the anterior abdominal wall
    B. the remnant of a fetal channel connecting the right atrium to the left atrium
    C. a fibrous remnant of a fetal channel connecting the left pulmonary artery to the aorta
    D. none of the above

12. In the human kidney, a renal papilla projects *directly* into the 12.____

    A. ureter
    B. minor calyx
    C. major calyx
    D. renal pyramid

13. The esophageal branches of the right vagus nerve in the lower thorax are found *mainly* on the _______ wall of the esophagus. 13.____

    A. left
    B. right
    C. posterior
    D. none of the above

14. The motor division of the trigeminal nerve leaves the skull through the 14.____

A. foramen ovale
B. foramen rotundum
C. inferior orbital fissure
D. superior orbital fissure

15. The common bile duct, the hepatic artery and the portal vein are found grouped in the 15.____

A. mesocolon
B. lesser omentum
C. greater omentum
D. gastrosplenic ligament

16. Ependymal cells constitute the tissue that 16.____

A. lines the ventricles of the brain
B. lines the ventricles of the heart
C. forms a part of the peripheral neuroglia
D. covers the nerve cell body in the ganglion

17. The histologic feature that MOST readily distinguishes the aorta is the presence of 17.____

A. a clearly visible external elastic membrane
B. distinct vasa vasorum in the tunica media
C. a relatively wide and distinct tunica adventitia
D. a tunica media composed primarily of elastic membranes

18. The difference between capillaries and sinusoids is that capillaries 18.____

A. contain blood whereas sinusoids contain plasma
B. have a constant lumen and a complete endothelial lining whereas sinusoids are irregular, tortuous tubes
C. have a muscular wall that can contract and shut off the circulation whereas sinusoids do not
D. are restricted to muscular tissue only whereas sinusoids are widely distributed in every organ

19. The temporalis muscle originates along the side of the skull and passes _______ the zygomatic arch and inserts into the _______. 19.____

A. medial, coronoid process of the mandible
B. lateral, coronoid process of the mandible
C. medial, medial side of the angle of the ramus
D. lateral, medial side of the angle of the ramus

20. In the spinal cord, white matter consists *mainly* of 20.____

A. perineurium
B. myelinated axons
C. nerve cell bodies
D. loose connective tissue

21. Electron microscopy has revealed that each cilium is girdled by the cell membrane and that it consists of filaments. 21.____
The *typical* arrangement of these structures is nine

A. double circumferential and two single centrally located microtubules
B. single circumferential and two double centrally located microtubules
C. single circumferential and two single centrally located microtubules
D. double circumferential and two double centrally located microtubules

22. Sensory loss in the skin overlying the parotid gland could be caused by damage to the _______ nerve. 22.____

A. great auricular
B. greater occipital
C. zygomaticotemporal
D. transverse cervical

23. An upward extension from the thyroid gland may be identified as a 23.____

A. remnant of the thyroglossal duct
B. pyramidal lobe
C. muscular slip
D. all of the above

24. The osteon is a cylinder of compact bone composed of 24.____

A. basal laminae
B. concentric lamellae
C. interstitial lamellae
D. circumferential lamellae

25. *Irritability* is defined as the 25.____

A. ability of a cell to contract when stimulated
B. property of protoplasm which enables a cell to move away from a painful stimulus
C. property of a stimulated nerve cell exhibiting electrical activity
D. property of protoplasm responsible for a cell's being sensitive to a stimulus

---

KEY (CORRECT ANSWERS)

1. A
2. A
3. A
4. C
5. C
6. A
7. A
8. D
9. C
10. C
11. C
12. B
13. C
14. A
15. B
16. A
17. D
18. B
19. A
20. B
21. A
22. A
23. D
24. B
25. D

TEST 2

DIRECTIONS: Each question or incomplete statement is followed by several suggested answers or completions. Select the one that BEST answers the question or completes the statement. *PRINT THE LETTER OF THE CORRECT ANSWER IN THE SPACE AT THE RIGHT.*

1. The middle cranial fossa is separated from the posterior cranial fossa *primarily* by the 1.____

   A. crista galli
   B. groove for the transverse sinus
   C. lesser wing of the sphenoid bone
   D. petrous part of the temporal bone

2. Cytoplasmic granules containing histamine can be found in the 2.____

   A. mast cell
   B. fibroblast
   C. eosinophil
   D. plasma cell

3. The common bile duct and the pancreatic duct join at the 3.____

   A. cystic duct
   B. hepatic duct
   C. cisterna chyli
   D. hepatopancreatic ampulla (of Vater)

4. The cellular organelle that contains many types of hydrolytic enzymes is the 4.____

   A. lysosome
   B. centrosome
   C. mitochondrion
   D. endoplasmic reticulum

5. The fibrillar component of mature dentin is 5.____

   A. elastin
   B. keratin
   C. collagen
   D. reticulin

6. The respiratory diaphragm is innervated by the ______ nerves. 6.____

   A. vagus
   B. phrenic
   C. splanchnic
   D. recurrent (inferior) laryngeal

7. The descending palatine artery is a branch of the ______ artery. 7.____

   A. pterygopalatine part of the maxillary
   B. first part of the facial
   C. ascending pharyngeal
   D. sphenopalatine

8. The crista terminalis is the line of junction between the primitive 8.____

   A. sinus venosus and the auricle
   B. ventricle and the conus arteriosus
   C. conus arteriosus and the right atrium
   D. truncus arteriosus and the left atrium

9. In the case of a slowly occluded inferior vena cava, a *useful* collateral route may develop involving the 9.____

A. several epigastric veins
B. total azygos system
C. both A and B above
D. neither A nor B above

10. Metaphase is a stage in mitotic division in which 10.____

A. cell constriction takes place
B. the nuclear chromatin is first dispersed
C. chromosomes line up at the equatorial plate
D. chromosomes migrate toward the polar ends of the cell

11. Increased resistance to pulmonary blood flow in the lungs would cause a strain on the 11.____

A. left atrium
B. right atrium
C. left ventricle
D. right ventricle

12. The bones that aid in forming the pterygopalatine fossa are the 12.____

A. palatine, maxillary, vomer
B. maxillary, temporal, palatine
C. sphenoid, palatine, maxillary
D. sphenoid, temporal, palatine

13. Which of the lymphoid tissues in the body are considered subepithelial and nonencapsulated? 13.____

A. Tonsils and thymus glands
B. Peyer's patches and tonsils
C. Thymus gland and lymph nodes
D. Lymph nodes and aggregated nodules

14. The growth hormone of the pituitary gland is produced by 14.____

A. the basophils
B. the acidophils
C. the chromophobe cells
D. all of the chromophil cells

15. The germinal center of a lymph nodule represents the 15.____

A. area of proliferation of lymphocytes
B. area of red pulp
C. central artery
D. medulla

16. The postganglionic parasympathetic cell bodies to the parotid gland are found within the _______ ganglion. 16.____

A. otic
B. ciliary
C. sphenopalatine
D. pterygopalatine

17. Lymphoid tissue of the spleen has the function of filtering 17.____

A. lymph *only*
B. blood *only*
C. tissue fluid
D. both lymph and blood

18. The articulating surface of the adult mandibular condyle is covered by 18.____

A. hyaline cartilage
B. typical perichondrium
C. a thin layer of synovial membrane
D. a dense layer of collagenous connective tissue

19. Endochondral ossification is a procedure in the development of bone in which 19.____

A. hyaline cartilage is transformed into bone
B. calcified cartilage is replaced by bone
C. osteocytes of perichondrium form bone
D. osteons with cartilage lamellae are formed

20. At the opening between the small and the large intestines is the 20.____

A. cardiac sphincter
B. pyloric sphincter
C. ileocecal valve
D. tricuspid valve

21. Which of the following statements indicates a true *similarity* between skin of the forearm and skin of the palm? 21.____

A. Both types contain sebaceous glands.
B. The stratum lucidum is present in each.
C. The stratum germinativum is present in each.
D. The thickness of the epidermis is about the same.

22. In the development of a neutrophil from the stem cell in red bone marrow, the 22.____

A. cytoplasm acquires chromatin granules
B. property of phagocytosis is gained
C. nucleus becomes more hyperchromatic
D. nucleus acquires its centrioles

23. In the pancreatic islets (Langerhans), the cell type which produces insulin is the 23.____

A. alpha
B. beta
C. delta
D. gamma

24. When the cell body of a neuron is destroyed, 24.____

A. all its fibers degenerate and die
B. afferent fibers serve as production sites for new cell bodies
C. new nerve cells develop from remaining cells to take the place of those lost
D. the sheath cells or surrounding neuroglia cells serve as guides or pathways for new neuron formation

25. When compared with the diameter of the lumen, the GREATEST proportion of thickness of smooth muscle is found in 25.____

A. large arteries
B. capillaries
C. arterioles
D. veins

KEY (CORRECT ANSWERS)

1. D
2. A
3. D
4. A
5. C

6. B
7. A
8. A
9. C
10. C

11. D
12. C
13. B
14. B
15. A

16. A
17. B
18. D
19. B
20. C

21. C
22. C
23. B
24. A
25. C

ANATOMIC SCIENCES
EXAMINATION SECTION
TEST 1

DIRECTIONS: Each question or incomplete statement is followed by several suggested answers or completions. Select the one that BEST answers the question or completes the statement. *PRINT THE LETTER OF THE CORRECT ANSWER IN THE SPACE AT THE RIGHT.*

1. The component of bone tissue that gives bone tensile strength is the 1.____

   A. elastic fibers
   B. calcified ground substance
   C. interconnecting canaliculi
   D. periosteal connective tissue
   E. collagenous fibrils of matrix

2. The cerebellar cortex is characterized histologically by which of the following types of cells? 2.____

   A. Basket B. Purkinje C. Pyramidal
   D. Martinotti E. Horizontal

3. If the spinal tract of the fifth cranial nerve were sectioned at the level of the caudal medulla, which of the following modalities would be MOST affected? 3.____

   A. Taste
   B. Proprioception
   C. Pain from the ipsilateral side of the face
   D. Light touch from the contralateral side of the face
   E. None of the above

4. Skeletal muscle enlarges with prolonged activity as a consequence of 4.____

   A. differentiation of myoblasts
   B. mitotic division of muscle fibers
   C. an increase in endomysial connective tissue
   D. an increase in sarcoplasm and in the number of myofibrils of existing muscle fibers
   E. none of the above

5. The thick myofilaments observed in transmission electron microscopic preparations of skeletal muscle are 5.____

   A. composed mainly of actin
   B. present only in the A band
   C. present in both A and I bands
   D. traversed or crossed by the Z band
   E. composed mainly of collagenous fibrils

6. From an anatomic standpoint, an emergency airway may be established MOST readily by opening into the trachea 6.____

A. between thyroid cartilages
B. at the level of the jugular notch
C. through the thyrohyoid membrane
D. through the median cricothyroid ligament
E. through the middle constrictor muscle of the pharynx

7. The organelle that binds and releases calcium during relaxation and contraction of skeletal muscle is a 7.____

A. nucleus
B. lysosome
C. mitochondrion
D. transverse tubule
E. sarcoplasmic reticulum

8. Right subclavian and right common carotid arteries arise from the 8.____

A. thoracic aorta
B. ascending aorta
C. arch of the aorta
D. pulmonary artery
E. brachiocephalic artery

9. The common bile duct, the hepatic artery, and the portal vein are found grouped in the 9.____

A. mesocolon
B. lesser omentum
C. greater omentum
D. gastrosplenic ligament
E. pancreatic duct

10. The greater peritoneal sac communicates with the lesser peritoneal sac by means of the 10.____

A. aortic hiatus
B. inguinal canal
C. epiploic foramen
D. lesser pelvic aperture
E. superior pelvic aperture

11. The posterior cervical triangle is bounded partly by the ______ muscle(s). 11.____

A. trapezius and subclavius
B. splenius capitis and trapezius
C. trapezius and sternocleidomastoid
D. clavicle and the longus colli
E. gluteus maximus

12. The PRIMARY histologic characteristic of the pancreas is 12.____

A. follicles filled with secretion
B. groups of special cells scattered among glandular alveoli
C. small groups of cells scattered between follicles
D. cells arranged in layers among which are special cells
E. secretion of bile

13. The middle constrictor muscle of the pharynx originates from the 13.____

A. hyoid bone
B. thyroid cartilage
C. pterygoid hamulus
D. pterygomandibular raphe
E. sphenoid and zygomatic bones

14. Pharyngotympanic (eustachian) tubes connect the nasopharynx with the 14.____

A. outer ear
B. middle ear
C. semicircular canals
D. vestibule of the inner ear
E. thyroid gland

15. Bacteria are frequently ingested by 15.____

A. mast cells
B. fibrocytes
C. small lymphocytes
D. basophilic leukocytes
E. neutrophilic leukocytes

16. Considering number and location, the parathyroid glands are usually ______ the thyroid gland. 16.____

A. single and dorsal to
B. single and embedded in the dorsum of
C. multiple and embedded in the dorsum of
D. multiple and just superior to
E. not related to

17. The arterial supply of the submandibular gland is from which branch of the external carotid artery? 17.____

A. Ascending pharyngeal
B. Superior thyroid
C. Maxillary
D. Facial
E. Mandibular

18. Which of the following blood elements is a fragment of megakaryocytic cytoplasm? 18.____

A. Platelet
B. Normoblast
C. Erythrocyte
D. Promyelocyte
E. Proerythroblast

19. The lateral boundary of the retropharyngeal space at the level of the oropharynx is the 19.____

A. carotid sheath
B. pterygomandibular raphe
C. medial pterygoid muscle and its fascia
D. stylopharyngeus muscle and its fascia
E. lateral pterygoid muscle and its fascia

20. The common hepatic artery is a branch of the ______ artery. 20.____

A. gastric
B. splenic
C. celiac (trunk)
D. superior mesenteric
E. carotid

21. Most of the antibodies in the body that act against bacterial antigens are produced by 21.____

A. T-lymphocytes
B. B-lymphocytes
C. macrophages
D. plasma cells
E. leukocytes

22. In the fetus, blood enters the common carotid arteries by means of the 22.____

A. aorta
B. pulmonary vein
C. pulmonary artery
D. ductus arteriosus
E. thebesian veins (venae cordis minimae)

23. Which of the lymphoid tissues in the body are considered subepithelial and nonencapsulated? 23.____

A. Thymus gland and lymph nodes
B. Lymph nodes and aggregated nodules
C. Pharyngeal tonsils and thymus gland
D. Peyer's patches and pharnygeal tonsils
E. Thyroid gland and lymph nodes

24. Of the following sites, most of the lymph is returned to the blood at the _____ vein(s). 24.____

A. right brachiocephalic
B. left external jugular
C. junction of left internal jugular and subclavian
D. junction of right internal jugular and subclavian
E. right external jugular

25. In the fetal heart, the foramen ovale connects the 25.____

A. pulmonary artery and the aorta
B. right and the left atria, permitting the flow of blood from right to left
C. right and the left atria, permitting the flow of blood from left to right
D. right and the left ventricles, permitting the flow of blood from right to left
E. right and the left ventricles, permitting the flow of blood from left to right

26. Which of the following muscles receives its motor supply from the facial nerve? 26.____

A. Masseter
B. Temporal
C. Buccinator
D. Lateral pterygoid
E. Tensor veli palatini

27. Identify the thalamus in the sketch at the right. 27.____

A. A
B. B
C. C
D. D
E. E

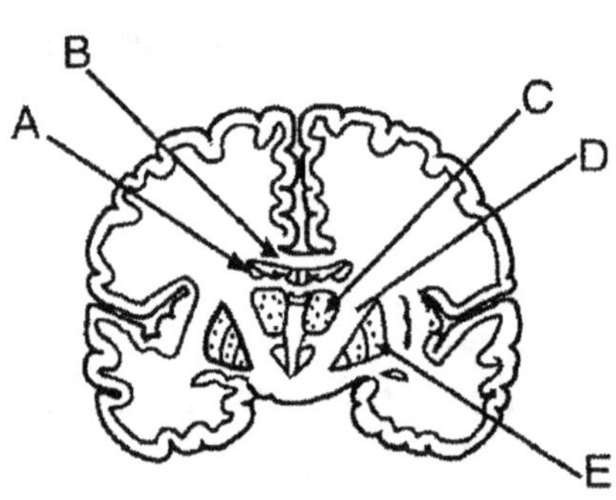

28. Second, third, and fourth right posterior intercostal veins drain from the right superior intercostal vein into the _____ vein. 28.____

A. azygos
B. hemiazygos
C. accessory hemiazygos
D. left brachiocephalic
E. left internal jugular

29. At a muscle-tendon junction, the union is made by 29.____

A. myofibrils connecting with collagenous fibrils of the tendon
B. an abundance of reticular fibers in the area of the junction
C. a continuity of connective tissue sheaths of the muscle with those of the tendon
D. a special thickening of sarcoplasm that unites with collagenous fibrils of the tendon
E. none of the above

30. In the sulcular epithelium, small spaces between cells in the stratum spinosum (prickle cell layer) are normally filled by 30.____

A. keratin
B. a small amount of tissue fluid
C. capillaries that course between cells to approach the free surface
D. collagen
E. none of the above

31. The bony floor of the nasal cavity is formed by the 31.____

A. palatine process of the maxilla and the vertical part of the palatine
B. palatine process of the temporal and the horizontal part of the palatine
C. vomer and the vertical part of the palatine
D. palatine process of the maxilla and the horizontal part of the palatine
E. vertical part of the palatine and the palatine process of the maxilla

32. Cells of the stratum granulosum of thick stratified squamous epithelium characteristically contain ______ granules. 32.____

A. melanin
B. keratin
C. keratohyalin
D. organelles that are
E. lipofuscin

33. A MAJOR sensory innervation of the temporomandibular joint is derived from the ______ nerve. 33.____

A. great auricular
B. auriculotemporal
C. inferior alveolar
D. temporal branches of the facial
E. superior alveolar

34. The middle nasal concha is part of which of the following bones? 34.____

A. Nasal
B. Vomer
C. Ethmoid
D. Palatine
E. Sphenoid

35. The external carotid artery contributes to the blood supply of the nasal cavity by way of the _____ arteries. 35.____

A. facial, superior labial, and angular
B. lingual, deep lingual, and internal nasal
C. occipital, ascending palatine, and posterior nasal
D. maxillary, sphenopalatine, and posterior lateral nasal
E. superficial temporal, transverse facial, and external nasal

---

KEY (CORRECT ANSWERS)

1. E
2. B
3. C
4. D
5. B

6. D
7. E
8. E
9. B
10. C

11. C
12. B
13. A
14. B
15. E

16. C
17. D
18. A
19. A
20. C

21. D
22. A
23. D
24. C
25. B

26. C
27. C
28. A
29. C
30. B

31. D
32. C
33. B
34. C
35. D

TEST 2

DIRECTIONS: Each question or incomplete statement is followed by several suggested answers or completions. Select the one that BEST answers the question or completes the statement. *PRINT THE LETTER OF THE CORRECT ANSWER IN THE SPACE AT THE RIGHT.*

1. The impulse-conducting mechanism in the heart is composed of 1.____

   A. autonomic nerve fibers
   B. bundles of collagenous fibers
   C. reticuloendothelial components
   D. modified cardiac muscle fibers
   E. elastic and reticular fibers *only*

2. Movement of the head about its vertical axis (rotation to right or left) occurs CHIEFLY at which of the following joints? 2.____

   A. Atlanto-axial
   B. Spheno-occipital
   C. Atlanto-occipital
   D. Third to seventh cervical vertebrae
   E. None of the above

3. Which of the following structures is formed from the FIRST branchial (visceral) arch? 3.____

   A. Hyoid bone
   B. Buccinator muscle
   C. Stylopharyngeus muscle
   D. Lateral pterygoid muscle
   E. Superior parathyroid gland

4. Lateral clefting of the lip results from the failure of merging of ______ processes. 4.____

   A. maxillary with mandibular
   B. maxillary
   C. maxillary and medial nasal
   D. medial and lateral nasal
   E. nasal septum with palatine

5. Which of the following cells is MOST likely to have an abundant amount of rough-surfaced endoplasmic reticulum? 5.____

   A. Osteocyte
   B. Macrophage
   C. Osteoblast
   D. Mesothelial cell
   E. Small lymphocyte

6. The ground substance of hyaline cartilage is basophilic because it contains 6.____

   A. phosphatases
   B. polypeptides
   C. orthophosphoric esters
   D. sulfated proteoglycans
   E. lipids

7. Tropocollagen is a protein molecule found in 7.____

   A. collagen and elastic fibers *only*
   B. elastic and reticular fibers *only*
   C. collagen and reticular fibers *only*
   D. collagen, elastic, and reticular fibers
   E. none of the above

8. Hyaline cartilage differs from bone in that hyaline cartilage 8.____

   A. cells lie in lacunae
   B. may grow interstitially
   C. may grow appositionally
   D. can become more highly calcified
   E. may not grow at all

9. The MOST prominent functional component in the tunica media of small arteries is 9.____

   A. elastic fibers
   B. smooth muscle
   C. striated muscles
   D. reticular fibers
   E. collagenous fibers

10. The nucleolus produces 10.____

   A. DNA
   B. transfer RNA
   C. ribosomal RNA
   D. messenger RNA
   E. none of the above

11. An organ with a retroperitoneal location that can be approached surgically without violating the continuity of the peritoneum is the 11.____

   A. ovary
   B. kidney
   C. spleen
   D. gallbladder
   E. lung

12. Which of the following are mobilized when a cell produces an excessive amount of protein? 12.____

   A. Lysosomes
   B. Mitochondria
   C. Lipofuscin granules
   D. Rough endoplasmic reticula
   E. All of the above

13. During endochondral ossification of a long bone of an extremity, the function of hyaline cartilage is to 13.____

   A. increase strength of the developing bone
   B. provide a region where bone can grow in length
   C. provide undifferentiated cells that will become osteoblasts
   D. form cores of trabeculae that compose most compact bone of the diaphysis
   E. obstruct the process of ossification

14. Most intrinsic muscles of the larynx receive their motor innervation from the 14.____

   A. laryngeal plexus
   B. inferior (recurrent) laryngeal nerve

C. external branch of the superior laryngeal nerve
D. internal branch of the superior laryngeal nerve
E. external and internal branches of the superior laryngeal nerve

15. In a relaxed state, transitional epithelium can be distinguished from stratified squamous epithelium because transitional epithelium contains 15.____

A. stratum corneum
B. flattened superficial cells
C. dome-shaped superficial cells
D. more visible ground substance
E. lymphocytes

16. It is possible to distinguish histologically between the stomach and the duodenum because of the presence of _______ only. 16.____

A. mucosal glands in the stomach
B. muscularis mucosa in the stomach
C. simple columnar epithelium lining the stomach
D. submucosal glands in the duodenum
E. smooth muscle in the external musculature of the duodenum

17. A disturbance in cartilage formation in a fetus results in deformities of 17.____

A. sphenoid and zygomatic bones
B. axial skeleton and the base of the skull
C. axial skeleton and the flat bones of the skull
D. petrous portion of the temporal bones and the parietal bones
E. cervical vertebrae

18. The alveolar bone proper (cribriform plate) USUALLY consists of _______ bone. 18.____

A. woven
B. bundle
C. lamellar
D. bundle and lamellar
E. brittle

19. Which of the following structures may be found within the posterior mediastinum? 19.____

A. Heart
B. Phrenic nerve
C. Thoracic duct
D. Arch of the aorta
E. Recurrent laryngeal nerve

20. The optic tracts consist of axons from which of the following cells? 20.____

A. Rod
B. Bipolar
C. Ganglion
D. Horizontal
E. All of the above

21. The large mass of gray matter that bulges into the floor and the lateral aspect of the lateral ventricle is the 21.____

A. hypothalamus
B. caudate nucleus
C. substantia nigra
D. amygdaloid complex
E. none of the above

22. The large ascending bundle of fibers in the medulla that is composed of second order neuron fibers conveying proprioception and discriminatory touch sensations to conscious levels is the 22.____

A. medial lemniscus
B. reticular formation
C. spinal trigeminal tract
D. inferior cerebellar peduncle
E. cardiac muscle

23. Which of the following forms of connective tissues has a preponderance of amorphous ground substance over fibers? 23.____

A. Loose
B. Cartilage
C. Reticular
D. Dense, regularly arranged
E. Dense, irregularly arranged

24. The lamina papyracea is located in the orbital 24.____

A. roof
B. floor
C. lateral wall
D. medial wall
E. all of the above

25. Which of the following articulate directly with the body of the sternum? 25.____

I. Clavicle
II. Eleventh rib
III. Manubrium
IV. First rib
V. Xiphoid process

The CORRECT answer is:

A. I, II, IV
B. II, IV, V
C. III, IV, V
D. III, V
E. I, II, III, IV, V

26. Obstruction of the cerebral aqueduct causes enlargement of the ______ ventricle. 26.____

I. third
II. fourth
III. lateral

The CORRECT answer is:

A. I *only*
B. I, II
C. I, III
D. II *only*
E. II, III

27. Which of the following abdominal viscera are retroperitoneal? 27.____

I. Aorta
II. Liver
III. Kidney
IV. Spleen
V. Pancreas
VI. Suprarenal

The CORRECT answer is:

A. I, II, III, IV
B. I, II, III, V
C. I, II, IV, VI
D. I, III, V, VI
E. II, IV, V, VI

28. Each of the following cell types secretes the substance with which it is paired EXCEPT 28.____

A. Sertoli's cells - testosterone
B. corpus luteum - progesterone
C. alpha cells of the pancreas - glucagon
D. chromaffin cells of the suprarenal - catecholamine
E. serous cells of the parotid gland - saliva

29. All of the following structures can be seen in a histologic examination of the adult parotid gland EXCEPT 29.____

A. striated ducts
B. serous demilunes
C. intercalated ducts
D. myoepithelial cells
E. granular serous cells

30. Which of the following arteries does NOT accompany the corresponding nerve throughout its course? 30.____

A. Lingual
B. Infraorbital
C. Inferior alveolar
D. Posterior superior alveolar
E. Inferior laryngeal

31. Which of the following structural changes is NOT encountered in passing along the respiratory system from the trachea to a respiratory bronchiole? 31.____

A. Decrease in goblet cells
B. Decrease in ciliated cells
C. Total loss of cartilage from the wall
D. Progressive change from stratified squamous to cuboidal epithelial lining
E. Increase in ciliated cells

32. Which of the following layers of the epidermis is LEAST cytodifferentiated? 32.____

A. Stratum basale
B. Stratum corneum
C. Stratum spinosum
D. Prickle-cell layer
E. Stratum granulosum

33. Which of the following tissues would be LEAST affected if the anterior lobe of the hypophysis were destroyed? 33.____

A. Thyroid epithelium
B. Medulla of the adrenal gland
C. Interstitial cells of the testis
D. Zona fasciculata of the adrenal gland
E. Spermatogenic epithelium of the testis

34. The secretion of which of the following endocrine glands is NOT essential to life? 34.____

A. Parathyroids
B. Adrenal cortex
C. Adrenal medulla
D. Anterior pituitary
E. Pancreatic islets (Langerhans)

35. Cell bodies of primary sensory neurons of mechanoreceptors in the periodontal ligament are found in which of the following brainstem nuclei? 35.___

A. Nucleus solitarius
B. Reticular formation
C. Descending nucleus of V
D. Chief sensory nucleus of V
E. Mesencephalic nucleus of V

KEY (CORRECT ANSWERS)

1. D
2. A
3. D
4. C
5. C

6. D
7. C
8. B
9. B
10. C

11. B
12. A
13. B
14. B
15. C

16. D
17. B
18. D
19. C
20. C

21. B
22. A
23. B
24. D
25. D

26. C
27. D
28. A
29. B
30. A

31. D
32. A
33. B
34. C
35. E

ANATOMIC SCIENCES
EXAMINATION SECTION
TEST 1

DIRECTIONS: Each question or incomplete statement is followed by several suggested answers or completions. Select the one that BEST answers the question or completes the statement. *PRINT THE LETTER OF THE CORRECT ANSWER IN THE SPACE AT THE RIGHT.*

1. The inter ______ septum of the ______ is where the foraminal ovale is located. 1.____

   A. atrial; adult
   B. atrial; embryo and fetus
   C. ventricular; adult
   D. ventricular; embryo and fetus
   E. auricular; adult

2. The temporalis muscle originates on the lateral surface of the skull and passes ______ to the zygomatic arch and inserts into the ______. 2.____

   A. medial; coronoid process of the mandible
   B. lateral; coronoid process of the mandible
   C. medial; medial side of the angle of the ramus
   D. lateral; medial side of the angle of the ramus
   E. medial; coronoid process of the maxilla

3. Variation of the size of the lumen of the bronchiole during inspiration and expiration is caused PRIMARILY by 3.____

   A. striated muscle and cartilage
   B. smooth muscle and elastic fibers
   C. the basement membrane and collagen fibers
   D. areolar connective tissue and cartilage
   E. the cell structure of the lumen of the bronchiole

4. The ______ is located at the opening between the small and the large intestines. 4.____

   A. cardiac sphincter
   B. pyloric sphincter
   C. ileocecal valve
   D. tricuspid valve
   E. bicuspid valve

5. Fordyce spots appearing on the mucous membrane of the cheek result from the presence of 5.____

   A. aberrant sweat glands
   B. aberrant sebaceous glands
   C. superficial salivary glands
   D. aberrant fatty accumulations
   E. none of the above

6. The cellular organelle that binds and releases calcium during relaxation and contraction of skeletal muscle is the 6.___

A. nucleus
B. lysosome
C. mitochondrion
D. transverse tubule
E. sarcoplasmic reticulum

7. Acidophils (alpha cells) of the hypophysis secrete 7.___

A. insulin
B. thyroxin
C. sex hormone
D. growth hormone
E. adrenalin

8. A child falls on a nail that penetrates the submental region in the midline. What is the FIRST muscle to be impaled? 8.___

A. Mylohyoid
B. Thyrohyoid
C. Hyoglossus
D. Genioglossus
E. Posterior digastric

9. Salivary, sweat, sebaceous, and von Ebner's glands all have in common the characteristic of being 9.___

A. simple
B. compound
C. exocrine
D. holocrine
E. merocrine

10. An active fibroblast is characterized by 10.___

A. multiple nucleoli
B. a bloated appearance
C. a thick plasma membrane
D. an unusually large nucleus
E. abundant endoplasmic reticulum

11. The white pulp of the spleen is composed PRIMARILY of 11.___

A. sinusoids
B. macrophages
C. lymphocytes
D. connective tissue
E. leukocytes

12. Serotonin is thought to be produced by ______ cells. 12.___

A. chief
B. Paneth's
C. mucous neck
D. enteroendocrine (argentaffin)
E. myoepithelial

13. Most of the postganglionic sympathetic nerve fibers of the head are derived from the 13.___

A. superior cervical ganglion alone
B. superior cervical ganglion and the vagus nerve
C. superior cervical ganglion and the glossopharyngeal nerve
D. inferior, middle, and superior cervical ganglia
E. inferior cervical ganglia alone

14. Production of bile takes place in the 14.____

A. Kupffer cells
B. gallbladder
C. hepatic duct
D. common bile duct
E. none of the above

15. Which of the following branches of the axillary artery USUALLY supplies the latissimus dorsi muscle? 15.____

A. Thoracodorsal
B. Thoracoacromial
C. Lateral thoracic
D. Circumflex scapular
E. Posterior humeral circumflex

16. The esophagus is subdivided into three portions on the basis of a transition in the 16.____

A. submucosa
B. adventitia
C. mucosal layer
D. muscularis externa
E. structure of the thoracic vertebrae

17. Basket (myoepithelial) cells are located in the 17.____

A. periodontal ligament
B. lumen of secretory acini
C. lamina propria of gingiva
D. lumen of intercalated ducts
E. spaces between the basal lamina and the secretory cell membrane

18. Most of the fibers ascending to or descending from the cerebral cortex traverse the 18.____

A. pyramids
B. internal capsule
C. medial lemniscus
D. cerebral peduncles
E. carotid artery

19. Which of the following represents the organelle that is typically composed of vesicles and of curved, flattened cisternae that are parallel to one another? 19.____

A. Centriole
B. Mitochondrion
C. Golgi complex
D. Rough endoplasmic reticulum
E. Smooth endoplasmic reticulum

20. Long bones of the skeleton INCREASE in length because of the 20.____

A. mitotic division of osteocytes
B. mitotic division of osteoblasts
C. resorption of primary bone by osteoclasts
D. appositional growth on the cartilaginous epiphyseal plate
E. interstitial growth in the cartilaginous epiphyseal plate

21. The thoracic splanchnic nerves to the celiac ganglion consist predominantly of 21.___

A. parasympathetic fibers
B. preganglionic visceral efferents
C. postganglionic visceral efferents
D. endoplasmic reticulum
E. osteocytes

22. The motor division of the trigeminal nerve leaves the skull through the 22.___

A. foramen ovale
B. foramen rotundum
C. inferior orbital fissure
D. superior orbital fissure
E. inferior and superior orbital fissure

23. The presence of valves characterizes 23.___

A. veins *only*
B. blood sinusoids *only*
C. lymphatic vessels *only*
D. veins and lymphatic vessels
E. blood sinusoids and blood capillaries

24. The visceral and parietal pericardia are continuous at the 24.___

A. pulmonary artery *only*
B. inferior vena cava *only*
C. veins and arteries entering and leaving the heart
D. bronchial artery *only*
E. phrenic nerve

25. In addition to the bronchus, the ______ form the root of the lung. 25.___

A. pulmonary artery and veins
B. pulmonary artery and azygos vein
C. bronchial arteries and veins
D. bronchial arteries and veins, and the phrenic nerve
E. visceral and parietal pericardia

26. In the sketch at the right which illustrates the head and neck region of a human embryo, the facial process labeled A gives rise to the 26.___

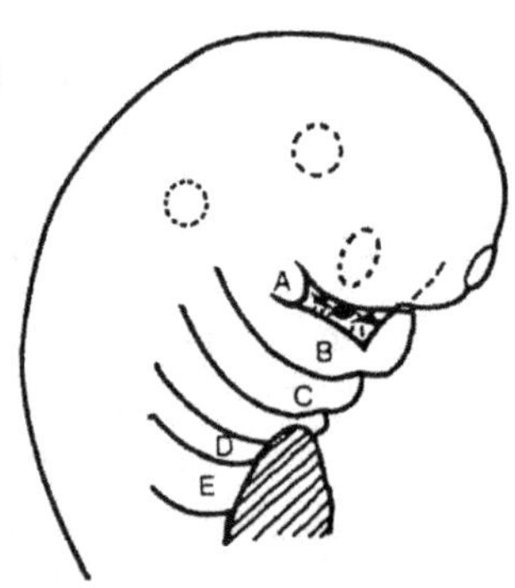

A. nasal septum
B. nasal conchae
C. incisive papilla
D. secondary palate
E. pterygoid plexus

27. The unpaired vessels contributing to the arterial circle of the brain include the _______ arteries. 27.____

A. internal carotid and vertebral
B. posterior and anterior cerebral
C. anterior cerebral and anterior communicating
D. anterior cerebral and posterior communicating
E. anterior communicating and basilar

28. The stratum _______ is TOTALLY lacking in thin skin. 28.____

A. corneum
B. lucidum
C. spinosum
D. germinativum
E. none of the above

29. The anterior interventricular (descending) artery is accompanied by the 29.____

A. small cardiac vein
B. middle cardiac vein
C. great cardiac vein
D. coronary sinus
E. lateral thoracic vein

30. In the circulating blood of an adult, which of the following leukocytes normally appears in the highest numbers? 30.____

A. Basophils
B. Monocytes
C. Eosinophils
D. Neutrophils
E. Lymphocytes

31. The jugular foramen transmits which cranial nerves? 31.____

A. VII, IX, XII
B. IX, X, XI
C. IX, XI, XII
D. X, XI, XII
E. IX *only*

32. The _______ supplies oxygenated blood to the capillary plexus of tissues surrounding a secondary bronchus. 32.____

A. pulmonary vein
B. pulmonary artery
C. bronchial artery
D. carotid artery
E. none of the above

33. Of the following structures, the _______ contacts the thyroid gland. 33.____

A. lingual nerve
B. phrenic nerve
C. thoracic duct
D. thyroarytenoid muscle
E. recurrent laryngeal nerve

34. Connective tissue proper is characterized as having 34.____

A. little tissue fluid
B. poor reparative ability
C. sensitivity as its main function
D. more intercellular material than cells
E. less intercellular material than cells

35. The ______ descends anteriorly to the root of the right lung and between the mediastinal pleura and the pericardium. 35.____

A. right vagus nerve
B. right greater splanchnic nerve
C. nerve that supplies the right half of the diaphragm
D. nerve that supplies pain fibers to alveoli of the right lung
E. left vagus nerve

KEY (CORRECT ANSWERS)

1. B
2. A
3. B
4. C
5. B
6. E
7. D
8. A
9. C
10. E
11. C
12. D
13. A
14. E
15. A
16. D
17. E
18. B
19. C
20. E
21. B
22. A
23. D
24. C
25. A
26. D
27. E
28. B
29. C
30. D
31. B
32. C
33. E
34. D
35. C

TEST 2

DIRECTIONS: Each question or incomplete statement is followed by several suggested answers or completions. Select the one that BEST answers the question or completes the statement. *PRINT THE LETTER OF THE CORRECT ANSWER IN THE SPACE AT THE RIGHT.*

1. Identify the thalamus in the drawing shown at the right. 1.____

   A. A
   B. B
   C. C
   D. D
   E. E

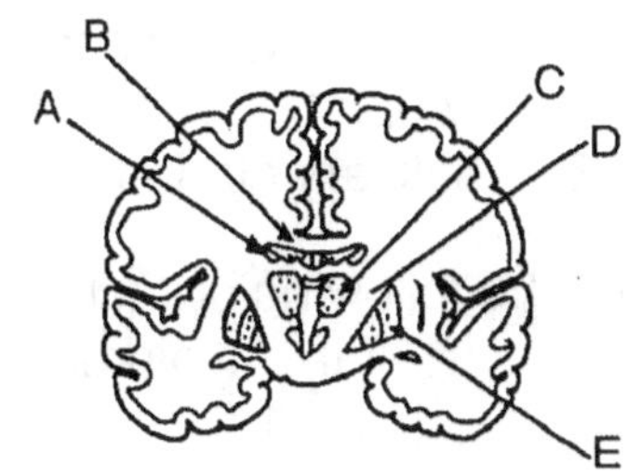

2. The ribonucleic acid involved in protein synthesis is found PRIMARILY in the 2.____

   A. nucleolus
   B. mitochondria
   C. Golgi apparatus
   D. fluid ground substance
   E. granular endoplasmic reticulum

3. The ductus venosus permits blood to flow from the ______ to the ______ the fetus. 3.____

   A. pulmonary vein; aorta
   B. pulmonary artery; aorta
   C. right atrium; left atrium
   D. umbilical vein; inferior vena cava
   E. umbilical vein; superior vena cava

4. The posterior cord of the brachial plexus gives rise to which of the following nerves? 4.____

   A. Radial
   B. Long thoracic
   C. Thoracoacromial
   D. Medial pectoral
   E. Lateral pectoral

5. The postcentral gyrus is located in the 5.____

   A. insula
   B. frontal lobe
   C. temporal lobe
   D. parietal lobe
   E. occipital lobe

6. The cell body of the efferent (motor) neuron of a spinal reflex arc is located in 6.____

   A. an autonomic ganglion
   B. the dorsal root ganglion (spinal ganglion)
   C. the anterior gray column (ventral horn) of the spinal cord
   D. the posterior gray column (dorsal horn) of the spinal cord
   E. none of the above

7. The MOST important organelle or component of a cell for oxidative processes is the 7.____

A. nucleus
B. nucleolus
C. mitochondrion
D. Golgi complex
E. endoplasmic reticulum

8. Lymph from lungs, bronchi, and trachea drains CHIEFLY into 8.____

A. mediastinal lymph nodes
B. deep cervical lymph nodes and vessels
C. superficial cervical lymph nodes and vessels
D. lymph nodes and the vessels paralleling internal mammary blood vessels
E. salivary glands

9. Of the following branches of the external carotid artery, the one that originates just below the level of the hyoid bone's greater cornu is the _______ artery. 9.____

A. facial
B. occipital
C. maxillary
D. superior thyroid
E. posterior auricular

10. The zona pellucida is associated with which of the following? 10.____

A. Corpus luteum
B. Corpus albicans
C. Oocyte in a mature follicle
D. Oocyte in an early primary follicle
E. None of the above

11. Which of the following muscles serves as the forearm's principal extensor? 11.____

A. Pronator teres
B. Brachioradialis
C. Triceps brachii
D. Coracobrachialis
E. Extensor carpi radialis longus

12. The middle pharyngeal constrictor muscle originates from the 12.____

A. hyoid bone
B. thyroid cartilage
C. pterygoid hamulus
D. pterygomandibular raphe
E. hyaline cartilage

13. Preganglionic parasympathetic fibers pass through which of the following structures? 13.____

A. Foramen ovale
B. Stylomastoid foramen
C. Foramen magnum and hypoglossal canal
D. Superior orbital fissure and petrotympanic fissure
E. Styloid process

14. The tendon of the tensor veli palatini muscle curves around the 14.____

A. angular spine
B. styloid process
C. pterygoid hamulus
D. lateral pterygoid plate
E. spine of the sphenoid

15. The zona reticularis is the *inner* layer of the 15.____

A. cortex of the thymus
B. medulla of the thymus
C. cortex of the suprarenal (adrenal)
D. medulla of the suprarenal (adrenal)
E. surface of the retina

16. Which of the following abdominal viscera are retroperitoneal? 16.____

I. Aorta
II. Liver
III. Kidney
IV. Stomach
V. Pancreas
VI. Suprarenal (adrenal)

The CORRECT answer is:

A. I, II, III, V
B. I, II, IV, VI
C. III, IV, V, VI
D. I, III, V, VI
E. II, IV, V, VI

17. The ______ empty into the right atrium. 17.____

A. pulmonary and bronchial veins
B. coronary sinus and pulmonary veins
C. superior and inferior venae cavae and coronary sinus
D. superior vena cava, coronary sinus, and hemiazygos vein
E. small cardiac vein

18. The connective tissue sheath that surrounds a muscle as a whole and is synonymous with the gross anatomic deep fascia is the 18.____

A. epimysium
B. endomysium
C. perimysium
D. periosteum
E. perichondrium

19. The external carotid artery contributes to the blood supply of the nasal cavity by way of the ______ arteries. 19.____

A. facial, the superior labial, and angular
B. lingual, the deep lingual, and internal nasal
C. occipital, the ascending palatine, and posterior nasal
D. maxillary, the sphenopalatine, and posterior lateral nasal
E. superficial temporal, the transverse facial, and external nasal

20. The branch of the ophthalmic artery that pierces the optic nerve is the 20.____

A. supraorbital
B. anterior ciliary
C. anterior ethmoidal
D. central artery of the retina
E. posterior ciliary

21. Which of the following is the MAJOR change in bone matrix during its mineralization? 21.____

A. Osteons enlarge
B. Cells develop processes
C. Water content decreases
D. Collagenous fibrils form
E. Ground substance aggregates

22. The internal thoracic artery gives rise to the _______ artery(ies). 22.____

A. highest intercostal
B. posterior intercostal
C. bronchial and esophageal
D. superior epigastric and musculophrenic
E. lowest intercostal

23. A lymph node 23.____

A. contains medullary cords
B. lacks afferent lymphatics
C. has crypts lined with stratified squamous epithelium
D. has efferent lymphatics leaving at multiple sites from the capsule
E. lacks medullary cords

24. Of the following organelles, _______ have a double-unit membrane. 24.____

I. Nucleus
II. Lysosome
III. Golgi complex
IV. Mitochondrion
V. Rough endoplasmic reticulum

The CORRECT answer is:

A. I, II, III
B. I and III *only*
C. I and IV *only*
D. I, IV, V
E. II, III, IV

25. Which of the following veins are normally concerned with drainage of the stomach? 25.____

I. Portal
II. Azygos
III. Splenic
IV. Internal iliac

The CORRECT answer is:

A. I and II *only*
B. I and III *only*
C. I, III, IV
D. II and III *only*
E. II, III, IV

26. The facial processes that contribute directly to the formation of the lips are the _______ and _______ processes. 26.____

I. maxillary; mandibular
II. maxillary; lateral nasal
III. maxillary; medial nasal
IV. medial; lateral nasal
V. lateral; medial palatine

The CORRECT answer is:

A. I, II
B. I, III
C. I, V
D. II, III
E. II, IV

27. Nutrients and oxygen reach the cells of compact bone by passing through the 27.____

I. lamellae
II. canaliculi
III. capillaries
IV. osseous matrix
V. Volkmann's canals

The CORRECT answer is:

A. I, II, V
B. I, III, V
C. I, IV, V
D. II, III, IV
E. II, III, V

28. During active inspiration, the 28.____

I. diaphragm descends
II. epiglottis closes
III. uvula swings superiorly
IV. rotation occurs at costo-vertebral articulations
V. lateral diameter of the thorax increases

The CORRECT answer is:

A. I, II, IV
B. I, IV, V
C. I, III, IV
D. II, III, V
E. II, III, IV

29. The _______ is NOT a branch of the maxillary artery. 29.____

A. deep temporal
B. middle meningeal
C. inferior alveolar
D. superficial temporal
E. posterior superior alveolar

30. Which of the following artery - foramen/fissure pairings is NOT correct? 30.____

A. Accessory meningeal - foramen ovale
B. Middle meningeal - foramen spinosum
C. Inferior alveolar - mandibular foramen
D. Anterior tympanic - petrotympanic fissure
E. Posterior superior alveolar - sphenopalatine foramen

31. Of the following laryngeal muscles, the ______ is NOT innervated by the recurrent laryngeal nerve. 31.____

A. cricothyroid
B. aryepiglottic
C. transverse arytenoid
D. lateral cricoarytenoid
E. posterior cricoarytenoid

32. The ______ is NOT contained in the posterior mediastinum. 32.____

A. thoracic duct
B. descending aorta
C. splanchnic nerve
D. hemiazygous vein
E. right recurrent laryngeal nerve

33. Of the following nerves, the ______ is NOT located in the wall of the cavernous sinus. 33.____

A. abducens
B. maxillary
C. trochlear
D. ophthalmic
E. oculomotor

34. Which of the following arteries is NOT derived from the celiac trunk or its branches? 34.____

A. Left gastric
B. Short gastric
C. Gastroduodenal
D. Left gastroepiploic
E. Inferior pancreaticoduodenal

35. All of the following structures lie superficial to the hyoglossus muscle EXCEPT the 35.____

A. lingual nerve
B. lingual artery
C. hypoglossal nerve
D. submandibular duct
E. nasolacrimal duct

KEY (CORRECT ANSWERS)

1. C
2. E
3. D
4. A
5. D

6. C
7. C
8. A
9. D
10. C

11. C
12. A
13. D
14. C
15. C

16. D
17. C
18. A
19. D
20. D

21. C
22. D
23. A
24. C
25. B

26. B
27. E
28. B
29. D
30. E

31. A
32. E
33. A
34. D
35. B

BIOCHEMISTRY / PHYSIOLOGY
EXAMINATION SECTION
TEST 1

DIRECTIONS: Each question or incomplete statement is followed by several suggested answers or completions. Select the one that *BEST* answers the question or completes the statement. *PRINT THE LETTER OF THE CORRECT ANSWER IN THE SPACE AT THE RIGHT.*

1. Protein metabolism in a normal man is *BEST* measured by the 1.____

   A. glucose/N ratio in urine
   B. respiratory quotient
   C. urea excretion
   D. uric acid excretion
   E. creatinine excretion

2. A presynaptic neuron may influence a postsynaptic neuron by 2.____

   A. exciting the latter to originate and conduct an impulse
   B. increasing the excitability of the latter
   C. inhibiting the action of the latter
   D. all of the above
   E. only *A* and *B* above

3. The normal hemoglobin concentration is about 15 gm./l00 ml. blood, and the normal arterial oxygen content is about 20 ml. O_2/100 ml. blood. An anemic individual breathing room air with a hemoglobin concentration of 10 gm./l00 ml. blood would have a 3.____

   A. *normal* arterial oxygen tension and normal arterial oxygen content
   B. *reduced* arterial oxygen tension, but a normal arterial oxygen content
   C. *reduced* arterial oxygen tension and an arterial oxygen content of 13.3 ml./l00 ml. blood
   D. *normal* arterial oxygen tension, but an arterial oxygen content of 13.3 ml./l00 ml. blood
   E. None of the above

4. A subject has a stroke volume of 70 cc. and a heart rate of 60 beats/min. His cardiac output (liters/min.) is 4.____

   A. 4.2
   B. 42
   C. 8.4
   D. 84
   E. none of the above

5. The biochemical mechanism by which epinephrine increases the breakdown of muscle glycogen is believed to involve 5.____

   A. activation of glycogen synthetase
   B. stimulation of cyclic AMP formation from ATP
   C. conversion of phosphorylase a to phosphorylase b
   D. stimulation of glucokinase

6. A substance which, when administered, *increases* lymph formation by increasing capillary permeability is 6.____

   A. salt
   B. urea
   C. water
   D. glucose
   E. histamine

7. The protein osmotic pressure of the blood is *important* because it 7.___

   A. *aids* in blood clotting
   B. *nourishes* the blood cells
   C. *prevents* the loss of erythrocytes from the blood
   D. *prevents* the excess loss of fluid from the capillaries
   E. *prevents* the entrance of tissue fluid into the capillaries

8. A histamine wheal is the result of a(n) 8.___

   A. rise in capillary blood pressure
   B. fall in plasma proteins
   C. decrease in interstitial pressure
   D. increase in capillary permeability
   E. All of the above

9. In a normal human, diuresis caused by ingestion of a large quantity of water results from a *decrease* in the 9.___

   A. tubular reabsorption of water
   B. diameter of efferent glomerular arterioles
   C. glomerular filtration rate
   D. glomerular filtration fraction
   E. None of the above

10. The formation of urine represents a process *important* to the 10.___

    A. regulation of acid-base balance and the formation of renin
    B. regulation of acid-base balance and normal osmotic pressures of intracellular fluids
    C. excretion of end-products of carbohydrate metabolism
    D. excretion of calcium
    E. All of the above

11. The **MAIN** centers for the control of respiration are in the 11.___

    A. cortex B. medulla C. thalamus D. cerebellum
    E. All of the above

12. Iron, a necessary dietary constituent, functions **PRIMARILY** 12.___

    A. in oxidation-reduction systems
    B. to maintain water and electrolyte balance
    C. in growth and repair of tissues
    D. to stimulate bone formation
    E. None of the above

13. A fall in blood pressure causes 13.___

    A. *increased* activity of the vasoconstrictor center and decreased activity of the cardio-inhibitory center
    B. *decreased* activity of the vasoconstrictor center and increased activity of the cardio-inhibitory center

C. *increased* activity of both centers
D. *decreased* activity of both centers
E. all of the above

14. The phenomenon referred to as Starling's law of the heart is explained as being related to the 14.____

A. greater diastolic volume of the ventricles
B. better nourishment of the heart muscle by the increased blood supply
C. ability of the heart to undergo isometric contraction
D. ability of the heart to undergo isometric relaxation
E. long refractory periods present in heart muscle

15. One of the chemical characteristics of collagen that makes it *unique* from other proteins is 15.____

A. its helical structure
B. its high glycine content
C. the presence of hydroxyproline
D. its low aromatic amino acid content
E. hydrogen bonding between polypeptide chains

16. An action potential in a nerve fiber is considered to be related to 16.____

A. the changed orientation of molecules in the membrane giving rise to a static potential difference
B. the entry of sodium ion followed by the exit of potassium ion
C. a breakdown of metabolic products resulting in different concentrations of potassium across the membrane
D. the flow of electrons across the membrane following change in membrane permeability
E. none of the above

17. Normal plasma calcium concentraton is, approximately, 17.____

A. 5 mg. per cent.
B. 10 mg. per cent.
C. 15 mg. per cent.
D. 20 mg. per cent.
E. 25 mg. per cent.

18. Autonomic postganglionic sympathetic nerve fibers which release acetylcholine at their endings are those leading to 18.____

A. the blood vessels in the splanchnic area
B. the circular muscles of the iris
C. the radial muscles of the iris
D. certain sweat glands
E. none of the above

19. Which of the following alterations in gastric function would result from bilateral vagotomy? 19.____

A. Increase in gastric secretion
B. Decrease in production of HCl and increase in production of pepsin
C. No effect on gastric secretion
D. Abolition of the cephalic phase of gastric secretion
E. No permanent effect on gastric motility

20. Which of the following groups contains ONLY enzymes secreted as zymogens? 20.__

A. Amylase, pepsin, trypsin
B. Lipase, nuclease, pepsin
C. Amylase, pepsin chymotrypsin
D. Chymotrypsin, trypsin, amylase
E. Pepsin, trypsin, chymotrypsin

21. Lack of which vitamin will produce cheilosis? 21.__

A. Biotin B. Thiamine C. Riboflavin
D. Nicotinic acid E. Pantothenic acid

22. Which of the following metallic ions is ESPECIALLY required in the blood clotting process? 22.__

A. Ba^{++} B. Na^{+} C. Ca^{++} D. Mg^{++} E. K^{+}

23. The effect of a vitamin C deficiency on the developing tooth is primarily on dentin and cementum. This can BEST be explained by which of the following statements? 23.__

A. Dentin is the most sensitive tissue in the body to a vitamin C deficiency.
B. Vitamin C influences the formation of collagen, the organic matrix found in dentin and cementum but not found in enamel.
C. Vitamin C has metabolic interrelations with other vitamins which have a greater influence on dentin and cementum than on enamel.
D. The vascular system is more important to these tissues than to the enamel, and in an avitaminosis C the vascular system is subject to hemorrhages.
E. None of the above

24. The PRIMARY structure of a protein is 24.__

A. an α-helix
B. peptidoglycan bonds
C. a specific sequence of α-amino groups
D. a specific sequence of amino acids linked by peptide bonds
E. all of the above

25. Normal prothrombin synthesis by the liver requires vitamin 25.__

A. A B. B complex C. C D. D E. K

KEY (CORRECT ANSWERS)

1. C
2. D
3. D
4. A
5. B
6. E
7. D
8. D
9. A
10. B
11. B
12. A
13. A
14. A
15. C
16. B
17. B
18. D
19. D
20. E
21. C
22. C
23. B
24. D
25. E

TEST 2

DIRECTIONS: Each question or incomplete statement is followed by several suggested answers or completions. Select the one that *BEST* answers the question or completes the statement. *PRINT THE LETTER OF THE CORRECT ANSWER IN THE SPACE AT THE RIGHT.*

1. In a poorly treated diabetic individual, the degree of ketosis is *closely* correlated with the blood level of 1.___

   A. amino acids
   B. free fatty acids
   C. lipoprotein triglycerides
   D. lipoprotein phospholipids
   E. none of the above

2. Proteins are able to buffer physiologic solutions over a wide range of pH because they 2.___

   A. are macromolecules of high molecular weight
   B. contain many functional groups with differing pKs
   C. have considerable secondary and tertiary structure which causes hydrogen ions to be sequestered
   D. have many peptide bonds which are very resistant to hydrolysis by hydrogen or hydroxyl ions
   E. None of the above

3. A hormone which lowers the blood calcium concentration is 3.___

   A. calcitonin
   B. calcikinase
   C. parathormone
   D. parathyrotropin
   E. all of the above

4. The *optimum* pH for an enzyme is the 4.___

   A. isoelectric point of the enzyme
   B. pH of most rapid reaction rate
   C. pH at which the enzyme is most soluble
   D. pH of most rapid denaturation of the enzyme
   E. None of the above

5. With decreased blood colloidal osmotic pressure, fluid will shift from the 5.___

   A. extracellular space to the intracellular space
   B. intracellular space to the interstitial space
   C. blood to the interstitial space
   D. interstitial space to blood
   E. None of the above

6. In direct calorimetry, the energy expenditure is determined by measuring the 6.___

   A. urinary nitrogen output
   B. oxygen consumption of the body
   C. amount of ingested carbohydrate
   D. total calories lost by evaporization of water from the body
   E. total calories lost through evaporation, radiation, conduction, and convection

7. When an impulse is carried by a chain of two or more neurons, the total transmission time is greater than the sum of the transmission times for each neuron because of 7.____

A. synaptic delay
B. inhibition
C. peripheral resistance
D. end-plate delay
E. None of the above

8. The plasma protein **MAINLY** responsible for antibody reactions is 8.____

A. globin
B. albumin
C. globulin
D. fibrinogen
E. prothrombin

9. The local of the *majority* of deoxyribonucleic acid of the cell is 9.____

A. nucleus
B. mitochondria
C. microsomes
D. nonparticular cyto-plasm
E. none of the above

10. Which of the following are essential fatty acids? 10.____

A. Acetic and oleic
B. Caprylic and caproic
C. Butyric and propionic
D. Linoleic and linolenic
E. Sterolic and palmitoleic

11. In considering the metabolic function of bone, which of the following functions could be considered the **MOST** prominent? 11.____

A. Sodium reservoir
B. Calcium reservoir
C. Buffering
D. Phosphate source
E. Fluoride reservoir

12. Which of the following **BEST** describes collagen? 12.____

A. The soluble fiber of ground substance
B. The most abundant protein in the body
C. A fibrous protein with a high content of tryptophan
D. A globular protein with a high content of hydroxyproline
E. None of the above

13. Bile salts promote digestion and absorption of fats by 13.____

A. converting all fatty acids to soaps
B. neutralizing the acid from the stomach
C. maintaining the optimal pH for lipase activity
D. forming water soluble complexes with fatty acids and glycerides
E. stimulating the secretion of pancreatic and intestinal juices

14. The annulospiral ending of the skeletal muscle spindle is stimulated when the 14.____

A. muscle is relaxed
B. muscle is stretched
C. intrafusal fibers are relaxed
D. gamma efferent fibers are inhibited
E. None of the above

15. The **MOST** distinctive functional difference between cardiac and skeletal muscle is the *greater* 15.___

A. force of contraction of cardiac muscle
B. refractory period of cardiac muscle
C. irritability of cardiac muscle
D. tone of skeletal muscle
E. None of the above

16. Parathyroid hormone secretion is regulated by a feedback mechanism directly controlled by 16.___

A. vitamin D
B. thyrocalcitonin
C. plasma ionic calcium level
D. plasma inorganic phosphorus level
E. hypothalamic secretion

17. In jaundice caused by obstruction of the biliary drainage system, 17.___

A. fecal bile pigment concentration is normal
B. serum bile pigment concentration is reduced
C. serum bile pigment concentration is normal
D. formation of bile pigment goes on as usual
E. None of the above

18. Hypothyroidism in the adult results in 18.___

A. thyrotoxicosis
B. increased BMR
C. osteitis fibrosa cystica
D. myxedema
E. none of the above

19. The digestion of food by salivary amylase continues for some time after the food has been swallowed. This results from the fact that 19.___

A. HCl in the stomach increases the digestive action of the amylase
B. contractions of the stomach help to distribute the amylase more evenly and, thus, facilitate its digestive action
C. amylase in the interior of the bolus is protected from the inactivating action of gastric HCl
D. absorption of water by the stomach concentrates the amylase and makes its action more effective
E. gastric mucin lubricates the bolus and assists the digestive action of amylase

20. At a constant dietary intake, the concentration of fluoride in the body fluids is regulated **PRINCIPALLY** by 20.___

A. hormonal factors
B. soft tissue uptake and release
C. equilibrium relations with bone and urinary excretion
D. the factor regulating intestinal absorption of ingested fluoride
E. none of the above

21. The rate of diffusion through a membrane is 21.___

A. directly proportional to the concentration gradient of the diffusing substance
B. inversely proportional to the thickness of the membrane

C. directly proportional to the permeability constant (K)
D. directly proportional to the area of the membrane
E. All of the above

22. During dark adaptation, 22.____

A. rhodopsin is being synthesized in the rods
B. rhodopsin is being synthesized in the cones
C. the red part of the spectrum becomes brighter
D. color vision becomes more intense
E. visual acuity is increased

23. Facultative reabsorption of water from the glomerular filtrate occurs MAINLY in the 23.____

A. collecting duct
B. proximal convoluted tubules by active transport
C. proximal convoluted tubules by passive transport
D. distal tubules in the presence of antidiuretic hormone
E. None of the above

24. The blood pressure in the aorta is *lowest* 24.____

A. at the end of ventricular systole
B. at the end of ventricular diastole
C. at the end of isometric contraction in the ventricle
D. when the second heart sound occurs
E. at the beginning of ejection of blood from the auricles

25. Substituting 100 percent oxygen for air could be of *considerable* value in treating 25.____

A. carbon monoxide poisoning
B. cyanide poisoning
C. methemoglobinemia
D. diabetic acidosis
E. hyperventilation

KEY (CORRECT ANSWERS)

1. B
2. B
3. A
4. B
5. C

6. E
7. A
8. C
9. A
10. D

11. B
12. B
13. D
14. B
15. B

16. C
17. D
18. D
19. C
20. C

21. E
22. A
23. D
24. C
25. A

BIOCHEMISTRY / PHYSIOLOGY
EXAMINATION SECTION
TEST 1

DIRECTIONS: Each question or incomplete statement is followed by several suggested answers or completions. Select the one that BEST answers the question or completes the statement. *PRINT THE LETTER OF THE CORRECT ANSWER IN THE SPACE AT THE RIGHT.*

1. Which of the following *usually* are associated with hyper-parathyroidism? A(n) 1.____

   A. *elevated* serum calcium and an elevated serum inorganic phosphate
   B. *elevated* serum calcium and a lowered serum inorganic phosphate
   C. *lowered* serum calcium and an elevated serum inorganic phosphate
   D. *lowered* serum calcium and a lowered serum inorganic phosphate
   E. *elevated* serum inorganic phosphate, the serum calcium remaining normal

2. In the oxidation of metabolites the hydrogen is oxidized to water through a series of steps involving a number of hydrogen acceptors. 2.____
   Which of the following is considered a hydrogen acceptor?

   A. NAD
   B. Nucleic acid
   C. Acetyl coenzyme A
   D. Glucose-6-phosphate
   E. Tetrahydrofolic acid

3. Which of the following vitamins is necessary for the production of prothrombin by the liver? 3.____

   A. Thiamine
   B. Vitamin K
   C. Vitamin D
   D. Vitamin B_{12}
   E. Ascorbic acid

4. Which of the following substances is neither actively absorbed nor actively secreted in the renal tubules? 4.____

   A. Water
   B. Glucose
   C. Sodium ion
   D. Hydrogen ion
   E. All of the above
   F. None of the above

5. Which of the following factors does NOT directly promote mineralization of bone? 5.____

   A. Vitamin A
   B. Vitamin D
   C. Gonadal hormones
   D. Parathyroid hormone

6. A change in resting heart rate in a normal human adult from 70 to 85 beats per minute is *predominantly* due to 6.____

   A. a decrease in vagal tone
   B. an increase in sympathetic tone
   C. Both of the above are equally important
   D. Neither of the above are important in the rate of change
   E. epinephrine release from the adrenal medulla

7. The predominant form in which CO_2 is transported in the blood is as 7.___

A. carbonic acid
B. carbaminohemoglobin
C. bicarbonate in the plasma
D. bicarbonate in the erythrocyte
E. CO_2 physically dissolved in the plasma

8. Venous return would be reduced during 8.___

A. a forced expiration with the glottis closed
B. rhythmic muscular exercise
C. plasma transfusion
D. blood transfusion
E. all of the above
F. none of the above

9. Biliverdin is converted directly to 9.___

A. urobilin B. bilirubin C. stercobilin
D. urobilinogen E. stercobilinogen

10. A patient ductus arteriosus would result in 10.___

A. pulmonary edema
B. mitral insufficiency
C. a decrease in cardiac work
D. a decreased PO_2 of the arterial blood

11. The way in which free fatty acids are transported in blood plasma is as 11.___

A. sodium salt
B. undissociated acid
C. a complex with albumin
D. a micelle complexed with bile salts
E. a major constituent of plasma lipoproteins

12. The MOST important buffers in interstitial fluid are 12.___

A. sucrose and proteins
B. bicarbonate and phosphate
C. polysaccharides and lipids
D. proteins and organic acids
E. hemoglobin and organic acids

13. Insulin secretion is influenced *principally* by the 13.___

A. thyroid hormone B. blood sugar level
C. pituitary hormones D. adrenocortical hormones

14. The vitamin important in tyrosine metabolism and in the formation of collagen is 14.___

A. thiamine B. riboflavin
C. β-carotene D. ascorbic acid

15. The glomerular filtration rate of the human kidney may be determined by measuring the plasma clearance of 15.____

A. PAH
B. urea
C. inulin
D. glucose
E. diodrast

16. If one divides the expired carbon dioxide by the oxygen consumed, one has calculated the 16.____

A. basal metabolic rate
B. oxygen exchange rate
C. respiratory quotient
D. respiratory dead space
E. partial pressure of carbon dioxide

17. The gastrocolic reflex serves the purpose of 17.____

A. moving the food materials through the pyloric sphincter
B. completing the final evacuation of the bowel in defecation
C. forcing the unabsorbed materials toward the descending colon and rectum
D. regurgitation of the irritating substances which might cause gastric disturbance in infants
E. diminishing the gastric tone associated with hunger pangs which occur whenever the entire gastrointestinal tract becomes empty

18. Stimulation of the sympathetic nervous supply to the gastrointestinal tract *generally* causes 18.____

A. inhibition of motility
B. increase in HCl secretion
C. ecbolic secretion by the pancreatic acini
D. an increase in the rate of colonic evacuation

19. Under physiologic conditions, the *lowest* partial pressure of oxygen is found in 19.____

A. normal atmospheric air
B. humidified atmospheric air
C. alveolar air
D. expired air
E. venous blood

20. A substance secreted by alveolar epithelium which contains phospholipids and serves to reduce the surface tension of alveolar fluids is 20.____

A. surfactant
B. scopolamine
C. sphingomyelin
D. suxamethonium
E. all of the above
F. none of the above

21. The oxygen dissociation curve for hemoglobin is shifted to the right by 21.____

A. increased CO_2
B. increased acid content
C. increased temperature
D. both A and B above
E. both B and C above
F. all of the above

22. The liver has many complex functions including each of the following EXCEPT 22.____

A. urea elimination
B. formation of bile
C. steroid conjugation
D. carbohydrate storage
E. prothrombin synthesis

23. All of the following factors increase stroke volume EXCEPT increased 23.____

A. venous return
B. arterial blood pressure
C. activity of skeletal *muscle pump*
D. concentration of plasma epinephrine
E. sympathetic tonus of venous blood vessels

24. Water in the human body functions in all of the following areas EXCEPT as 24.____

A. being primarily responsible for maintaining acid-base balance
B. a reactant or product in many chemical reactions
C. a medium in which chemical reactions take place
D. a transport medium for nutrients and wastes
E. an aid in maintaining body temperature

25. The PRINCIPAL action of injected insulin is to 25.____

A. *increase* glucose clearance by kidney
B. *decrease* intestinal absorption of glucose
C. *increase* penetration of glucose into muscle and fat cells
D. *decrease* penetration of glucose into muscle and fat cells

KEY (CORRECT ANSWERS)

1. B
2. A
3. B
4. A
5. D

6. A
7. C
8. A
9. B
10. D

11. C
12. B
13. B
14. D
15. C

16. C
17. C
18. A
19. E
20. A

21. F
22. A
23. B
24. A
25. C

TEST 2

DIRECTIONS: Each question or incomplete statement is followed by several suggested answers or completions. Select the one that BEST answers the question or completes the statement. *PRINT THE LETTER OF THE CORRECT ANSWER IN THE SPACE AT THE RIGHT.*

1. Which of the following is internally consistent data corresponding to a compensated alkalosis? 1.___

	HCO_3 mEq./1.	H_2CO_3 mEq./1.	pH
A.	40	1.3	7.3
B.	26	1.3	7.4
C.	32	2.0	7.3
D.	20	1.2	7.3
E.	None of the above		

2. In which of the following conditions is there a low oxygen *partial pressure* in arterial blood? 2.___

   A. Anemia
   B. Carbon monoxide poisoning
   C. Hypovolemia due to hemorrhage
   D. Tetany due to hyperventilation
   E. A shunt which allows blood to flow from the pulmonary artery to the pulmonary vein
   F. All of the above
   G. None of the above

3. Which of the following dietary components are *specifically* involved in the synthesis of hemoglobin? 3.___

   I. Sodium
   II. Potassium
   III. Iron
   IV. Copper
   V. Phosphate
   VI. Selenium

   The CORRECT combination is:

   A. I, II B. I, II, C. III, IV
   D. III, VI E. IV, V

4. Which of the following compounds are iron containing? 4.___

   I. Hemoglobin
   II. Cytochromes
   III. Aldolase
   IV. Phosphorylase b
   V. Ferritin

   The CORRECT combination is:

   A. I *only* B. I, II, V C. I, III, V
   D. II, IV E. III, IV

5. Inhibition of acetylcholinesterase at a neuromuscular junction causes 5.____

A. the resting potential of the muscle fiber to increase in magnitude
B. prolongation of the end-plate potential
C. the critical membrane potential of the muscle fiber to move to a value nearer the resting potential
D. increased liberation of acetycholine from neuronal terminals

6. In the conversion of pro-insulin to insulin, 6.____

A. disulfide bonds are formed
B. disulfide bonds are broken
C. the peptide chain is lengthened
D. a segment of the polypeptide chain is removed

7. Which of the following is internally consistent data for plasma corresponding to a respiratory acidosis? 7.____

	HCO_3 mEq./1.	H_2CO_3 mEq./1.	pH
A.	40	1.3	7.3
B.	26	1.3	7.4
C.	32	2.0	7.3
D.	20	1.2	7.3

E. None of the above

8. Which of the following is the normal consequence of a single impulse traveling down a motor axon? 8.____

A. A single motor unit discharge
B. Contraction of one muscle fiber
C. A subthreshold generator potential
D. A muscle action potential without contraction
E. Brief repetitive firing of the innervated muscle fibers

9. A number of factors can potentially increase the caries rate. Which of the following results in an increased rate? 9.____

A. Hereditary lack of a chelating agent required to hold the calcium within tooth structure
B. Decalcification of the teeth during pregnancy and lactation
C. Ingestion of detergent foods between meals
D. A meticulous dental hygiene program
E. None of the above

10. By what route will a patient seated in a dental chair lose the GREATEST amount of heat when the office temperature is 90° F., relative humidity is 22 percent, and an electric fan is running nearby? 10.____

A. Radiation
B. Conduction
C. Convection
D. Evaporation

11. Which of the following compounds is presently considered to be *directly* involved in the action of hormones on their target cells? 11.___

A. ATP
B. UTP
C. AMP (adenosine-5'-monophosphate)
D. UDPG (uridine diphosphoglucose)
E. Cyclic AMP (adenosine 3', 5' monophosphate)

12. Certain amino acids need not be present in the diet of an animal because of its ability to synthesize them at an adequate rate. Principal sources of carbon for these amino acids include: 12.___

I. Methylene folic acid derivatives
II. Metabolism of carbohydrates
III. Metabolism of fatty acids
IV. Carbon dioxide
V. Nucleic acids

The CORRECT combination is:

A. I, II
B. I, III
C. I, IV
D. II, III
E. II, IV
F. III, V
G. IV, V

13. Urinary neutral 17-ketosteroids have their origin in the: 13.___

I. Testis
II. Ovarian follicle
III. Adrenal cortex
IV. Corpus luteum

The CORRECT combination is:

A. I *only*
B. I, III, IV
C. I, III
D. III *only*
E. III, IV
F. All of the above

14. Which of the following hormones *directly* influence mineral metabolism? 14.___

I. Testerone
II. Parathyroid
III. Corticosterone
IV. Aldosterone
V. Somatotropin (growth hormone)

The CORRECT combination is:

A. I, III
B. I, II, III
C. II, IV, V
D. II, IV
E. III, V

15. Which of the following is NOT considered a type of connective tissue fiber? 15.___

A. Elastin
B. Chitin
C. Reticulin
D. Collagen

16. Which of the following is an allosteric effector of an enzymic reaction? 16.___

A. Competitive inhibitor
B. Uncompetitive inhibitor
C. Denaturant of the enzyme
D. Substance which binds to the substrate
E. Substance which affects enzymic activity by binding to a site other than the active site

17. How much water does dentin contain? ______ percent. 17.____

A. Less than 1
B. 1-5
C. 5-10
D. 15-25
E. 35

18. Which of the following reactions would NOT be influenced directly by the absence of nicotinic acid? 18.____

A. Conversion of citrulline to arginine
B. Conversion of pyruvate to acetyl coenzyme A
C. Conversion of acetyl coenzyme A to fatty acids
D. Oxidation of glucose by way of the pentose mono-phosphate pathway
E. Conversion of glutamate to alpha-ketoglutarate under catalysis by glutamic dehydrogenase

19. Protein digestion is accomplished by a series of specifically acting enzymes. Which of the following would accomplish the final step to render the material absorbable? 19.____

A. Aminopolypeptidase
B. Carboxypolypeptidase
C. Dipeptidase
D. Pepsin
E. Trypsin

20. Which substance, secreted into the intestine, converts a zymogen to an active enzyme? 20.____

A. Trypsinogen
B. Enterokinase
C. Bile pigments
D. Carboxypeptidase
E. Cholesterol esters

21. Consider one side of a membrane A, and the other side B. The membrane is permeable to water and there is water on each side of the membrane. Hydrostatic pressure is the same on each side. 21.____
Water will flow from side B to side A when a nonpermeant solute is dissolved on

A. side A, in greater concentration than on side B
B. side B, in greater concentration than on side A
C. side B, but not at all on side A
D. both sides in equal concentration

22. The primary translation of the genetic code from nucleotide language to amino acid language is accomplished by 22.____

A. ribonuclease
B. RNA polymerase
C. reverse transcriptase
D. peptidyl transferase
E. tRNA aminoacyl synthetase

23. Linolenic acid and arachidonic acids are essential dietary fatty acids for the human. They serve as precursors to the important biochemical structures 23.____

A. prostaglandins
B. steroid hormones
C. lecithin and other phospholipids
D. isoprenoid chains required for cholesterol and vitamin A synthesis

24. Enzymes can alter 24.___

A. the equilibrium of a reaction but not its rate
B. both the equilibrium and the rate of a reaction
C. the rate of a reaction but not the equilibrium
D. any of the above depending upon the enzyme in question
E. any of the above depending upon whether there is a linear sequence of D-amino acids
F. any of the above depending upon whether the enzymes themselves are permanently altered during the course of catalyzing a reaction

25. The citric acid cycle is initiated by the condensation of 25.___

A. NAD and succinate
B. pyruvate and citrate
C. acetyl coenzyme A and pyruvate
D. acetyl coenzyme and oxaloacetate
E. acetyl coenzyme and oxalosuccinate

KEY (CORRECT ANSWERS)

1.	E	11.	E
2.	E	12.	D
3.	C	13.	C
4.	B	14.	C
5.	B	15.	B
6.	D	16.	E
7.	C	17.	D
8.	A	18.	A
9.	E	19.	C
10.	D	20.	B

21. A
22. E
23. A
24. C
25. D

BIOCHEMISTRY / PHYSIOLOGY
EXAMINATION SECTION
TEST 1

DIRECTIONS: Each question or incomplete statement is followed by several suggested answers or completions. Select the one that BEST answers the question or completes the statement. *PRINT THE LETTER OF THE CORRECT ANSWER IN THE SPACE AT THE RIGHT.*

1. The NORMAL physiologic stimulus for the Hering-Breuer reflex is 1.____

   A. inflation of the lung
   B. reduced pH in arterial blood
   C. reduced oxygen tension in arterial blood
   D. increased arterial carbon dioxide tension
   E. decreased arterial carbon dioxide tension

2. The calcified tissue with the HIGHEST ash content is 2.____

   A. bone B. enamel C. dentin
   D. calculus E. cementum

3. The change from a pulsatile flow in the arteries to a nonpulsatile flow in the capillaries is the result of 3.____

   A. short length of the capillaries
   B. an increased volume of the capillary bed
   C. short length of the arterioles as compared with the capillaries
   D. high resistance in the arterioles and elasticity of large arteries

4. The IMMEDIATE site of action of epinephrine in the process of glycogenolysis is 4.____

   A. conversion of ADP to AMP
   B. activation of adenyl cyclase
   C. activation of phosphoprotein kinase
   D. inhibition of phosphoprotein phosphatase
   E. conversion of phosphorylase b to phosphorylase a

5. One of the PRINCIPAL characteristics of a sensory receptor is that it 5.____

   A. allows for conduction in one direction only
   B. insulates the nerve from other forms of stimuli
   C. does not permit adaptation to the stimulus
   D. has a low threshold for a certain type of adequate stimulus

6. During dark adaptation, rhodopsin is being 6.____

   A. broken down B. synthesized
   C. converted into vitamin A D. converted into photopsin
   E. None of the above

7. The role of the liver in edema may be the result of 7.____

A. a decrease in aldosterone secretion
B. a decrease in secretion of vasopressin
C. diminished albumin synthesis
D. both A and B above
E. both A and C above
F. all of the above

8. Angular stomatitis (cheliosis) can be experimentally produced by placing a volunteer on a diet that is deficient in 8.____

A. E_2 or B_6
B. B_{12} or biotin
C. niacin or riboflavin
D. B_1 or L-ascorbic acid
E. pantothenic acid or folic acid

9. The energy requirement for contracting striated muscle is supplied *largely* from the 9.____

A. oxidation of fatty acids and acetoacetate
B. oxidation of acetyl coenzyme A in the tricarboxylic acid cycle
C. oxidative-decarboxylation of pyruvic acid to acetyl coenzyme A
D. anaerobic transformation of glucose from glycogen to lactic acid

10. A deficiency in vitamin D during the posteruptive period of the teeth will produce a(n) 10.____

A. insignificant modification of the teeth
B. increased calcium to phosphorus (Ca:P) ratio in the serum
C. hypoplasia of permanent incisors limited essentially to the enamel
D. enamel hypoplasia involving permanent first molars but not permanent incisors
E. increased caries susceptibility that can be reversed by supplementary vitamin D intake

11. The process of DNA replication is said to be semiconservative.
This means that the daughter molecules formed are 11.____

A. antiparallel
B. single stranded
C. synthesized in small pieces
D. complementary with respect to base composition
E. composed of one strand from the parent molecule and one strand which has been newly synthesized

12. Evidence that DNA is the genetic material has been shown by experiments in 12.____

A. denaturation
B. hybridization
C. transformation
D. x-ray crystallography
E. none of the above

13. The PR interval in the electrocardiogram is an index of the 13.____

A. period of maximal ejection of ventricular systole
B. conduction time between the atria and ventricles
C. length of auricular contraction
D. period of isometric relaxation
E. length of auricular filling

14. The following information is available on a patient: oxygen consumption, 250 ml./min.; blood pressure, 130/80; heart rate, 60; arterial oxygen content, 20 cc./100ml.; venous oxygen content, 15 cc./100ml. 14.____
His cardiac output is ______ liters/minute.

A. 1.5
B. 3.6
C. 5.0
D. 6.2
E. 9.0

15. Blood carrying 7.5 grams of oxygenated hemoglobin and 7.5 grams of reduced hemoglobin per 100 cc. would be 15.____

A. anemic
B. cyanotic
C. hydremic
D. anhydremic
E. histotoxic

16. The stimulating effect of low arterial O_2 tension on respiration is produced CHIEFLY through an effect on the 16.____

A. carotid bodies
B. carotid sinuses
C. expiratory center
D. inspiratory center
E. nerve endings in the alveoli

17. Keratosulfate occurs PRIMARILY in 17.____

A. bile
B. blood
C. liver
D. urine
E. cartilage

18. An increase in strength of a suprathreshold stimulus to a receptor causes its afferent fiber to transmit 18.____

A. a faster impulse
B. a slower impulse
C. an impulse of larger amplitude
D. an impulse of smaller amplitude
E. two or more impulses as a volley

19. The portion of the electrocardiogram corresponding to activation of the atria is the 19.____

A. P wave
B. T wave
C. PR interval
D. PRS complex
E. QT interval

20. Tyrosine is a precursor in the biosynthesis of the biologically active agent 20.____

A. serotonin
B. histamine
C. nicotinamide
D. acetylcholine
E. norepinephrine

21. Serum which causes agglutination of the cells in BOTH type A and type B blood must belong to type ______ blood 21.____

A. O
B. A
C. B
D. AB

22. The loops of Henle are responsible for the 22.____

A. acidification of the urine
B. almost complete reabsorption of amino acids
C. reabsorption of most of the glomerular filtrate
D. formation of most of the ammonium ion excreted in the urine
E. establishment of an osmotic gradient within the medulla of the kidney

23. The reabsorption of sodium chloride is controlled in the kidney tubules by ______ hormone. 23.____

A. thyrotropic
B. antidiuretic
C. an adrenal cortical
D. an adrenal medullary

24. The plasma protein MOST readily affected by nutritional protein deficiency is 24.____

A. albumen
B. α -globulin
C. β-globulin
D. γ -globulin
E. fibrinogen

25. A class of RNA involved in protein synthesis is 25.____

A. transfer RNA
B. messenger RNA
C. 5 S ribosomal RNA
D. 16 S ribosomal RNA
E. all of the above
F. none of the above

KEY (CORRECT ANSWERS)

1. A
2. B
3. D
4. B
5. D
6. B
7. C
8. A
9. D
10. A
11. E
12. C
13. B
14. C
15. B
16. A
17. E
18. E
19. A
20. E
21. A
22. E
23. C
24. A
25. E

TEST 2

DIRECTIONS: Each question or incomplete statement is followed by several suggested answers or completions. Select the one that BEST answers the question or completes the statement. *PRINT THE LETTER OF THE CORRECT ANSWER IN THE SPACE AT THE RIGHT.*

1. The sensory organs concerned with maintenance of skeletal muscle tonus are 1.____

   A. Golgi's tendon organs   B. pacinian corpuscles
   C. the gamma efferents   D. the muscle spindles

2. Normal storage of iron in the liver is almost entirely in the form of 2.____

   A. ferritin   B. transferrin   C. hemosiderin
   D. apoferritin   E. ceruloplasmin

3. The MAXIMUM frequency of effective nerve stimulation is limited by the length of the 3.____

   A. chronaxie
   B. negative after potential
   C. relative refractory period
   D. absolute refractory period
   E. utilization time of stimulus

4. After taking part in fat digestion and absorption, the bulk of the bile salts are 4.____

   A. excreted in the urine
   B. excreted in the feces
   C. reabsorbed into the lymph
   D. destroyed by bacteria in the colon
   E. reabsorbed into the portal circulation

5. Biologic oxidation enzymes occur in the cell PRIMARILY as 5.____

   A. soluble enzymes of the cytoplasm
   B. highly organized multienzyme units in the mitochondria
   C. partly in the microsomes and partly in the mitochondria
   D. components of the cell wall
   E. components of the nuclear membrane

6. A man's dead space is 200 ml., his tidal volume is 600 ml., and he breathes at the rate of 100 breaths per minute. 6.____
   His alveolar ventilation is ______ ml./min.

   A. 2000   B. 3000
   C. 3560   D. 4000
   E. 6000

7. The gate control theory of pain perception implies that 7.____

   A. there are three neurons from the periphery to the sensory cortex subserving pain
   B. large fiber activation serves to inhibit pain perception
   C. substantial gelatinosa cells function by producing postsynaptic inhibition of small and large fibers
   D. small fibers trigger a central control mechanism to open the gate

8. The kidney enzyme MOST actively involved in regulation of acid-base balance and conservation of sodium in the body is 8.____

A. lipase
B. aldolase
C. glutaminase
D. transaminase
E. succinic dehydrogenase

9. The enzyme involved in the production of hydrochloric acid by the gastric parietal cell is 9.____

A. pepsin
B. amylase
C. secretin
D. gastrin
E. carbonic anhydrase

10. Inulin clearance is 120 cc./min. Clearance of substance X is 40 cc./min. Plasma concentration of X is 0.5 mg./cc. 10.____
The amount of X reabsorbed by the tubule is ______ mg./min.

A. 20
B. 40
C. 60
D. 80
E. 120

11. Iodine is PRIMARILY important in the biochemical synthesis of 11.____

A. thyroxin
B. adrenalin
C. enamel matrix
D. parathyroid hormone
E. organic matrix of bone

12. Epinephrine when injected may cause 12.____

A. increase in blood sugar
B. decrease in blood sugar
C. increase in blood calcium
D. decrease in metabolic rate
E. retention of sodium chloride

13. The light-sensitive component of the retina consists of a complex between a protein AND 13.____

A. a derivative of vitamin A
B. a derivative of vitamin C
C. thiamine pyrophosphate
D. sphingomyelin
E. none of the above

14. Edema is a condition in which there occurs 14.____

A. abnormally low hemoglobin
B. an increased plasma oncotic pressure
C. an increased blood pressure
D. a localized accumulation of interstitial fluid
E. inflammation of tissue cells

15. The protein which is MAINLY responsible for the colloidal osmotic pressure of the plasma is 15.____

A. albumin
B. fibrinogen
C. lipoprotein
D. alpha globulin
E. gamma globulin

16. Dissociation of oxyhemoglobin with release of oxygen increases with increasing 16.____

A. partial pressure of O_2
B. partial pressure of CO_2
C. alkalosis
D. chloride concentration
E. bicarbonate concentration

17. The blood from bleeding ginglval tissue contains an enzyme whose action would result in the accelerated release of carbon dioxide from saliva. 17.____
The enzyme is

A. amylase
B. esterase
C. catalase
D. peroxidase
E. carbonic anhydrase

18. Corpus luteum secretion is stimulated by 18.____

A. FSH
B. LH
C. estrogen
D. LTH
E. progesterone

19. Ribonucleic acid and deoxyribonucleic acid differ in type of 19.____

A. sugars
B. purines
C. pyrimidines
D. both A and B above
E. both A and C above

20. Formation and excretion of ammonium ion by the distal tubule of the kidney is a mechanism for conservation of 20.____

A. sodium
B. water
C. acidity
D. calcium
E. potassium

21. During pregnancy, certain plasma proteins are increased and may cause a(n) 21.____

A. *increase* in tissue fluid formation resulting from an increase in intravascular hydrostatic pressure
B. *increase* in tissue fluid formation resulting from a decrease in intravascular hydrostatic pressure
C. *decrease* in tissue fluid formation resulting from an increase in intravascular osmotic pressure
D. *decrease* in tissue fluid formation resulting from a decrease in intravascular osmotic pressure

22. The MOST biologically important physicochemical property of connective tissue which is regulated by its mucopolysaccharide molecules is 22.____

A. viscosity
B. buffering capacity
C. solubility in dilute acids
D. supersaturation with calcium ions

23. The circulation of fluid between the capillaries and the interstitial spaces is increased 23.____

A. when the arterial blood pressure falls
B. in hyperproteinemia
C. with increased cellular metabolism
D. during vasoconstriction of the arterioles

24. The PRINCIPAL sensory relay station in the brain is the 24.____

A. thalamus
B. cerebellum
C. sensory cortex
D. substantia nigra

25. Stimulation of the carotid sinus baroreceptors will cause a DECREASE in blood pressure because 25.____

A. parasympathetic impulses to the blood vessels will be increased
B. there will be central inhibition of the cardiac inhibitory center
C. epinephrine release will cause vasodilation in skeletal muscles
D. parasympathetic impulses to the heart will be increased and the vasomotor center will be inhibited

KEY (CORRECT ANSWERS)

1. D
2. A
3. D
4. E
5. B

6. D
7. B
8. C
9. E
10. B

11. A
12. A
13. A
14. D
15. A

16. B
17. E
18. D
19. E
20. A

21. C
22. A
23. C
24. A
25. D

MICROBIOLOGY / PATHOLOGY

EXAMINATION SECTION

TEST 1

DIRECTIONS: Each question or incomplete statement is followed by several suggested answers or completions. Select the one that BEST answers the question or completes the statement. *PRINT THE LETTER OF THE CORRECT ANSWER IN THE SPACE AT THE RIGHT.*

1. The tensile strength of a healing wound depends upon 1.____

   A. wound hormones
   B. adequate fluid intake
   C. activation of fibrinolysis
   D. formation of collagen fibers
   E. erythropoietin stimulation of bone marrow

2. The organism which causes Rocky Mountain spotted fever is perpetuated in nature *mainly* in 2.____

   A. lice
   B. mites
   C. ticks
   D. humans
   E. rabbits

3. Reed-Sternberg cells are pathognomonic of 3.____

   A. typhoid fever
   B. Hodgkin's disease
   C. Burkitt's lymphoma
   D. anterior poliomyelitis
   E. von Recklinghausen's disease

4. Two important "post-streptococcal" diseases are 4.____

   A. impetigo and osteolyelitis
   B. puerperal fever and anthrax
   C. scarlet fever and erysipelas
   D. pharyngitis and the common cold
   E. rheumatic fever and glomerulonephritis

5. Margination of leukocytes refers to 5.____

   A. crowding of the cells into an axial stream
   B. lining up of the cells along the wall of a dilated vessel
   C. an increase in the number of cells at the margin of a wound
   D. abnormal motility of the cells
   E. none of the above

6. A darkfield microscope would be useful in examining blood for 6.____

   A. treponema
   B. actinomyces
   C. streptococcus
   D. mycobacterium
   E. bacillus anthracis spores

7. The indiscriminate use of broad-spectrum antibiotics is CONTRAINDICATED because they frequently 7.___

   A. are extremely nephrotoxic
   B. cause psychogenic symptoms
   C. produce dependency reactions
   D. induce anaphylactoid reactions
   E. interfere with indigenous biota

8. Although the exact mechanism of the formation of calculus is not understood, it is known that the organic matrix of calculus in humans includes 8.___

   A. an abundance of microorganisms
   B. *only* an occasional microorganism
   C. *only* the by-products of bacterial metabolism
   D. a fusospirochetal complex
   E. no living microorganisms

9. Hemorrhage may occur in patients with severe liver disease because of a deficiency in 9.___

   A. prothrombin
   B. thromboplastin
   C. gamma globulin
   D. calcium ions in the serum
   E. none of the above

10. Measles is transmitted from one person to another via 10.___

   A. feces
   B. fomites
   C. insect bites
   D. contaminated water supply
   E. respiratory droplets

11. Hematemesis refers to 11.___

   A. nasal hemorrhage
   B. vomiting of blood
   C. blood in the stool
   D. blood in the urine
   E. coughing up blood from the lungs

12. When a rejected allograft is followed by a second allograft from the same donor, the 12.___

   A. graft takes
   B. second rejection occurs more rapidly than the first
   C. second rejection occurs more slowly than the first
   D. second rejection occurs in 50 percent of the cases
   E. none of the above

13. In the replication of viral particles, the host cell provides 13.____

A. genetic information, and the virus provides synthetic enzymes
B. nutrients, and the virus provides metabolic enzymes
C. metabolic enzymes, and the virus provides genetic information
D. genetic information, and the virus incorporates nutrients
E. none of the above

14. The substrate on which streptococcus mutans acts to produce dextrans and levans is 14.____

A. glucose
B. sucrose
C. fructose
D. glycogen
E. amylopectin

15. Mutations are due to changes in 15.____

A. amino acid sequence of deoxyribonuclease
B. amino acid sequence of ribonuclease
C. RNA nucleotide sequence
D. DNA nucleotide sequence
E. cell wall peptidoglycan

16. Epithelial pearls and intercellular bridges observed in an infiltrating malignancy are diagnostic of 16.____

A. adenocarcinoma
B. anaplastic carcinoma
C. squamous cell carcinoma
D. undifferentiated carcinoma
E. transitional cell carcinoma

17. Reducing the number of infectious agents on headrests and operating light handles to an acceptable level is called 17.____

A. asepsis
B. attenuation
C. disinfection
D. sterilization
E. none of the above

18. An antibacterial substance found in saliva, tears and egg white is 18.____

A. albumin
B. isozyme
C. amylase
D. lysozyme
E. betalysin

19. A virus which causes two distinct diseases in different age groups is 19.____

A. influenza
B. measles
C. smallpox
D. varicella
E. Newcastle disease

20. Staphylococci *typically* occur in 20.____

A. pairs
B. chains
C. tetrads
D. irregular clusters
E. palisade arrangement

21. A protoplast is BEST characterized as a bacterial cell 21.____

A. with a cell wall but free of a capsule
B. containing a cell wall and a capsule
C. free of a cell wall and a capsule
D. uniquely sensitive to penicillin
E. none of the above

22. A 65-year-old male who demonstrates urinary retention or difficulty in voiding his bladder *most likely* has 22.____

A. malignant neoplasm of the ureter
B. carcinoma of the prostate
C. benign prostatic hyperplasia
D. bladder metastasis of bronchogenic carcinoma
E. none of the above

23. Of the following, the MOST radiosensitive cell is the 23.____

A. lymphocyte
B. nerve cell
C. muscle cell
D. cartilage cell
E. endothelial cell

24. On the basis of histogenesis and transitions observed in clinical cases, there appears to be a relationship between lymphocytic lymphoma and 24.____

A. lymphadenitis
B. lymphoepithelioma
C. lymphocytic leukemia
D. infectious lymphocytosis
E. infectious mononucleosis

25. Dystrophic calcification of tissue or cells is 25.____

A. secondary to pituitary hypoplasia
B. associated with high blood calcium
C. associated with high blood phosphorus
D. secondary to disease of the tissue affected
E. none of the above

KEY (CORRECT ANSWERS)

1. D
2. C
3. B
4. E
5. B

6. A
7. E
8. A
9. A
10. E

11. B
12. B
13. C
14. B
15. D

16. C
17. C
18. D
19. D
20. D

21. C
22. C
23. A
24. C
25. D

TEST 2

DIRECTIONS: Each question or incomplete statement is followed by several suggested answers or completions. Select the one that BEST answers the question or completes the statement. *PRINT THE LETTER OF THE CORRECT ANSWER IN THE SPACE AT THE RIGHT.*

1. A positive skin test in an individual who has had tuberculosis is an example of 1.____

   A. atopy
   B. autoimmunity
   C. hypersensitivity
   D. passive immunity
   E. none of the above

2. Rough pneumococci grown in the presence of DNA from smooth pneumococci develop capsules. This is known as 2.____

   A. mutation
   B. conjugation
   C. translation
   D. transduction
   E. transformation

3. The *most likely* mechanism for the increased occurrence of drug-resistant microorganisms is 3.____

   A. R factor transfer of resistance
   B. increased mutation rate
   C. diet of the host
   D. lysogeny
   E. none of the above

4. A disease of childhood characterized by mental retardation, delayed growth and delayed tooth eruption is associated with a deficiency of 4.____

   A. oxytocin
   B. growth hormone
   C. thyroid hormone
   D. testicular hormone
   E. mineralocorticoids

5. A person's blood is mixed separately with A antiserum, B antiserum and Rh positive antiserum. No clumping or agglutination of the red cells occurs. This person has type _______ blood and is Rh _______. 5.____

   A. O, positive
   B. O, negative
   C. AB, positive
   D. AB, negative
   E. A, positive

6. The mechanism of action of quaternary ammonium compounds is against the 6.____

   A. metachromatic granules
   B. cytoplasmic membrane
   C. cell wall
   D. flagella
   E. DNA

7. In general, rickettsia and viruses have in common 7.____

   A. size
   B. filterability
   C. growth environment
   D. method of reproduction
   E. resistance to antibiotics

8. Selective cytotoxicity denotes a drug action which 8.____

   A. is easily tested in vitro
   B. affects parasites more strongly than host cells
   C. substitutes a poisonous analogue for an essential nutrient
   D. is limited to bacteria and does not include protozoa
   E. destroys the cell with no effect on the nucleus

9. For uniform staining reaction, morphology and biochemical activity, it is advisable to study bacterial cultures during the _______ phase. 9.____

   A. lag
   B. death
   C. stationary
   D. logarithmic
   E. none of the above

10. Endotoxins differ from exotoxins in that endotoxins 10.____

   A. are proteins
   B. are heat labile
   C. are highly antigenic
   D. activate complement by the alternate pathway
   E. can be converted into toxoids by treatment with formalin

11. Transformation of mucous-secreting bronchial epithelium to squamous epithelium is an example of 11.____

   A. aplasia
   B. anaplasia
   C. dysplasia
   D. metaplasia
   E. hyperplasia

12. The term "nephrosis" *generally* implies renal disease which *primarily* involves the 12.____

   A. tubules
   B. glomeruli
   C. renal papillae
   D. renal artery
   E. interstitial connective tissue

13. The mechanism by which most fungi cause disease is 13.____

   A. endotoxin production
   B. exotoxin production
   C. lecithinase production
   D. coagulase production
   E. hypersensitivity

14. Hypochromic microcytic anemia is characteristic of 14.____

   A. sprue
   B. aplastic anemia
   C. pernicious anemia
   D. iron-deficiency anemia
   E. none of the above

15. The pulmonary neoplasm to which the endocrine effect of hyperparathyroidism is attributed is 15.____

   A. squamous cell carcinoma
   B. medullary carcinoma
   C. oat cell carcinoma
   D. pheochromocytoma
   E. adenocarcinoma

16. The medium of choice for growing MOST fungi is 16.____

A. blood agar
B. tissue culture
C. Sabouraud's agar
D. thioglycollate medium
E. nutrient agar containing lactophenol cotton blue

17. The chemotactic accumulation of mononuclear cells which occurs at the sites where immune complexes are deposited is *most probably* the result of 17.____

A. C3
B. IgA
C. IgD
D. IgE
E. sensitized lymphocytes

18. Bronchopneumonia is characterized by 18.____

A. inflammation of a bronchus only
B. organization of alveolar exudate
C. patchy distribution of lobular inflammation
D. uniform involvement of the lobe associated with the inflamed bronchus
E. none of the above

19. Massive necrotizing lesions of the palate in a patient with poorly-controlled diabetes mellitus are *frequently* related to 19.____

A. mucormycosis
B. blastomycosis
C. coccidoidomycosis
D. histoplasmosis
E. cryptococcosis

20. A lysogenic bacterium is one that 20.____

A. lyses red cells
B. produces properdin
C. harbors a temperate bacteriophage
D. produces lecithinase when incubated anaerobically
E. produces spheroplasts when incubated anaerobically

21. The effectiveness of autoclaving is BEST determined by 21.____

A. indicators that change color at elevated temperatures
B. thermocouples (temperature recording devices)
C. culturing the water reservoir
D. culturing bacterial spores
E. none of the above

22. A patient with shingles (herpes zoster) is *most likely* to have had a previous episode of 22.____

A. smallpox
B. chickenpox
C. autoimmune disease
D. respiratory syncytial virus infection
E. trauma to the spinal cord or the nerve roots

23. Herpes simplex virus type 1 is *usually* associated with 23.____

A. neural lesions
B. genital lesions
C. cervical carcinoma
D. oral and ocular lesions
E. none of the above

24. The essential antigen in diplococcus pneumoniae which determines both its virulence and its specific type is the 24.____

A. somatic carbohydrate
B. flagellar carbohydrate
C. thermolabile leukocidin
D. capsular polysaccharide
E. nucleoprotein structure

25. In Bruton's agammaglobulinemia, adequate host defense mechanisms exist for resistance to 25.____

A. virus infections
B. fungal infections
C. bacterial infections
D. nonpathogenic bacteria
E. none of the above

KEY (CORRECT ANSWERS)

1. C
2. E
3. A
4. C
5. B

6. B
7. C
8. B
9. D
10. D

11. D
12. A
13. E
14. D
15. C

16. C
17. A
18. C
19. A
20. C

21. D
22. B
23. D
24. D
25. A

MICROBIOLOGY / PATHOLOGY

EXAMINATION SECTION
TEST 1

DIRECTIONS: Each question or incomplete statement is followed by several suggested answers or completions. Select the one that BEST answers the question or completes the statement. *PRINT THE LETTER OF THE CORRECT ANSWER IN THE SPACE AT THE RIGHT.*

1. Which of the following statements concerning the microbiologic aspects of periodontal disease in humans is NOT substantiated by scientific data? 1.____

   A. Periodontal disease is contagious in humans.
   B. Adequate oral hygiene results in remission of gingivitis.
   C. As bacterial plaque accumulates, gingivitis is manifested.
   D. When oral hygiene is stopped, gingival inflammation is produced.
   E. There is a quantitative rather than a qualitative change in the oral flora.

2. The agent of which of the following diseases is NOT transmitted from person to person by droplets or droplet spray? 2.____

   A. Pneumonia
   B. Diphtheria
   C. Meningitis
   D. Whooping cough
   E. Equine encephalitis

3. Which of the following USUALLY causes a systemic infection? 3.____

   A. Trichophyton
   B. Epidermophyton
   C. Microsporum
   D. Coccidioides
   E. Aspergillus

4. Which of the following is useful in differentiating between Salmonella typhi and Escherichia coli? 4.____

   A. Urease test
   B. Test for motility
   C. Fermentation of lactose
   D. Phenylalanine deaminase
   E. Production of acid from glucose

5. What kind of immunity would result in a susceptible person given tetanus antitoxin? 5.____

   A. Natural, active
   B. Natural, passive
   C. Artificial, active
   D. Artificial, passive
   E. A combination of A and C above

6. Elevation of serum acid phosphatase levels is likely to be seen in which of the following? Carcinoma of the 6.____

   A. colon
   B. breast
   C. stomach
   D. uterine cervix
   E. prostate gland

7. A six-year-old boy has minute white specks on the oral mucosa opposite the first molars. A bluish-to-red ring surrounds these spots. He also has a *cold,* and his eyes are red and runny. There is a blotchy reddish rash behind his ears and on his face. This child has 7.____

A. eczema
B. measles
C. chickenpox
D. scarlet fever
E. Rocky Mountain spotted fever

8. Fungi produce disease in man by 8.____

A. hypersensitivity
B. enzyme production
C. exotoxin production
D. endotoxin production
E. stimulation of high antibody titers

9. A reduction in acid secretion by the stomach, an increased tendency toward gastric carcinoma, atrophic glossitis and myelin degeneration of peripheral nerves are characteristic findings with 9.____

A. thalassemia
B. agranulocytosis
C. sickle cell anemia
D. pernicious anemia
E. polycythemia vera

10. An endocrine disease characterized by increased susceptibility to infection, increased fatigability, recessive inheritance and polyuria is 10.____

A. acromegaly
B. Grave's disease
C. diabetes mellitus
D. Cushing's disease
E. Hashimoto's disease

11. The MOST important pathologic changes of carbon monoxide poisoning takes place in the 11.____

A. brain
B. adrenal
C. pituitary
D. myocardium
E. none of the above

12. The MOST important result of portal cirrhosis is 12.____

A. atrophy of spleen
B. obstruction of portal circulation
C. tendency to form angiomas of liver
D. decrease in plasma protein formation
E. none of the above

13. An iron-containing pigment derived from normal breakdown of hemoglobin is 13.____

A. hemosiderin
B. hematoidin
C. bilirubin
D. hematin
E. melanin

14. Most rickettsial diseases are severe human infections because the organisms 14.____

A. produce potent exotoxins
B. are particularly destructive to cutaneous tissues
C. are primarily neurotropic and cause extensive damage in certain CNS centers
D. have predilection for endothelial cells and smooth muscle cells of small blood vessels
E. none of the above

15. Enzymes which can be detected ONLY in the presence of their specific substrate are 15.____

A. inductive
B. digestive
C. nonspecific
D. constitutive
E. none of the above

16. A viral disease with oral manifestations is 16.____

A. anthrax
B. diphtheria
C. leishmaniasis
D. herpangina
E. moniliasis

17. In the process of necrosis, a reduction in size and a condensation of nuclear material is known as 17.____

A. karyolysis
B. pyknophrasia
C. karyorrhexis
D. pyknosis
E. none of the above

18. Oral protozoa are found to INCREASE in the oral cavity when 18.____

A. periodontitis becomes more advanced
B. patient's teeth are severely stained
C. carious lesions increase
D. all of the above
E. none of the above

19. Of the conditions listed below, the MOST frequent cause of conspicuous hemosiderin pigmentation of the lung is 19.____

A. hemochromatosis
B. pulmonary infarction
C. hemorrhagic pneumonia
D. passive pulmonary congestion
E. hemolytic disease of the newborn

20. Negri bodies are histologic structures characteristically found in 20.____

A. rabies
B. herpes zoster
C. rheumatic fever
D. herpes simplex
E. infectious mononucleosis

21. Ten days after he was hospitalized for a large incapacitating myocardial infarct, a 50-year-old man suddenly developed paralysis of the right side of his body. 21.____
The BEST explanation for his brain damage would be

A. rupture of a congenital aneurysm of the circle of Willis
B. brain abscess from necrosis of the myocardium
C. detachment of a bacterial embolus from the pulmonic valve

D. detachment of a mural thrombus from the right ventricle
E. detachment of a mural thrombus from the left ventricle

22. Rubeola, pertussis, poliomyelitis, and mumps have in common the fact that all are 22.____

A. air-borne diseases
B. vector-borne diseases
C. characterized by a toxemia
D. primarily diseases of infants
E. prevented by acute immunization

23. A virus which persists in the oral tissues throughout the life of most individuals is ______ virus. 23.____

A. rubella
B. varicella
C. herpes zoster
D. herpes simplex
E. none of the above

24. Contraction, organization, canalization, and resorption are all terms relating to the possible fate of a(n) 24.____

A. infarct
B. furuncle
C. thrombus
D. hematoma
E. fat embolus

25. One of the distinguishing characteristics of ALL viruses is 25.____

A. absence of nucleic acids
B. growth in cell-free medium
C. adaptability to external environment
D. constant route of infection
E. failure to grow in the absence of living cells

KEY (CORRECT ANSWERS)

1. A
2. E
3. D
4. C
5. D
6. E
7. B
8. A
9. D
10. C
11. A
12. B
13. A
14. D
15. A
16. D
17. D
18. A
19. D
20. A
21. E
22. E
23. D
24. C
25. E

TEST 2

DIRECTIONS: Each question or incomplete statement is followed by several suggested answers or completions. Select the one that BEST answers the question or completes the statement. *PRINT THE LETTER OF THE CORRECT ANSWER IN THE SPACE AT THE RIGHT.*

1. Which of the following is the BEST procedure to select encapsulated Streptococcus (Diplococcus) pneumoniae? 1.____

   A. Growth of bacteria in whole rabbit blood
   B. Growth of bacteria on blood agar plates containing excessive catalase
   C. Injection of bacteria into mice and harvesting I.P. fluid after death
   D. Growth of bacteria on media containing specific streptococcus antiserum
   E. None of the above

2. An infarct is MOST frequently characterized by what type of necrosis? 2.____

   A. Fat B. Caseation C. Gangrenous
   D. Coagulation E. Liquefaction

3. Which of the following cell types is MOST likely associated with antibody formation? 3.____

   A. Basophil B. Monocyte C. Eosinophil
   D. Neutrophil E. Plasma cell

4. What tumor of low malignancy originates in the skin, grows slowly, seldom metastasizes, but may cause great destruction of underlying structures? 4.____

   A. Dermatofibroma B. Scleroderma
   C. Melanoma D. Basal cell carcinoma
   E. Epidermoid carcinoma

5. What type leukocyte appears first and is present in GREATEST numbers in an inflammatory focus soon after tissue injury has occurred? 5.____

   A. Plasma cell B. Neutrophil C. Eosinophil
   D. Lymphocyte E. Monocyte

6. Which of the following histologic characteristics is pathognomonic for Hodgkin's disease? 6.____

   A. Reed-Sternberg cells
   B. Obliteration of the follicular pattern
   C. Enlargement of the germinal centers
   D. Langhans' giant cells
   E. None of the above

7. Generally, resistance of a bacterium to killing by heat is influenced by time and temperature employed in growth of the culture.
   ANOTHER factor is the ability of the organism to 7.____

   A. form spores
   B. withstand acid pH
   C. produce protoplasts
   D. undergo transformation
   E. grow at elevated temperatures

8. A berry aneurysm may result in 8.____

A. cerebrovascular accident
B. sudden, tearing chest pain
C. symptomless swelling of the leg
D. focus of radiolucency in a long bone
E. none of the above

9. The characteristic appearance of viral pneumonia is that of ______ pneumonia. 9.____

A. lobar
B. broncho
C. lobular
D. interstitial
E. none of the above

10. Perleche is a disease caused by a 10.____

A. virus
B. fungus
C. bacterium
D. rickettsia
E. none of the above

11. The PRINCIPAL antibacterial action of penicillin is an impairment of 11.____

A. DNA synthesis
B. histone formation
C. cell permeability
D. protein synthesis
E. cell wall synthesis

12. Amphotericin B, griseofulvin, and nystatin are often USEFUL in the treatment of 12.____

A. streptococcal infections
B. fungi diseases
C. viral diseases
D. tuberculosis
E. cancer

13. Primary systemic amyloidosis may be manifested in the mouth by 13.____

A. macroglossia
B. oropharyngeal vesicles
C. papules on buccal mucosa
D. enlarged sublingual glands
E. none of the above

14. Metastasis is LIKELY in which of the following neoplasms? 14.____

A. Adenoma
B. Melanoma
C. Chondroma
D. Papilloma
E. All of the above

15. Which of the following is an example of delayed hyper-sensitivity? 15.____

A. Atopy
B. Arthus' reaction
C. Contact dermatitis
D. Active anaphylaxis
E. Schultz-Dale reaction

16. Amyloid deposition may be associated with which of the following? 16.____

I. Chronic osteomyelitis
II. Acute suppurative osteomyelitis
III. Periostitis
IV. Multiple myeloma

The CORRECT answer is:

A. I, III
B. I, IV
C. II, III
D. II, IV
E. III, IV

17. Growth of which of the following neoplasma is OFTEN influenced by hormones? 17.____

I. Glioma
II. Breast carcinoma
III. Prostatic carcinoma
IV. Renal cell carcinoma

The CORRECT answer is:

A. I, II
B. I, III
C. I, IV
D. II, III
E. II, IV

18. Which of the following can result from syphilis? 18.____

I. Paresis
II. Locomotor ataxia
III. Condyloma latum
IV. Mesaortitis
V. Mucocutaneous eruptions

The CORRECT answer is:

A. I, II, III
B. I, II, IV
C. I, II, V
D. II *only*
E. All of the above

19. A phenol coefficient of 5.0 for an unknown disinfectant would dictate that 19.____

A. the disinfectants are equally effective
B. phenol is five times more effective against bacteria than the unknown compound
C. the unknown disinfectant is five times as effective as phenol against all bacteria
D. phenol is required at five times the concentration of the unknown for equal disinfection
E. under the test conditions a dilute solution of phenol is more effective than a concentrated unknown

20. Protozoa actively pathogenic for man include: 20.____

I. Entamoeba gingivalis
II. Leishmania donovani
III. Plasmodium malariae
IV. Trichomonas tenax
V. Entamoeba histolytica

The CORRECT answer is:

A. I, II, III
B. I, IV, V
C. II, III, IV
D. II, III, V
E. III, IV, V

21. IgE would be involved in 21.____
    I. Hives
    II. Hay fever
    III. Anaphylactic shock
    IV. Lupus erythematosus

The CORRECT answer is:

A. I, II B. I, III C. I, IV
D. II, III E. III, IV

22. Which of the following may be seen in multiple myeloma? 22.____
    I. Hypercalcemia
    II. Amyloidosis
    III. Bence Jones protein
    IV. Abnormal distribution of immunoglobulins
    V. Anemia

The CORRECT answer is:

A. I, II, III B. I, III C. I, III, V
D. II, IV, V E. All of the above

23. The tensile strength of a healing would depends upon 23.____

A. wound hormones
B. adequate fluid intake
C. activation of fibrinolysis
D. formation of collagen fibers
E. erythropoletin stimulation of bone marrow

24. Which of the following statements is(are) CORRECT? 24.____
    I. Sterilization means the destruction of infectious forms of life.
    II. Disinfection means the destruction of all forms of life.
    III. A germicide is an agent used to eliminate infectious contamination without actually destroying it.
    IV. Sanitation means the destruction of living organisms.
    V. Steam under pressure (autoclaving) is the least effective method of sterilization.

The CORRECT answer is:

A. I, II B. I, II, III C. I, II, III, IV
D. All of the above E. None of the above

25. Which of the following statements is(are) CORRECT? 25.____
    I. Dental caries is a term for the process commonly referred to as decay of tooth.
    II. Dental caries or dental decay is a specific disease which brings about the dissolution, and disintegration of the hard structures of the tooth - enamel, cementum, and dentin.
    III. Dental caries is the most widespread disease affecting the human race.
    IV. The incidence of the disease is greatest during childhood and young manhood.
    V. It attacks deciduous teeth the same as it attacks permanent teeth.

The CORRECT answer is:

A. I, II B. I, II, III C. I, II, III, IV
D. All of the above E. None of the above

KEY (CORRECT ANSWERS)

1.	C	11.	E
2.	D	12.	B
3.	E	13.	A
4.	D	14.	B
5.	B	15.	C
6.	A	16.	B
7.	A	17.	D
8.	A	18.	E
9.	D	19.	D
10.	B	20.	D

21. A
22. E
23. D
24. E
25. D

MICROBIOLOGY / PATHOLOGY

EXAMINATION SECTION
TEST 1

DIRECTIONS: Each question or incomplete statement is followed by several suggested answers or completions. Select the one that BEST answers the question or completes the statement. *PRINT THE LETTER OF THE CORRECT ANSWER IN THE SPACE AT THE RIGHT.*

1. Chronic inflammatory reactions are characterized by the presence of lymphocytes in the exudate and by 1.____

   A. production of mucin
   B. production of fibrin
   C. permeation of serum
   D. proliferation of granulation tissue

2. A hypoparathyroid patient is likely to exhibit tetany because the 2.____

   A. muscle protein is altered
   B. blood has a low concentration of serum calcium
   C. blood has a low concentration of serum phosphorus
   D. patient develops degenerative central nervous system lesions

3. Staphylococci are characteristically grouped in 3.____

   A. pairs B. chains
   C. tetrads D. irregular clusters
   E. palisade arrangement

4. Rickettsia are distinguishable from viruses because viruses contain 4.____

   A. DNA; rickettsia contain RNA
   B. RNA; rickettsia contain DNA
   C. either RNA or DNA; rickettsia contain both RNA and DNA
   D. both RNA and DNA; rickettsia contain either RNA or DNA
   E. either RNA or DNA; rickettsia contain neither RNA nor DNA

5. Persons having anti-A and anti-B isoagglutinins in their serum belong in the blood group 5.____

   A. A B. B C. AB D. O

6. The Lancefield streptococcus group MOST likely to contain strains pathogenic for man is 6.____

   A. A B. B C. D D. E E. H

7. The microorganism which has been isolated MOST frequently from infected tooth pulps is 7.____

   A. yeast B. antinomyces C. streptococci
   D. lactobacilli E. staphylococci

8. Intensification of the normal red color of tissues in an area of acute inflammation is the result of 8.____

   A. liberation of fibrin
   B. increased amount of blood in the area
   C. extravasation of blood into tissue spaces
   D. accumulation of large numbers of neutrophils
   E. damage to capillary endothelium resulting in edema

9. The leading cardiac cause of death in the United States is 9.____

   A. mitral stenosis
   B. coronary heart disease
   C. myocarditis (all causes)
   D. hypertensive cardiovascular disease
   E. congenital anomalies

10. A positive tuberculin test means that the patient 10.____

   A. has active tuberculosis
   B. has a subclinical infection
   C. is susceptible to tuberculosis
   D. has an immunity to tuberculosis as a result of a past infection
   E. has a hypersensitivity to the tubercle bacillus and its products

11. Scarlet fever is an acute disease caused by 11.____

   A. viridans streptococci releasing toxin
   B. Salmonella typhosa with endotoxin release
   C. group A streptococci releasing erythrogenic toxin
   D. a mixture of streptococci and staphylococci with coagulase production

12. Cretinism is the result of a metabolic disturbance related to 12.____

   A. hypothyroidism
   B. hyperthyroidism
   C. hypoparathyroidism
   D. hyperparathyroidism
   E. hyperfunction of anterior pituitary

13. Desensitization against pollen is accomplished by injecting 13.____

   A. histamine and histamine analogues
   B. antihistaminic drugs
   C. pollens or pollen antigens
   D. antibodies specific against pollens
   E. none of the above

14. Prolonged ischemia to an organ or tissue results in 14.____

   A. atrophy
   B. neoplasia
   C. metaplasia
   D. hyperplasia

15. A femoral osteosarcoma would MOST likely metastasize to 15.____

A. retroperitoneal lymph nodes
B. inguinal lymph nodes
C. femoral lymph nodes
D. the lungs
E. the jaws

16. Infectious hepatitis DIFFERS from serum hepatitis in that serum hepatitis 16.____

A. has a shorter incubation period
B. is more highly contagious
C. is transmitted solely by the oral-fecal route
D. is associated with the presence of Australia antigen in the patient's serum

17. The majority of antibodies have a half-life CLOSEST to 17.____

A. 20 minutes
B. 1 hour
C. 1 day
D. 1 week
E. 1 month
F. 1 year

18. Rheumatic fever is a disease which 18.____

A. can result from a transient bacteremia by viridans streptococci
B. is preceded by a Group A streptococcal infection of the heart
C. develops as a sequela to Group A streptococcal infections
D. affects the glomeruli of the kidney
E. all of the above

19. The Snyder test is used for the 19.____

A. diagnosis of mucous patches in the mouth
B. correlation of acidogenic bacteria and caries
C. isolation of Lactobacillus acidophilus
D. detection of dental caries
E. erosion of enamel in deciduous teeth

20. Adenomas are benign tumors arising from 20.____

A. cartilage
B. adipose tissue
C. glandular tissue
D. connective tissue
E. covering epithelium

21. Ribonucleic acid is considered to be the chemical basis for heredity in poliomyelitis virus because 21.____

A. it is the only nucleic acid present
B. ultraviolet light induces mutations
C. DNA is infective under appropriate conditions
D. viral infectivity is destroyed by deoxyribonuclease

22. The presence of glossitis, pallor, macrocytic anemia, hyperplasia of the bone marrow, achlorhydria, atrophy of the gastric mucosa, and focal degenerative lesions of the dorsal and lateral columns of the spinal cord in a person older than middle-age suggests the individual has had a deficiency of vitamin 22.____

A. A
B. B_1
C. B_6
D. B_{12}
E. C

23. The frequency of transient bacteremia has been shown to be HIGHEST in patients with 23.____

A. pulpectomies
B. recurrent aphthae
C. epulis fissuratum
D. root canal therapy
E. multiple extractions

24. Antibiotics are obtained from growth of 24.____

A. fungi and virus
B. bacteria and fungi
C. tissue cell culture
D. mycoplasma and rickettsiae
E. bacteria, fungi, and spirochetes

25. A fungal disease which may be confused with tuberculosis because it produces pulmonary calcifications is 25.____

A. amebiasis
B. candidiasis
C. blastomycosis
D. actinomycosis
E. histoplasmosis

KEY (CORRECT ANSWERS)

1. D
2. B
3. D
4. C
5. D

6. A
7. C
8. B
9. B
10. E

11. C
12. A
13. C
14. A
15. D

16. D
17. E
18. C
19. B
20. C

21. A
22. D
23. E
24. B
25. E

TEST 2

DIRECTIONS: Each question or incomplete statement is followed by several suggested answers or completions. Select the one that BEST answers the question or completes the statement. *PRINT THE LETTER OF THE CORRECT ANSWER IN THE SPACE AT THE RIGHT.*

1. Avirulent Corynebacterium diphtheriae can be converted to the virulent form by 1.____

   A. plasmids
   B. transfer of F factors
   C. specific bacteriophage
   D. purified diphtheria toxin
   E. DNA from a toxigenic culture

2. Vegetations on the heart valves in acute bacterial endocarditis USUALLY consist of 2.____

   A. swelling caused by inflammatory edema
   B. scar tissue containing masses of bacteria
   C. fused platelets, fibrin, and masses of bacteria
   D. areas where healing and calcification have occurred

3. Fragmentation of nuclei in necrotic cells is referred to as 3.____

   A. pyknosis
   B. karyolysis
   C. algor mortis
   D. karyorrhexis
   E. cloudy swelling

4. The mechanism of action of quaternary ammonium compounds is against the 4.____

   A. metachromatic granules
   B. cytoplasmic membrane
   C. cell wall
   D. flagella
   E. DNA

5. The reason for heating serum used in the complement fixation test to 56° C for 20-30 minutes is to inactivate 5.____

   A. antigen
   B. antibody
   C. complement
   D. any bacteria present

6. A viral disease which is stress-influenced, causes local oral lesions, and may also cause central nervous system disease is 6.____

   A. rabies
   B. smallpox
   C. yellow fever
   D. poliomyelitis
   E. herpetic stomatitis

7. Fibroma, chondroma, myxoma, and lipoma are all examples of 7.____

   A. choristomas
   B. hamartomas
   C. mixed tumors
   D. malignant neoplasms
   E. connective tissue tumors

8. For a bacterium to be seriously considered in the etiology of dental caries, it must 8.____

   A. exist regularly in the dental plaque
   B. produce extracellular amylopectins

C. be lethal for germ-free animals
D. produce intracellular dextrans
E. secrete collagenase

9. The radiosensitivity of tissue is MOST closely related to 9.____

A. the mitotic rate of tissue
B. the RNA content of the cytoplasm
C. the nuclear cytoplasmic ratio
D. ionization density of the primary irradiation
E. the size of the cells that make up the tissue

10. Hyperplasia is a condition in which there is 10.____

A. an increase in the size of a part, organ, or cell
B. a decrease in the size of a part, organ, or cell
C. an increase in the number of individual tissue elements or cells in a given organ
D. a congenital defective formation in which there is incomplete development of an organ or part
E. the production of one type of adult tissue by cells which normally produce tissue of another type

11. Shingles is caused by ______ virus. 11.____

A. rubella
B. herpes zoster
C. herpes simplex
D. Newcastle disease

12. The dermotropic viral diseases include 12.____

A. smallpox, chicken pox, and measles
B. hepatitis, mumps, and yellow fever
C. rabies, encephalitis, and encephalomyelitis
D. influenza, common cold, and primary atypical pneumonia

13. Absence of an organ because of failure of the anlage to develop is referred to as 13.____

A. aplasia
B. atrophy
C. anaplasia
D. hypoplasia
E. dysplasia

14. Several mediators of the inflammatory response are known to be activated or released in the host by antigen-antibody reactions. 14.____
One such mediator of inflammation is

A. IgA
B. histamine
C. epinephrine
D. formic acid
E. cardiolipin

15. An in utero complication arising from rubella infection OFTEN results in 15.____

A. jaundice
B. pneumonia
C. paralysis
D. chronic kidney disease
E. congenital malformations

16. The type of necrosis MOST commonly seen in tuberculosis is 16.____

A. hyaline
B. caseous
C. fibrinous
D. gummatous
E. liquefaction

17. An acute diffuse inflammation is synonymous with 17.____

A. polyposis
B. cellulitis
C. serous exudate
D. agranulocytosis
E. granulation tissue

18. The dermatomycoses are IMPORTANT fungal diseases because the 18.____

A. infections tend to resist most forms of therapy
B. organisms are primarily found in the soil
C. organisms frequently cause epidemics
D. infections are often fatal
E. all of the above

19. Gout is an example of a disturbance in the metabolism of 19.____

A. calcium
B. purines
C. cholesterol
D. carbohydrates

20. Rough pneumococci grown in the presence of DNA from smooth pneumococci develop capsules. 20.____
This is known as

A. mutation
B. conjugation
C. translation
D. transduction
E. transformation

21. Research on experimental caries in gnotobiotic animals has indicated that the majority of oral microorganisms capable of producing smooth surface dental caries with high carbohydrate diets are species of the genus 21.____

A. Veillonella
B. Streptococcus
C. Fusobacterium
D. Lactobacillus
E. Actinomyces

22. Organisms that cause gas gangrene have a metabolism which is predominantly 22.____

A. lipolytic
B. proteolytic
C. saccharolytic
D. psychronophilic

23. Acute osteomyelitis may be caused by many microorganisms, but statistically the one MOST frequently encountered is 23.____

A. gonococcus
B. enterococcus
C. streptococcus
D. staphylococcus

24. Squamous cell carcinoma is a predominant type of malignant neoplasm in all of the following EXCEPT 24.____

A. bronchus
B. esophagus
C. lower lip
D. cervix uteri
E. corpus uteri

25. Oral or pharyngeal lesions are NOT found in 25.____

A. dysentery
B. diphtheria
C. candidiasis
D. . scarlet fever
E. Ludwig's angina

KEY (CORRECT ANSWERS)

1. C
2. C
3. D
4. B
5. C

6. E
7. E
8. A
9. A
10. C

11. B
12. A
13. A
14. B
15. E

16. B
17. B
18. A
19. B
20. E

21. B
22. B
23. D
24. E
25. A

PHARMACOLOGY EXAMINATION SECTION TEST 1

DIRECTIONS: Each question or incomplete statement is followed by several suggested answers or completions. Select the one that *BEST* answers the queston or completes the statement. *PRINT THE LETTER OF THE CORRECT ANSWER IN THE SPACE AT THE RIGHT.*

1. A prescription order for 2-PAM indicates an attempt to antagonize 1.____

   A. boric acid ingestion
   B. insulin overdose
   C. petroleum distillate
   D. digitalis toxicity
   E. cholinesterase inhibitors

2. The ingestion of 1 milligram per day of folic acid is known to mask the clinical symptoms of which of the following? 2.____

   I. Iron-deficiency anemia
   II. Pernicious anemia
   III. Anoxic anemia

   The *CORRECT* answer is:

   A. Ionly
   B. II *only*
   C. I and III
   D. II and III
   E. I, II, and III

3. Vomiting should *NEVER* be induced after the ingestion of *which* of the following toxic substances? 3.____

   I. Strychnine
   II. Sulfuric acid
   III. Aspirin

   The *CORRECT* answer is:

   A. I *only*
   B. III only
   C. I and II
   D. II and III
   E. I, II, and III

4. Symptoms that suggest digitalis toxicity include *which* of the following? 4.____

   I. Hyperkalemia
   II. Yellow-greenish vision
   III. Nausea and vomiting

   The *CORRECT* answer is:

   A. I only
   B. III only
   C. I and II
   D. II and III
   E. I, II, and III

5. The toxic manifestation of drugs that are used in cancer chemotherapy are *MOST* frequently seen in 5.____

   A. old cells since the blood supply is reduced
   B. liver cells because of their high metabolic activity
   C. cells of the G.I. tract because they are rapidly dividing
   D. cells on the surface of organs since they are more exposed
   E. kidney cells because they receive a high percentage of the total blood flow

6. Spironolactone (Aldactone) is frequently prescribed concurrently with thiazide diuretics *MAINLY* because Spironolactone 6.____

   A. enhances potassium excretion
   B. promotes potassium retention
   C. enhances uric acid excretion
   D. promotes uric acid retention
   E. reduces the hypotensive activity of the thiazide

7. A patient who is experiencing ventricular extrasystoles following a myocardial infarction *MOST* likely would be given 7.____

   A. digitoxin B. quinidine C. lidocaine
   D. propranolol E. spironolactone

8. Subsequent to surgery, a patient develops thrombophlebitis. To prevent further formation of thrombi, the recommended orally administered drug is 8.____

   A. protamine sulfate B. vitamin K_1 C. menadione
   D. heparin E. warfarin

9. The oral antimicrobial agent of choice for the treatment of urinary tract infections caused by pseudomonas organisms is 9.____

   A. carbenicillin B. polymyxin B C. gentamicin
   D. ampicillin E. sulfisoxazole

10. Of the following, *which* is the drug of choice for the *initial* treatment of a patient with mild essential hypertension (e.g., diastolic pressure approximately 100 millimeters of mercury)? 10.____

   A. Guanethidine (Israel in)
   B. Pentolinium (Ansolysen)
   C. Hydrochlorothiazide (HydroDIURIL)
   D. Intravenous reserpine
   E. Diazoxide (Hyperstat I.V)

11. A teenage female patient has mild cyclic fluid retention. The *MOST* appropriate diuretic dose of HydroDIURIL for her to take every morning is 11.____

   A. 2.5 mg. B. 25 mg. C. 100 mg. D. 250 mg. E. 500 mg.

12. Which of the following is the *MOST* appropriate daily hypotensive dose of reserpine? 12.____

   A. 0.25 mg. B. 1 mg. C. 5 mg. D. 25 mg. E. 50 mg.

13. The commonly accepted reason for tetracycline's beneficial action in the treatment of acne is based upon the drug's ability to 13.____

   A. increase hepatic metabolism of circulating fats
   B. increase excretion of circulating fats
   C. decrease intestinal absorption of dietary fats
   D. decrease free fatty acid production within the follicle
   E. dilate follicle pores to permit better drainage

14. In prescribing "alternate day therapy" for a patient who is taking corticosteroids, a physician's rationale is *MOST* likely *which* of the following? 14.____

A. The patient's cost will be reduced
B. There will be fewer gastrointestinal effects
C. Inhibition of ACTH release will be minimized
D. It is more convenient for the patient
E. There are fewer chances for drug interactions to occur

15. A report in the literature indicates that propranolol depresses renin release from the juxtaglomerular apparatus.
This action, if clinically significant, is *MOST* closely associated with the use of propranolol in treating 15.____

A. migraine
B. asthma
C. tachycardia
D. hypertension
E. angina

Question 16,

DIRECTIONS: Read the following paragraph and then answer the question that follows.

Caffeine stimulates gastric acid secretion and reduces the competence of the lower esophageal sphincter in man. These effects of caffeine have been used as evidence that regular coffee should not be used by patients with peptic ulcer disease or gastrointestinal reflux. We compared the dose-response relations of caffeine, regular coffee, and decaffeinated coffee for gastric acid secretion and sphincter pressure in normal subjects. Decaffeinated coffee gave a maximal acid response of 16.5 - 2.6 milliequivalents per hour (mean - S.E.), which was similar to that of regular coffee, 20.9 - 3.6 milliequivalents per hour, both values being higher than that of caffeine, 8.4 - 1.3, on a cup-equivalent basis. Sphincter pressure showed minimal changes in response to caffeine, but was significantly increased by both regular and decaffeinated coffee.

16. Which of the following is the *MOST* appropriate interpreta-tion of the data given? 16.____

A. Caffeine is safe to use in ulcer patients
B. Clinical recommendations based upon the known G.I. effects of caffeine may bear little relation to the actual observed action of coffee or decaffeinated coffee
C. Caffeine alone should not be compared with regular coffee or decaffeinated coffee in clinical investigations
D. The results of this study suggest that both regular and decaffeinated coffee are less potent stimulants of gastric acid secretion than caffeine alone
E. The experimental design was not rigorous enough to draw any conclusions

17. A *PRIMARY* symptom of an incontinent patient is 17.____

A. intermittent claudication
B. an impacted bowel
C. frequent urination
D. partial impotency
E. severe mental depression

18. The clinical significance of achlorhydria is that it usually suggests that the patient also has 18.___

A. aplastic anemia
B. pernicious anemia
C. Cooley's anemia
D. duodenal ulcers
E. gastric ulcers

19. The efficacious route of administration for procaine penicillin G is 19.___

A. topical
B. oral
C. subcutaneous
D. intravenous
E. intramuscular

20. Which of the following drugs must be given with extreme caution to patients who have a known orythrocytic glucose-6-phosphate dehydrogenase deficiency? 20.___

A. Indomethacin
B. Nitrofurantoin
C. Penicillin
D. Warfarin
E. Isoniazid

21. Following oral dosing of griseofulvin, enhanced absorption of the anti-infective agent can occur if the patient 21.___

A. takes antacids containing calcium
B. takes B-complex vitamins
C. drinks large amounts of water
D. takes the drug within 2 hours of a meal
E. eats foods rich in fat

22. Succinylcholine, a neuromuscular blocking agent, is used as a preanesthetic medication because its duration of action is 22.___

A. short, due to rapid oxidation in the liver
B. *short,* due to a high affinity for plasma albumin binding sites
C. *short,* due to rapid hydrolysis by plasma esterases
D. *long,* due to relatively slow hydrolysis by plasma esterases
E. *long,* due to the body's low concentration of hepatic metabolizing enzymes

23. Among pediatric patients between 1 and 3 years of age, the *MOST* prominent factor concerned with drug toxicity is 23.___

A. improperly developed absorption surfaces
B. inadequate circulatory systems
C. incompletely developed microsomal enzyme systems
D. incompletely developed plasma albumin
E. incompletely developed excretory mechanisms

24. In the event of carbon monoxide poisoning, a *rational* first-aid measure is to 24.___

A. administer alcohol
B. administer amyl nitrite by inhalation
C. administer dimercaprol (BAL)
D. have the victim exercise to avoid losing consciousness
E. allow the victim to breathe fresh air

25. The *MOST* important antidotal measure in treating barbiturate toxicity is to 25.____

A. keep the patient standing upright
B. support respiration
C. apply ice packs to the patient's forehead
D. give an oil-retention enema at once
E. inject morphine p.r.n. pain

KEY (CORRECT ANSWERS)

1. E
2. B
3. C
4. D
5. C

6. B
7. D
8. E
9. A
10. C

11. B
12. A
13. D
14. C
15. D

16. B
17. C
18. B
19. E
20. B

21. E
22. C
23. C
24. E
25. B

TEST 2

DIRECTIONS: Each question or incomplete statement is followed by several suggested answers or completions. Select the one that *BEST* answers the question or completes the statement. *PRINT THE LETTER OF THE CORRECT ANSWER IN THE SPACE AT THE RIGHT.*

1. When deferoxamine is used in the treatment of iron toxicity, the antagonism represents 1.____

   A. chelation with iron to promote its excretion by the kidney
   B. oxidation of iron to form an insoluble complex
   C. displacement of iron from plasma protein binding sites
   D. reaction with bone matrix to induce deposition of iron in bone
   E. stimulation of microsomal enzymes to reduce iron levels

2. Which of the following oral hypoglycemic agents does *NOT* act *primarily* by stimulating endogenous insulin release? 2.____

   A. Acetohexamide B. Phenformin C. Chlorpropamide
   D. Tolazamide E. Tolbutamide

3. Which of the following chemotherapeutic agents is a folic acid antagonist? 3.____

   A. Tetracycline B. Methotrexate C. Chloramphenicol
   D. Isoniazid E. Quinine

4. Which of the following agents is used to diagnose pheochromocytoma? 4.____

   A. Phentolamine (Regitine)
   B. Dehydrocholate (Decholin Sodium)
   C. Tolbutamide (Orinase)
   D. Sodium aminohippurate
   E. Metyrapone (Metopirone)

5. A patient complaining of gastric upset is admitted to the hospital to undergo tests for achlorhydria. Of the following, the diagnostic agent of choice is 5.____

   A. diphenhydramine hydrochloride (Benadryl)
   B. dehydrocholate (Decholin Sodium)
   C. phentolamine (Regitine)
   D. bromsulphalein (BSP)
   E. betazole hydrochloride (Histalog)

6. Forms of insulin that can be administered by intravenous infusion include *which* of the following? 6.____

   I. Isophane (NPH)
   II. Regular (Iletin)
   III. Insulin zinc (lente)

   The *CORRECT* answer is:

   A. I *only* B. II *only* C. *I* and III
   D. II and III E. I, II, and III

7. Agents that would be suitable for a patient who has a known allergy to aspirin include which of the following? 7.____

I. Acetaminophen
II. Propoxyphene
III. Phenacetin

The *CORRECT* answer is:

A. II *only*
B. III only
C. I and II
D. I and III
E. I, II, and III

8. Of the following, which sulfonamide is used as a pre-operative medication to sterilize the bowel prior to abdominal surgery? 8.____

A. Sulfisoxazole
B. Sulf amethoxazole
C. Phthalylsulfathiazole
D. Sulfadiazine
E. Triple sulfas

9. Which of the following oral hypoglycemic agents has the *LONGEST* biological half-life? 9.____

A. Acetohexamide
B. Phenformin
C. Chlorpropamide
D. Tolazamide
E. Tolbutamide

10. Patients receiving metronidazole (Jlagyl) for trichomonal infections should be cautioned to *avoid* the ingestion of 10.____

A. certain cheeses
B. alcohol
C. milk
D. penicillin
E. anticholinergics

11. The antibacterial action of raethenamine mandelate (Mandelamine) is *increased* by the concurrent administration of 11.____

A. physiological saline
B. sodium benzoate
C. ammonium chloride
D. sodium bicarbonate
E. acetylsalicylic acid

12. A patron taking levodopa for parkinsonism should be advised *against* concurrent administration of vitamin preparations that contain 12.____

A. folicacid
B. vitaminB_2
C. vitaminB1
D. vitamin6_{12}
E. vitamin B_6

13. Ibuprofen is *BEST* classified as a(n) 13.____

A. anti-inflammatorya gent
B. antiarrhythmic agent
C. hypotensive agent
D. anticholinergic
E. diuretic

14. Methapyrilene, a common component of OTC sleep preparations, can be classified pharmacologically as a(n) 14.____

A. hypnotic
B. sympathomimetic
C. parasympathornimetic
D. analgesic
E. antihistaminic

15. Which of the following agents is considered the prototype of predominant beta-adrenergic antivation? 15.___

A. Phenylephrine
B. Propranolol
C. Epinephrine
D. Isoproterenol
E. Norepinephrine

16. In adults, the *MOST* common side-effect associated with Benadryl is 16.___

A. gastrointestinal distress
B. sedation
C. xerostomia
D. blurred vision
E. excitation

17. Which of the following conditions *CONTRAINDICATES* the local instillation of corticosteroids, such as Decadron, into the eye? 17.___

A. Glaucoma
B. Night blindness
C. Allergies to pollen
D. Astigmatism
E. Conjunctivitis

18. Diuril must be used with caution in persons *with* 18.___

A. hyperkalemia
B. hypernatremia
C. hypertension
D. hyperkinesis
E. hyperuricemia

19. Phenylephrine (Neo-Synephrine) acts as a nasal decongestant by 19.___

A. causing a local anesthetic action
B. blocking at the synaptic ganglia
C. constricting blood vessels by alpha-adrenergic stimulation
D. dilating blood vessels by beta-adrenergic stimulation
E. blocking nuscarinic receptors

20. Isoproterenol (Isuprel) stimulates the heart, in part, by 20.___

A. blocking the vagal reflex
B. stimulating the cardioaccelerator center in the medulla
C. blocking the Renshaw cells in the spinal cord
D. stimulating the beta-adrenergic receptors in the heart
E. inhibiting the effect of epinephrine on alpha-adrenergic receptors

21. The agent of choice for treating acute attacks of gout is 21.___

A. allopurinol
B. probenecid
C. phenylbutazone
D. sulfinpyrazone
E. colchicine

22. A prescription for 3.5 grams of ampicillin and 1 gram of probenecid to be taken as a single oral dose is *MOST* likely for the treatment of 22.___

A. cystitis
B. rheumaticfever
C. gonorrhea
D. impetigo
E. ulcerativecolitis

23. Drugs that are appropriate for a person who requests medication for motion sickness include *which* of the following? 23.____
    I. Dimenhydrinate
    II. Meclizine
    III. Dexamethasone
    The *CORRECT* answer is:

    A. I *only*
    B. II *only*
    C. I and II
    D. II and III
    E. I, II, and III

24. A daily dose of 160 milligrams of propranolol (Inderal) is *likely* to be used for the treatment of 24.____

    A. angina
    B. atherosclerosis
    C. asthma
    D. myalgia
    E. gout

25. Benztropine mesylate (Cogentin) is indicated for treatment of 25.____

    A. gouty arthritis
    B. petit mal epilepsy
    C. wide-angle glaucoma
    D. Parkinson's disease
    E. myasthenia gravis

KEY (CORRECT ANSWERS)

1.	A	11.	C
2.	B	12.	E
3.	B	13.	A
4.	A	14.	E
5.	E	15.	D
6.	B	16.	B
7.	E	17.	A
8.	C	18.	E
9.	C	19.	C
10.	B	20.	D

21. E
22. C
23. C
24. A
25. D

PHARMACOLOGY

EXAMINATION SECTION
TEST 1

DIRECTIONS: Each question or incomplete statement is followed by several suggested answers or completions. Select the one that *BEST* answers the question or completes the statement. *PRINT THE LETTER OF THE CORRECT ANSWER IN THE SPACE AT THE RIGHT.*

1. Which of the following drugs does *NOT* possess an action common to the other four? 1.____

   A. Caffeine
   B. Ephedrine
   C. Strychnine
   D. Amphetamine
   E. Scopolamine

2. Generally, each of the following factors is important in assuring maximum effeetive absorption of a drug from the gastrointestinal tract *EXCEPT* 2.____

   A. high degree of ionization of the drug
   B. high lipid solubility of the drug
   C. particle size of the drug administered
   D. size of the drug molecule
   E. None of the above

3. All of the following pairs of drugs are opposite in their pharmacological action on smooth muscle of intestine *EXCEPT* 3.____

   A. morphine and papaverine
   B. neostigmine and atropine
   C. amphetamine and ephedrine
   D. acetylcholine and epinephrine
   E. None of the above

4. Hydrochlorothiazide has all of the following actions in man *EXCEPT* 4.____

   A. a hypotensive effect
   B. mobilization of edema fluid
   C. increased excretion of potassium
   D. increased excretion of uric acid
   E. increased excretion of sodium

5. Each of the following is useful as an antihypertensive agent *EXCEPT* 5.____

   A. reserpine
   B. amyl nitrite
   C. hydralazine
   D. chlorothiazide
   E. alpha-methyldopa

6. Each of the following local anesthetics is a benzoic acid ester *EXCEPT* 6.____

   A. procaine
   B. tetracaine
   C. piperocaine
   D. mepivacaine
   E. ethyl aminobenzoate

7. Which of the following statements *BEST* describes the toxicity of most drugs? 7.___

   A. Toxicity is unpredictable and random.
   B. Toxicity and therapeutic effect always arise from different mechanisms.
   C. Toxicity is not produced by the average dose listed in the U. S. PHARMACOPEIA.
   D. Toxicity is often an extension of the desired drug effect.
   E. Toxicity is predictable and consistent.

8. Organophosphate insecticides and nerve gases inhibit the action of which of the following enzymes? 8.___

   A. Adenylate cyclase
   B. Monoamine oxidase
   C. Phosphodieterase
   D. Acetylcholinesterase
   E. None of the above

9. Which of the following forms of drug toxicity is particularly associated with the halogenated hydrocarbon general anesthetics? 9.___

   A. Liver damage
   B. Myocardial atrophy
   C. Peripheral neuritis
   D. Severe hypertension
   E. None of the above

10. Which of the following statements is *TRUE* regarding the use of the barbiturates in treating convulsions due to local anesthesia? 10.___

    A. Barbiturates are incapable of terminating local anesthetic convulsions.
    B. Barbiturates may delay return to consciousness and are synergistic with respiratory and cardiovascular depressant effects of local anesthetics.
    C. Premedication with the barbiturates may prevent the convulsions due to local anesthetics.
    D. All of the above
    E. None of the above

11. How is the therapeutic index of a drug calculated? 11.___

    A. The therapeutic dose is divided by the toxic base
    B. Half the toxic dose is divided by half the therapeutic dose
    C. The maximum tolerated dose is divided by the minimum therapeutic dose
    D. The lethal dose for 50 percent of animals is divided by the therapeutic dose for 50% of animals
    E. The toxic base is divided by the therapeutic dose

12. The systemic activity of the ester (procaine) types of local anesthetics is terminated *PRIMARILY* by 12.___

    A. elimination by the kidney
    B. storage in adipose tissue
    C. metabolism in the liver only
    D. metabolism in the liver and by pseudocholinesterase in the plasma
    E. all of the above

13. A patient receiving propranolol has an acute asthmatic attack while undergoing treatment. The *MOST* useful agent for management of the condition is 13.____

A. morphine B. epinephrine C. phentolamine
D. aminophylline E. norepinephrine

14. Anithistaminic compounds exert their effect by 14.____

A. chemically neutralizing histamine
B. competing with histamine for peripheral receptor sites
C. preventing the release of histamine in injured tissues
D. preventing the antigen-antibody reaction upon exposure to an allergen
E. chemically freeing histamine

15. A patient states that he has been taking mecamylamine regularly for the past year. Oral examination is *most likely* to reveal 15.____

A. ptyalism B. xerostomia
C. palatal petechiae D. gingival hypertrophy
E. bullous lesions on the buccal mucosa

16. Prolonged therapeutic administration of cortisone induces 16.____

A. hypoglycemia
B. hypofunction of the adrenal cortex
C. hypofunction of the adrenal medulla
D. hyperfunction of the pituitary gland
E. hyperfunction of the thyroid gland

17. Which of the following statements are *TRUE* regarding general anesthetics? 17.____
A. All are gases at room temperature.
B. Speed of induction is inversely related to blood solubility.
C. Effects are dependent upon attaining a critical partial pressure in the CNS.
D. All are associated with a decrease in central synaptic activity.
E. All are explosive.
The *CORRECT* answer is:

A. I, II, III B. I, IV, V C. II, III, IV
D. III, IV E. III, IV, V

18. Which of the following are side-effects of anti-anxiety drugs such as diazepam? 18.____
I. Drug dependence similar to the barbiturates
II. Ataxia
III. Impaired mechanical abilities
IV. Drowsiness
V. Hypnosis
The *CORRECT* answer is:

A. I, II, V B. I, III, IV C. II, III, IV
D. III, IV, V E. All ofthe above

19. Which of the following drugs may cause adverse reactions when administered in the presence of the monoamine oxidase inhibitors? 19.____

I. Epinephrine
II. Amphetamine
III. Tyramine
IV. Penicillin
V. Aspirin

A. I, II, III, IV
B. I, II, III
C. II, IV, V
D. III, IV, V
E. All of the above

20. Scopolamine is often used for premedication prior to administration of a general anesthetic because it 20.____

A. *increases* heart rate
B. *decreases* heart rate
C. *decreases* blood pressure
D. *decreases* the possibility of laryngospasm by inhibiting salivation
E. *retards* liver metabolism of the general anesthetic agent

21. The activity of benzalkonium chloride is markedly antagonized by 21.____

A. soap
B. sodium nitrite
C. sodium chloride
D. cetylpyridinium chloride
E. alkylbenzyldimethyl ammonium chloride

22. Inadvertently, an overdose of morphine is administered to a patient. To treat this condition, it is appropriate to administer 22.____

A. oxygen and inject naloxone hydrochloride
B. caffeine sodium benzoate intravenously
C. doxapram intramuscularly
D. nalorphine and epinephrine intramuscularly
E. none of the above

23. The *single MOST* useful agent in resuscitation is 23.____

A. oxygen
B. an endotracheal tube
C. a respiratory stimulant
D. aromatic spirits of ammonia
E. 1:1000 epinephrine for injection

24. The advantages of nitrous oxide sedation over intravenous sedation include: 24.____

I. Shorter recovery time
II. Less respiratory depression
III. The ability to discharge the patient without an escort
IV. The ability to alter the depth of sedation from moment to moment
V. Lack of toxicity and allergenicity of the agent

The *CORRECT* answer is:

A. I, II, III
B. I, IV
C. II, III, IV
D. III, IV, V
E. All of the above

25. Which of the following is *NOT* true regarding combined oral contraceptives? 25.____

A. Inhibit ovulation
B. Stimulate pituitary secretion of FSH and LH
C. Chemically contain an estrogen and a progestin
D. Produce endometrial changes resembling pregnancy
E. Are contraindicated in the presence of estrogen-dependent cancers

---

KEY (CORRECT ANSWERS)

1. E
2. A
3. C
4. D
5. B
6. D
7. D
8. D
9. A
10. B
11. D
12. D
13. D
14. B
15. B
16. B
17. C
18. E
19. B
20. D
21. A
22. A
23. A
24. E
25. B

TEST 2

DIRECTIONS: Each question or incomplete statement is followed by several suggested answers or completions. Select the one that *BEST* answers the question or completes the statement. *PRINT THE LETTER OF THE CORRECTANSWER IN THE SPACE AT THE RIGHT.*

1. Tolerance is *LEAST* likely to develop with use of 1.____

   A. LSD B. heroin C. marihuana
   D. methadone E. amphetamines

2. The *MOST* important pharmacologic action of drugs which suppress cardiac arrhythmias is 2.____

   A. blockade of the vagus nerve
   B. stimulation of cardiac ATP-ase activity
   C. blockade of the beta-adrenergic receptor
   D. stimulation of the alpha-adrenergic receptor
   E. increased refractory period of cardiac muscle

3. Adrenergic neuron blocking drugs, such as guanethidine, are useful *PRIMARILY* in the treatment of 3.____

   A. mental disease B. cardiac arrest
   C. cholinergic crisis D. paroxysmal tachycardia
   E. essential (primary) hypertension

4. A patient on anticonvulsant therapy exhibits marked gingival hypertrophy. This patient, *MOST* likely, is regularly taking 4.____

   A. primidone B. mephobarbital
   C. phenacemide D. phenobarbital
   E. diphenylhydantoin

5. When methohexital is used to induce general anesthesia, the initial effect wears off within a short time and the patient awakens. This occurs because the drug is 5.____

   A. detoxified B. biotransformed
   C. eliminated from the body D. redistributed from the brain
   E. None of the above

6. At a pH of 7.8, lidocaine (pKa = 7.8) will exist in 6.____

   A. the ionized form
   B. the unionized form
   C. an equal mixture of ionized and unionized forms
   D. all of the above
   E. none of the above

7. The blood level of a drug is determined by its: 7.____

   I. Rate of absorption
   II. Rate of excretion
   III. Dose
   IV. Rate of metabolism
   V. Route of administration

The *CORRECT* answer is:

A. I, II, III B. I, II, V C. I, IV
D. II, III, IV E. All of the above

8. The inhalation of amyl nitrite may result in: 8.____
   I. Coronary artery dilation
   II. Peripheral arteriolar dilation
   III. Bradycardia
   IV. Increased motility of the small bowe
   V. A decrease in arterial blood pressure

   The *CORRECT* answer is:

   A. I, II, IV B. I, II, V C. I, III, IV
   D. II, III, V E. III, IV, V

9. An intravenous injection of epinephrine will cause: 9.____
   I. A constriction of cutaneous vascular beds
   II. An increase in cardiac rate
   III. An increase in the activity of the intestinal musculature
   IV. A depression of the central nervous system
   V. An increased blood sugar level

   The *CORRECT* answer is:

   A. I, II, III B. I, II, V C. I, IV, V
   D. II, III, IV E. III, IV, V F. All of the above

10. Which of the following drugs are categorized as "controlled" drugs under the Controlled Substances Act? 10.____
    I. Codeine
    II. Pentobarbital
    III. Meprobamate
    IV. Oxycodone

    The *CORRECT* answer is:

    A. I, II, III B. I, III, IV C. I, IV
    D. II, III, IV E. All of the above

11. The cholinergic effect of pilocarpine is due to 11.____

    A. reversible inactivation of acetylcholinesterase at the postganglionic synapse
    B. irreversible inactivation of acetylcholinesterase at the postganglionic synapse
    C. direct action upon the cholinergic receptor site
    D. stimulation of release of acetylcholine from the nerve terminal
    E. none of the above

12. An enzyme involved in the inactivation of epinephrine in the body is 12.____

    A. cholinesterase
    B. choline acetylase
    C. carbonic anhydrase
    D. cytochrome oxidase
    E. catechol-o-methyltransferase

13. The *first* clinically useful and systemically effective anti-infective agent was 13.____

A. penicillin B. sulfanilamide C. tetracycline
D. streptomycin E. bacitracin

14. The drugs phenformin, tolbutamide, and acetohexamide have in common the fact that they 14.____

A. prevent symptoms of metaphase
B. are anti-inflmmatory
C. reduce blood pressure in the hypertensive patient
D. are antithyroid drugs generally used before thyroid surgery
E. are hypoglycemic agents which may induce cardiovascular disease

15. If a patient requiring an extraction reports that he is on bishydroxyeoumarin therapy, the laboratory test *MOST* valuable in evaluating the surgical risk is 15.____

A. clotting time B. bleeding time
C. sedimentation rate D. complete blood count
E. plasma prothrombin time

16. Which of the following drugs is *MOST* commonly employed in an attack of angina pectoris? 16.____

A. Sodium nitrate B. Epinephrine
C. Theophylline D. Nitroglycerin
E. Isosorbide dinitrate

17. Which of the following antibiotics may cause discoloration of the teeth of the newborn if administered to the mother in the third trimester of pregnancy? 17.____

A. Penicillin B. Tetracycline C. Streptomycin
D. Clindamycin E. Erythromycin

18. Which of the following is the *BEST* substitute drug for a patient allergic to penicillin? 18.____

A. Lincomycin B. Tetracycline C. Sulfonamide
D. Erythromycin E. Ampicillin

19. Which of the following properties may be attributed to warfarin? 19.____

I. Interferes in the *in vivo* synthesis of Factor VII
II. Related structurally to vitamin K
III. Inhibits formation of prothrombin in vivo
IV. Immediate onset of anticoagulant activity
V. Hematological activity is reversed by whole blood administration

The *CORRECT* answer is:

A. I *only* B. I, II, III, V C. I, III, IV
D. II, IV, V E. All of the above

Questions 20-25.

DIRECTIONS: The information contained in Questions 20-25 consists of two main parts: a statement and a reason for the statement. *Which* of the following evaluations *BEST* describes each question?

A. Both statement and reason are correct and related
B. Both statement and reason are correct but not related
C. The statement is correct but the reason is not
D. The statement is not correct but the reason is an accurate statement
E. Neither statement nor reason is correct

20. Epinephrine is contraindicated in treating the vascular collapse of chlorpromazine toxicity *because* chlorpromazine blocks the vasoconstricting properties of epinephrine. 20.____

21. The liver affects the excretion rate of a drug *because* the liver is capable of chemically changing a drug to its lipid insoluble form. 21.____

22. Tincture of iodine is not used as a local anti-infective agent over large areas of the body *because* tincture of iodine causes many allergic reactions and is destructive of skin. 22.____

23. Neostigmine can be useful in treating an overdose of d-tubucurarine *because* neostigmine increases the release of acetylcholine from motor nerve endings. 23.____

24. Many nonprescription "sleeping tablets" contain an antihistamine because some antihistamines are effective against motion sickness. 24.____

25. Dimercaprol (BAL) is effective in early poisoning by mercuric salts *because* it forms a chelate with mercury. 25.____

KEY (CORRECT ANSWERS)

1. C
2. E
3. E
4. E
5. D
6. C
7. E
8. B
9. B
10. E
11. C
12. E
13. B
14. E
15. E
16. D
17. B
18. D
19. B
20. A
21. A
22. A
23. C
24. B
25. A

PHARMACOLOGY

EXAMINATION SECTION

TEST 1

DIRECTIONS: Each question or incomplete statement is followed by several suggested answers or completions. Select the one that BEST answers the question or completes the statement. *PRINT THE LETTER OF THE CORRECT ANSWER IN THE SPACE AT THE RIGHT.*

1. The diuresis seen after adequate digitalis therapy in a patient with congestive heart failure results from 1.____
   A. a direct action of digitalis on glomeruli of the kidney
   B. increased efficiency of the heart and increased renal blood flow
   C. decreased water reabsorption caused by a direct tubular action
   D. an inhibition of antidiuretic hormone output
   E. decreased efficiency of the heart and decreased renal blood flow

2. The action of local anesthetic drugs on nerve fibers resulting in blockage of impulse conduction is 2.____
   A. a decrease in action potential duration
   B. a decrease in magnitude of resting membrane potential
   C. prevention of the depolarization phase of the action potential
   D. a decrease in the rate of repolarization of the membrane
   E. an increase in magnitude of resting membrane potential

3. The PRINCIPAL therapeutic action of the glucocorticoids is 3.____
   A. antidiuretic
   B. antianabolic
   C. anti-infective
   D. antihypertensive
   E. anti-inflammatory

4. If the pH of an area is lower than normal body pH, the concepts involved for the membrane theory of local anesthetic activity would predict that the local anesthetic activity would be 4.____
   A. greater, due to an increase in the free-base form of the drug
   B. greater, due to an increase in the cationic form of the drug
   C. less, due to an increase in the free-base form of the drug
   D. less, due to a decrease in the free-base form of the drug
   E. none of the above

5. The PRIMARY effect produced by digitalis at therapeutic dose levels is a(n) 5.____
   A. slowing of the cardiac rate
   B. decrease in the venous pressure
   C. decrease in cardiac enlargement
   D. increase in the force of myocardial contraction
   E. increase in the venous pressure

6. Which of the following pertain to general anesthesia induced by thiopental? 6.____
   I. Fast induction
   II. Long duration of anesthesia
   III. Predisposition to laryngospasm
   IV. Decreased secretions
   The CORRECT answer is:
   A. I, III
   B. I, IV
   C. II, III
   D. III, IV
   E. All of the above

7. Which of the following therapeutic measures would be appropriate in attempting to ensure the recovery of a patient in coma (with six respiratory movements per minute) as a result of an overdose of pentobarbital? 7.____
   I. Artificial respiration
   II. Administration of oxygen
   III. Injection of nikethamide as an analeptic drug
   IV. Removal of secretions from nasopharynx and trachea
   V. Administration of neomycin by intramuscular injection
   VI. Intravenous infusion of electrolytes to maintain electrolyte balance
   The CORRECT answer is:
   A. I, II, III, V
   B. I, II, IV, V
   C. I, II, IV, VI
   D. I, III, IV, VI
   E. II, III, V, VI
   F. III, IV, V, VI

8. Which of the following are TRUE regarding the therapeutic index? 8.____
   I. Expresses the relationship between efficacy and toxicity of a drug
   II. The lower the number, the safer the drug
   III. Expresses the margin of safety of the drug
   IV. Determined by comparing ED_{30} and LD_{50} for a drug
   V. Identical for drugs belonging to the same general group (sedatives, antibiotics, etc.)
   The CORRECT answer is:
   A. I, II, III
   B. I, III, IV
   C. I, IV, V
   D. II, IV, V
   E. III, IV, V

9. Alpha adrenergic drugs are used in combination with local anesthetics to: 9.____
   I. Stimulate myocardial contraction
   II. Reduce vascular absorption of the local anesthetic
   III. Increase the rate of liver metabolism of the local anesthetic
   IV. Increase the concentration of the local anesthetic at its receptor site
   V. Antagonize the vasodilatory effects of the local anesthetic
   The CORRECT answer is:
   A. I, II, III
   B. II, III, IV
   C. II, IV, V
   D. III, IV, V
   E. IV, V

10. The side effects associated with the rauwolfia derivatives (e.g., reserpine) are: 10.____
   I. Tachycardia
   II. Nasal stuffiness
   III. Postural hypotension
   IV. Potentiation of barbiturate and narcotic agents
   V. Xerostomia

The CORRECT answer is:
A. I, II, IV
B. I, III, V
C. I, V
D. II, III, IV
E. All of the above

11. The FIRST sensations usually lost after local anesthetic administration are: 11.____
I. Touch
II. Pressure
III. Pain
IV. Temperature
V. Skeletal muscle movement
The CORRECT answer is:
A. I, II
B. I, III
C. II, III
D. III, IV
E. III, V

12. Which of the following are TRUE regarding neuroleptic analgesia? 12.____
I. Combination of an anti-psychotic agent and a Schedule II narcotic
II. May induce general anesthesia
III. Contraindicated in patients with impaired respiration
IV. Low therapeutic index
The CORRECT answer is:
A. I, II, III
B. I, IV
C. II, III, IV
D. II, IV
E. All of the above

13. Which of the following drugs of abuse produce little, if any, physical dependence? 13.____
I. Marijuana
II. Barbiturates
III. Amphetamine
IV. Cocaine
V. Heroin
The CORRECT answer is:
A. I, II, III
B. I, III, IV
C. I, IV
D. II,III, V
E. III, IV, V

14. Which of the following reduce skeletal muscle tone by action of the central nervous system? 14.____
I. Chlordiazepoxide
II. Mephenesin
III. Meprobamate
IV. Diazepam
The CORRECT answer is:
A. I, II, III
B. I, III
C. II, IV
D. III, IV
E. All of the above

15. Which of the following are TRUE regarding ethyl alcohol? 15.____
I. Diuretic
II. Respiratory depressant
III. Selectively concentrates in the brain
IV. 30% excreted by the kidney
V. No tolerance development
The CORRECT answer is:
A. I, II
B. I, II, III
C. I, IV, V
D. II, IV, V
E. II, V

Questions 16-25.

DIRECTIONS: Questions 16 through 25 are to be answered on the basis of the following case.

Mrs. Martin is scheduled in the office for minor periodontal surgery. She has a documented history of rheumatic heart disease, but is not receiving any prophylactic antibiotic therapy. Her medical history reveals narrow angle glaucoma and acute intermittent porphyria (porphyrism). She is anxious regarding her dental procedure and pharmacosedation procedures are deemed necessary. She has no known drug allergies.

16. In view of Mrs. Martin's rheumatic heart condition, the prophylactic antibiotic of choice to be administered orally is 16.____
    A. erythromycin B. penicillin V C. cephalexin
    D. lincomycin E. ampicillin

17. This prophylactic antibiotic therapy should begin _____ prior to the dental procedure. 17.____
    A. immediately B. one hour C. four hours
    D. one day E. two days

18. Due to Mrs. Martin's history of porphyrism, which of the following drug groups is contraindicated for pharmacosedation? 18.____
    A. Minor tranquilizers B. Antihistamines C. Barbiturates
    D. Narcotics E. None of the above

19. Which of the following pharmacosedation agents are contraindicated in the presence of glaucoma? 19.____
    I. Meperidine II. Scopolamine III. Diazepam
    IV. Pentobarbital V. Morphine
    The CORRECT answer is:
    A. I, II, III B. II, III, IV C. II, IV
    D. III, IV, V E. III, V

20. Considering Mrs. Martin's history of glaucoma and porphyrism, which of the following pharmacosedation techniques is PREFERRED? 20.____
    A. Intravenous secobarbital B. Intravenous diazepam
    C. Nitrous oxide-oxygen D. Intravenous thiopental
    E. None of the above

21. Because Mrs. Martin's postoperative discomfort is expected to be minimal, aspirin is advised for analgesia. Which of the following are TRUE regarding aspirin in therapeutic doses? 21.____
    I. Active form is salicylic acid
    II. Has antipyretic properties
    III. Produces central nervous system depressant effects
    IV. Produces central nervous system stimulant effects
    V. Retards platelet (thrombocyte) function

The CORRECT answer is:
A. I, II, III
B. I, II, V
C. I, III
D. II, III, IV
E. III, IV, V

22. A SIGNIFICANT mechanism by which aspirin produces its analgesic and anti-inflammatory effects is 22.____
A. antagonism of histamine
B. inhibition of prostaglandin synthesis
C. local anesthetic effect on pain fibers
D. release of adrenal steroids from the adrenal cortex
E. synaptic inhibition in the dorsal column of the spinal cord

23. Mrs. Martin calls the office with complaints suggesting a diffuse cellulitis and lymphadenopathy. A superinfection with a penicillinase-producing staphylococcus is immediately suspected. 23.____
Which of the following antibiotics is the drug of choice in treating this condition?
A. Chloramphenicol
B. Cephalexin
C. Penicillin G
D. Erythromycin
E. Polymyxin B

24. If this superinfection were to be confined to the gastrointestinal tract as a staphylococcal enteritis, which of the following antibiotics would be the drug of choice to be administered topically? 24.____
A. Bacitracin
B. Polymyxin B
C. Erythromycin
D. Lincomycin
E. Benzathine penicillin

25. If Mrs. Martin developed severe gastrointestinal upset from aspirin, which of the following analgesics would be ACCEPTABLE substitutes? 25.____
I. Pentazocine
II. Empirin® Compound
III. Acetaminophen
IV. Darvon® Compound-65
V. Codeine

The CORRECT answer is:
A. I, II, III
B. I, III
C. I, III, V
D. II, IV, V
E. II, V

KEY (CORRECT ANSWERS)

1.	B	11.	D
2.	C	12.	E
3.	E	13.	B
4.	D	14.	E
5.	D	15.	A
6.	A	16.	B
7.	C	17.	B
8.	B	18.	C
9.	C	19.	A
10.	D	20.	C

21. B
22. B
23. B
24. A
25. C

TEST 2

DIRECTIONS: Each question or incomplete statement is followed by several suggested answers or completions. Select the one that BEST answers the question or completes the statement. *PRINT THE LETTER OF THE CORRECT ANSWER IN THE SPACE AT THE RIGHT.*

1. Which of the following xanthine derivatives produces the BEST bronchodilation? 1.____
   A. Caffeine B. Theobromine C. Theophylline
   D. All of the above E. None of the above

2. The cardiac glycosides will reduce the concentration of which ion in an active heart muscle? 2.____
   A. Sodium B. Bromide C. Calcium
   D. Chloride E. Potassium

3. Pre-treatment with which of the following drugs will potentiate the ability of an intravenous injection of acetylcholine to lower blood pressure? 3.____
   A. Methacholine B. Epinephrine C. Pilocarpine
   D. Physostigmine E. Pralidoxime

4. Which of the following drugs might act by biotransformation into a FALSES adrenergic neurotransmitter? 4.____
   A. Alpha-methyldopa B. Hydralazine C. Phentolamine
   D. Dibenamine® E. Reserpine

5. An excess of which of the following hormones may be associated with increased sensitivity to epinephrine? 5.____
   A. Testosterone B. Parathyroid C. Insulin
   D. Thyroid E. None of the above

6. Which of the following procedures would be expected to increase the incidence and the severity of reactions to local anesthetic agents? 6.____
   A. Aspiration prior to injection
   B. Premedication with a barbiturate
   C. Rapid injection of the anesthetic solution
   D. Use of a vasoconstrictor agent along with the local anesthetic agent
   E. Aspiration after injection

7. Potassium is one of the most important and prevalent ions in the mammalian species. Which of the following statements about this ion are TRUE? 7.____
   I. It is the principal intracellular cation.
   II. High concentrations of the chloride salt can be safely injected intravenously.
   III. It is necessary for normal function of nerve and muscle.
   IV. It is the principal ion responsible for edema.
   The CORRECT answer is:
   A. I, II, III B. I, III C. I, III, IV
   D. II, III E. II, IV

8. Which of the following factors should be considered in adjusting the dose of a drug administered to a specific patient? 8.____

I. Age II. Sex III. Weight
IV. Disease state V. Emotional state

The CORRECT answer is:

A. I, II, III B. I, II, V C. I, III, V
D. III, IV, V E. All of the above

9. Which of the following statements is TRUE regarding prescriptions? 9.____

A. A dentist may legally prescribe only those drugs useful in a dental office.
B. Federal law prohibits the doctor's prescribing a drug over the phone to a pharmacist.
C. Drugs must be prescribed in dosage unit amounts greater than ten.
D. It is ethical and legal to prescribe a placebo.
E. Prescriptions may be signed by a dental assistant as long as the dentist initials the prescription.

10. Which of the following drug groups is currently the mainstay of treatment in depressive psychoneurotic disease? 10.____

A. Amphetamines
B. Phenothiazines
C. Benzodiazepines
D. Monoamine oxidase inhibitors
E. Tricylic (imipramine-like) antidepressants

11. The mechanism of action by which the fluoride ion when taken orally reduces dental caries is 11.____

A. inhibition of bacterial enzymes located in dental plaque
B. alteration in developing tooth morphology
C. alteration in developing tooth collagen matrix
D. alteration in tooth eruption pattern
E. production of less soluble fluorohydroxyapatite

12. The sulfonamides act by 12.____

A. suppressing bacterial protein synthesis
B. inhibiting cytoplasmic bacterial membrane formation
C. inducing the formation of "lethal" bacterial proteins
D. inducing folic acid deficiency by competition with para-aminobenzoic acid
E. releasing bacterial protein synthesis

13. The MOST serious and life-threatening blood dyscrasia associated with drug toxicity is 13.____

A. aplastic anemia B. agranulocytosis
C. thrombocytopenia D. hemolytic anemia
E. megaloblastic anemia

14. "Epinephrine reversal" of blood pressure can BEST be demonstrated by injecting epinephrine intravenously following pretreatment with 14.____
   A. atropine
   B. neostigmine
   C. guanethidine
   D. phenoxybenzamine
   E. dichloroisoproterenol

15. During a visit, a patient develops a severe, acute bronchial asthmatic attack. He should IMMEDIATELY receive 15.____
   A. cortisone
   B. epinephrine
   C. tripelennamine
   D. 90 percent oxygen, 10 percent CO_2
   E. none of the above

16. Derivatives of 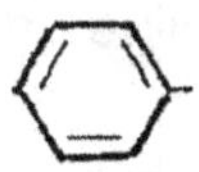 CH_2 CH_2 NH_2 are 16.____
   A. adrenergic drugs
   B. cholinergic drugs
   C. anticholinesterases
   D. cholinergic blocking agents
   E. synaptic transmitters in sympathetic ganglia

17. Which of the following statements are TRUE regarding the occupation theory of drug-receptor interaction? 17.____
   I. The affinity of a drug is dependent on its intrinsic activity.
   II. The maximum effect of the drug occurs when all receptors are occupied.
   III. An antagonist has affinity for the receptor but less intrinsic activity than its agonist.
   IV. The effect of the drug is proportional to the number of receptors occupied.
   V. It does not follow the law of mass action.

   The CORRECT answer is:
   A. I, II, III
   B. II, III
   C. II, III, IV
   D. II, IV
   E. III, IV, V

18. Concomitant administration of which of the following drugs tends to increase the depressant actions of morphine? 18.____
   I. Phenothiazines
   II. Barbiturates
   III. Alcohol
   IV. Monoamine oxidase inhibitors
   V. Tranquilizers

   The CORRECT answer is:
   A. I, II
   B. I, II, III
   C. II, IV, V
   D. III, IV, V
   E. All of the above

Questions 19-25.

DIRECTIONS: The information contained in Questions 19 through 25 consists of two main parts: A STATEMENT and a REASON FOR THE STATEMENT. Which of the following evaluations BEST describes each question?

A. Both statement and reason are correct and related.
B. Both statement and reason are correct but not related.
C. The statement is correct but the reason is not.
D. The statement is not correct but the reason is an accurate statement.

19. Atropine is a competitive inhibitor of acetylcholine at parasympathetic postganglionic autonomic sites because atropine and acetylcholine have the same affinity for all cholinergic receptor sites. 19.____

20. Penicillin is bactericidal because it inhibits the enzymatic processes responsible for determining the final three-dimensional structure of the bacterial cell wall. 20.____

21. Guanethidine can result in an initial sympathomimetic effect when administered intravenously because guanethidine, by rapidly inhibiting monoamine oxidase, produces an increase in intraneuronal norepinephrine. 21.____

22. Some patients are abnormally sensitive to succinylcholine because these individuals are congenitally deficient in pseudocholinesterase. 22.____

23. Hydrogen peroxide is useful in the management of necrotizing ulcerative gingivitis because hydrogen peroxide can result in the hypertrophy of the filiform papillae of the tongue. 23.____

24. Adenylate cyclase and cyclic AMP are thought to be intimately involved with the β-adrenergic receptor because increased tissue levels of cyclic AMP are seen in almost all cases of β-adrenergic stimulation. 24.____

25. Atropine in therapeutic doses can produce tachycardia because atropine has a depressant action on the myocardium. 25.____

KEY (CORRECT ANSWERS)

1. C
2. E
3. D
4. A
5. D

6. C
7. B
8. E
9. D
10. E

11. E
12. D
13. A
14. D
15. B

16. A
17. C
18. E
19. A
20. A

21. C
22. A
23. B
24. A
25. C

PHARMACOLOGY

EXAMINATION SECTION
TEST 1

DIRECTIONS: Each question or incomplete statement is followed by several suggested answers or completions. Select the one that BEST answers the question or completes the statement. *PRINT THE LETTER OF THE CORRECT ANSWER IN THE SPACE AT THE RIGHT.*

1. The drug of choice for prophylaxis against subacute bacterial endocarditis for the patient sensitive to penicillin is 1.____

   A. lincomycin
   B. ampicillin
   C. tetracycline
   D. streptomycin
   E. erythromycin

2. The mechanism by which 70 percent ethyl alcohol may act as a disinfectant is attributed to 2.____

   A. a metabolic degradation product of ethyl alcohol
   B. the lack of alcohol dehydrogenase in bacterial cells
   C. the interference of ethyl alcohol with carbohydrate metabolism
   D. the inebriating effect of ethyl alcohol on cells
   E. the ability of ethyl alcohol to denature proteins

3. d-tubocurarine is used in conjunction with general anesthesia to 3.____

   A. relax skeletal muscles
   B. prevent respiratory failure
   C. prevent a fall in blood pressure
   D. hasten the emergence from anesthesia
   E. increase the duration of anesthesia

4. When a laryngospasm occurs during general anesthesia, the drug of choice is 4.____

   A. atropine
   B. phenytoin
   C. meprobamate
   D. methantheline
   E. succinylcholine

5. Alcoholic euphoria results from 5.____

   A. *increased* activity of the cerebrum
   B. *increased* activity of thalamic areas
   C. *increased* activity of limbic synapses
   D. *decreased* activity of medullary centers
   E. *removal* of inhibitory effect of the cortex

6. Chlorothiazide administration results in a(n) 6.____

   A. *increased* urinary output of sodium
   B. *decreased* urinary output of chloride
   C. *increased* urinary output of glucose
   D. *decreased* urinary output of potassium
   E. *increased* urinary output of uric acid

7. Increasing the dose of a drug by a factor of 10 will INCREASE the response by a factor of 7.____

A. 10 B. 20 C. 100 D. 1,000 E. x

8. Symptoms which may be characterized as allergic manifestations during penicillin therapy are 8.____

A. deafness, dizziness, and acute anemia
B. crystalluria, nausea and vomiting, and anaphylactic shock
C. oliguria, hematuria, bronchoconstriction, and cardiovascular collapse
D. dermatitis, stomatitis, bronchoconstriction, and cardiovascular collapse
E. none of the above

9. Alpha or beta adrenergic blocking drugs, such as phentolamine and propranolol, act by 9.____

A. inhibiting synthesis of norepinephrine
B. increasing the metabolism of norepinephrine
C. competitive inhibition of postjunctional adrenergic receptors
D. a local anesthetic effect on the adrenergic nerve terminal
E. depleting norepinephrine from adrenergic nerve terminals

10. The analgesic effect of aspirin may be related to its suppression of the synthesis of 10.____

A. histamine
B. serotonin
C. bradykinin
D. prostaglandin
E. gamma-aminobutyric acid

11. The pressor action of epinephrine is reversed by 11.____

A. atropine
B. papaverine
C. neostigmine
D. phentolamine
E. propranolol

12. Drug-metabolizing enzymes are present *mainly* in liver 12.____

A. nuclei
B. lysosomes
C. microsomes
D. mitochondria
E. cell membranes

13. Termination of the action of procaine is accomplished *primarily* by 13.____

A. conjugation of the liver
B. the action of plasma amidase
C. hydroxylation in the liver
D. the action of plasma pseudocholinesterase
E. excretion in unchanged form by the kidney

14. The phenomenon in which two drugs produce opposite effects on a physiologic system but do NOT act at the same receptor site is 14.____

A. potentiation
B. chemical antagonism
C. competitive antagonism
D. physiologic antagonism
E. noncompetitive antagonism

15. When digitalis is used in atrial fibrillation, the therapeutic objective is to 15.____

A. inhibit vagal impulses to the heart
B. decrease the rate of A-V conduction
C. abolish cardiac decompensation
D. produce a decrease in the rate of atrial contraction
E. convert fibrillation to a normal sinus rhythm

16. An adrenergic drug, such as epinephrine, can be expected to 16.____

A. constrict bronchioles, systemic arterioles and cerebral arterioles
B. increase heart rate, blood pressure and myocardial contractile force
C. increase G.I. peristalsis and skeletal muscle tone, and dilate the bronchiolar smooth muscle
D. shunt blood from viscera and skin to muscles, and produce miosis without cycloplegia
E. increase body temperature, BMR and glucogenesis

17. The action of the ultra-short acting barbiturates is terminated *primarily* by the process of 17.____

A. oxidation
B. redistribution
C. renal excretion
D. plasma protein binding
E. conjugation with sulfate

18. The MAJOR therapeutic indication for the use of sulfonarnides is 18.____

A. tuberculosis
B. typhoid fever
C. urinary tract infections
D. fungal infections of the foot
E. fungal infections of the oral cavity

19. The antipsychotics are currently believed to produce their effect on the CNS by blocking the receptor for 19.____

A. dopamine
B. serotonin
C. epinephrine
D. aspartic acid
E. norepinephrine

20. A sudden INCREASE in the blood level of drug A after administration of drug B could result from 20.____

A. binding of drug A by drug B
B. chelation of drug A by drug B
C. competition for the same receptor sites
D. induction of hepatic microsomal enzymes
E. displacement of drug A by drug B from protein-binding sites

21. Spironolactone diuresis is the result of 21.____

A. increased potassium excretion
B. direct aldosterone antagonism
C. inhibition of carbonic anhydrase
D. inhibition of antidiuretic hormone release
E. increase in glomerular filtration rate

22. Oral contraceptives prevent conception *primarily* by 22.____

A. inducing abortion
B. preventing ovulation
C. a spermatocidal effect
D. causing a cessation of menses
E. preventing implantation of the fertilized ovum in the endometrial wall

23. The MOST important organ system involved in the excretion of a drug and its metabolites is the 23.____

A. lung
B. liver
C. kidney
D. gallbladder
E. gastrointestinal tract

24. Prilocaine hydrochloride four percent is supplied in a 1.8 ml. cartridge. It is recommended that 600 mg. NOT be exceeded in a two-hour period.
This amount is contained in *approximately* ______ cartridges. 24.____

A. 4 B. 8 C. 12 D. 16 E. 20

25. The current drug of choice for the treatment of the manic phase of manic-depressive psychosis is 25.____

A. amphetamine
B. imipramine
C. pargyline
D. reserpine
E. lithium

KEY (CORRECT ANSWERS)

1. E
2. E
3. A
4. E
5. E

6. A
7. E
8. D
9. C
10. D

11. D
12. C
13. D
14. D
15. B

16. B
17. B
18. C
19. A
20. E

21. B
22. B
23. C
24. B
25. E

TEST 2

DIRECTIONS: Each question or incomplete statement is followed by several suggested answers or completions. Select the one that BEST answers the question or completes the Statement. *PRINT THE LETTER OF THE CORRECT ANSWER IN THE SPACE AT THE RIGHT.*

1. When given together, the ability of two drugs to produce a response greater than either administered alone is termed 1.____

   A. synergism
   B. induction
   C. cumulation
   D. antagonism
   E. tachyphylaxis

2. Local anesthetics induce convulsions by effects on the 2.____
   I. cerebellum
   II. limbic system
   III. basal ganglia
   IV. cerebral cortex
   V. reticular activating system

   The CORRECT answer is:

   A. I, II, III B. I, V C. II, III, IV D. II, IV E. III, IV, V

3. Onset and duration of action of a drug is determined by its 3.____
   I. ability to cross membranes
   II. rate of liver metabolism
   III. degree of ionization at the urinary pH
   IV. route of administration
   V. affinity for the receptor site

   The CORRECT answer is:

   A. I, II, III, V B. I, IV C. II, III, IV D. III, IV, V
   E. all of the above

4. The adrenal steroids may be used to treat 4.____
   I. rheumatoid arthritis
   II. leukemia tuberculosis
   III. collagen diseases
   IV. Gushing disease

   The CORRECT answer is:

   A. I, II, III B. I, II, IV C. II, III, IV D. III, IV, V E. IV, V

5. The likelihood of adverse reactions to local anesthetics will be DECREASED by 5.____
   I. using an aspirating syringe
   II. injecting the anesthetic slowly
   III. taking a careful patient history
   IV. using less potent, less toxic local anesthetics
   V. limiting the amount of local anesthetics used

   The CORRECT answer is:

   A. I, II B. I, II, III C. I, II, IV D. IV, V
   E. all of the above

6. The various penicillins DIFFER in 6._____
   I. mechanism of action
   II. degree of oral absorption
   III. resistance to enzymatic degradation by penicillinase
   IV. antibacterial spectrum
   V. structural formula

   The CORRECT answer is:

   A. I, II, IV
   B. I, III, V
   C. II, III, IV
   D. II, III, IV, V
   E. III, IV, V

7. The ability of a given drug to pass through membranes is determined by the 7._____
   I. pka of the drug
   II. pH of the membrane surface
   III. lipid solubility of the drug
   IV. relative amounts of ATP in the membrane
   V. level of activity of pinocytosis in the membrane

   The CORRECT answer is:

   A. I, II
   B. I, II, III
   C. II, III, IV
   D. III, IV, V
   E. IV, V

8. Reserpine acts to 8._____
   I. block the passage of the nerve action potential in the postganglionic nerve fibers
   II. inhibit monoamine oxidase
   III. inhibit catechol-O-methyltransferase
   IV. deplete norepinephrine from the adrenergic neuron
   V. prevent re-uptake of norepinephrine by storage granules in the nerve terminal

   The CORRECT answer is:

   A. I, II
   B. I, II, III
   C. II, III, IV
   D. III, IV, V
   E. IV, V

9. Which of the following statements regarding anaphylaxis caused by drugs are TRUE? 9._____
   I. Administering drugs by the oral route diminishes the likelihood of anaphylaxis.
   II. Many, but not all, symptoms of anaphylaxis can be mimicked by injection of histamine.
   III. Anaphylaxis can appear within minutes after drug administration.
   IV. Immediate manifestations of anaphylaxis are effectively treated with epinephrine.
   V. Delayed manifestations of anaphylaxis are effectively treated with adrenal corticosteroids.

   The CORRECT answer is:

   A. I, II, III, IV
   B. I, II, IV
   C. I, III, V
   D. II, IV, V
   E. All of the above

10. Which of the following are contraindications to the use of oral contraceptives? 10.____

I. History of thromboembolic disease
II. Hyperthyroidism
III. History of breast cancer
IV. Peptic ulcer
V. Undiagnosed genital bleeding

The CORRECT answer is:

A. I, II, III
B. I, III, V
C. I, IV
D. II, III, IV
E. III, IV, V

11. Which of the following drugs produce an effect comparable to stimulation of the parasympathetic nervous system? 11.____

I. Pilocarpine
II. Physostigmine
III. Muscarine
IV. Amphetamine
V. Ergotamine

The CORRECT answer is:

A. I, II
B. I, II, III
C. II, IV, V
D. III, IV, V
E. IV, V

12. Which of the following statements are TRUE of the barbiturates? 12.____

I. They suppress REM sleep.
II. The cause of death in overdosage is respiratory depression.
III. They are metabolized primarily in the liver.
IV. In sedative doses, they are myocardial depressants.
V. In sedative doses, they have significant alpha-adrenergic blocking effects.

The CORRECT answer is:

A. I, II, III
B. I, III, V
C. II, III, IV
D. III, IV, V
E. IV, V

13. Which of the following statements are TRUE regarding the generic form of a drug? 13.____

I. A drug usually has more than one generic name.
II. Prescribing a drug by its generic name allows the pharmacist to dispense any comparable brand name preparation.
III. The generic preparation is generally less expensive than comparable brand name preparations.
IV. A narcotic, by law, must be prescribed by its generic name.
V. A generic preparation generally contains less of the pharmacologically active agent than comparable brand name preparations.

The CORRECT answer is:

A. I, II
B. I, II, III, V
C. II, III
D. II, III, IV
E. III, V

14. Which of the following are TRUE regarding the intravenous agent ketamine? It 14.____
    I. produces hypnosis and true anesthesia
    II. produces "dissociative anesthesia"
    III. may produce tonic and clonic convulsions
    IV. is now used primarily in children
    V. may produce delirium, hallucinations, and schizoid reactions

The CORRECT answer is:

A. I, II, III
B. I, III, V
C. I, IV, V
D. II, III, IV, V
E. II, V

15. Which of the following are *absolute* or *relative* contraindications to the use of morphine? 15.____
    I. Bronchial asthma
    II. Myocardial infarction
    III. Head injury
    IV. Patient history of drug abuse
    V. Chronic pain from terminal cancer

The CORRECT answer is:

A. I, II, III
B. I, III, IV
C. I, III, IV, V
D. I, IV, V
E. II, IV, V

16. Which of the following statements are TRUE regarding the cholinergic receptor? 16.____
    I. The muscarinic receptor is located in the effector organs which receive post-ganglionic parasympathetic fibers.
    II. No muscarinic receptors are found in the CNS.
    III. Muscarinic receptors are preferentially blocked by atropine.
    IV. Nicotinic receptors are located only at autonomic ganglia.
    V. The cholinergic receptor is closely related in structure to acetylcholinesterase.

A. I, II, III
B. I, III, V
C. II, III, IV
D. II, V
E. III, IV, V

17. Which of the following drugs may cause miosis? 17.____
    I. Morphine
    II. Pilocarpine
    III. Physostigmine
    IV. Reserpine
    V. Phenoxybenzamine

The CORRECT answer is:

A. I *only*
B. I, II, III
C. II, III
D. IV, V
E. All of the above

18. Which of the following are TRUE regarding the effects of digitalis on congestive heart failure? It 18.___

I. *decreases* heart rate through vagal and extravagal mechanisms
II. *increases* the efficiency of the failing myocardium
III. *increases* the force of myocardial contraction
IV. *increases* residual diastolic volume
V. *reduces* renal blood flow

The CORRECT answer is:

A. I, II, III
B. I, IV
C. II, III
D. III, IV
E. III, IV, V

19. Which of the following statements regarding drugs of abuse are TRUE? 19.___

I. All act on the CNS to produce depression, stimulation or mood-alteration.
II. All produce some degree of psychologic dependence.
III. All produce some degree of physiologic dependence.
IV. All produce drug disposition tolerance but not pharmacodynamic tolerance.
V. None of the drugs of abuse possesses any therapeutic pharmacologic properties.

The CORRECT answer is:

A. I, II
B. I, II, III
C. I, IV, V
D. II, III, IV
E. II, IV, V

20. Which of the following are endogenous catecholamines? 20.___

I. Epinephrine
II. Isoproterenol
III. Ephedrine
IV. Phenylephrine
V. Norepinephrine

The CORRECT answer is:

A. I, II, III, IV
B. I, II, V
C. I, V
D. II, V
E. IV, V

21. Which of the following are TRUE regarding pentazocine? 21.___

I. Requires DEA registration to prescribe
II. Prepared only as a parenteral analgesic
III. Partial agonist of the opioid receptor
IV. Equianalgesic with codeine
V. May induce dysphoria and mental aberrations

The CORRECT answer is:

A. I, II, IV B. I, III, V C. I, V D. II, III, IV E. III, IV, V

22. Which of the following statements are TRUE regarding the barbiturates? They 22.____
    I. significantly elevate pain thresholds
    II. are metabolized by the liver
    III. are classified according to duration of action.
    IV. depress all levels of the CNS
    V. produce death by cardiovascular depression

    The CORRECT answer is:

    A. I, II, III
    B. I, IV
    C. II, III, IV
    D. II, V
    E. III, IV, V

23. Which of the following drugs possess additive depressant effects on the central nervous system when given with another depressant? 23.____
    I. Antianxiety drugs
    II. Alcohol Barbiturates
    III. Narcotics
    IV. Antipsychotics

    The CORRECT answer is:

    A. I, II, III, V
    B. II, III
    C. II, III, IV
    D. IV, V
    E. All of the above

24. Which of the following penicillins are readily INACTIVATED by stomach acids? 24.____
    I. Penicillin G
    II. Phenoxymethyl penicillin
    III. Methicillin
    IV. Ampicillin
    V. Cloxacillin

    The CORRECT answer is:

    A. I, II
    B. I, III
    C. II, IV
    D. II, V
    E. III, IV

25. Which of the following drugs are useful in the treatment of hypertension? 25.____
    I. Sodium chloride
    II. Ephedrine
    III. Thiazide diuretics
    IV. Reserpine
    V. Alpha-methyldopa

    The CORRECT answer is:

    A. I, II, III
    B. I, III, V
    C. II, III, IV
    D. II, IV
    E. III, IV, V

KEY (CORRECT ANSWERS)

1. A
2. D
3. E
4. B
5. E

6. D
7. B
8. E
9. E
10. B

11. B
12. A
13. C
14. D
15. B

16. B
17. E
18. A
19. A
20. C

21. E
22. C
23. E
24. B
25. E

CLINICAL CHEMISTRY

EXAMINATION SECTION
TEST 1

DIRECTIONS: Each question or incomplete statement is followed by several suggested answers or completions. Select the one that *BEST* answers the question or completes the statement. *PRINT THE LETTER OF THE CORRECT ANSWER IN THE SPACE AT THE RIGHT.*

1. *Which one* of the following solutions has the *LOWEST* pH above neutrality? 1.____

   A. Sodium bicarbonate
   B. 1N sodium hydroxide
   C. Potassium hydroxide
   D. 1N sodium carbonate

2. *Which* substance is miscible with water? 2.____

   A. Toluene
   B. Alcohol
   C. Chloroform
   D. Immersion oil

3. Assume that a urine sample was measured with a hydrometer, and the value was found to be 1.036. Of the following, the *MOST* likely explanation is that the urine sample 3.____

   A. was taken over a 24-hour period
   B. contained too many dissolved substances
   C. contained erythrocytes
   D. was too dilute

4. Thirty-seven degrees centigrade *MOST* closely approximates *which one* of the following temperatures? 4.____

   A. Temperature at which water freezes
   B. Temperature at which water boils
   C. Normal refrigerator temperature
   D. Normal body temperature

5. The weight of the container or paper used on a balance to hold the specimen is called 5.____

   A. zero weight
   B. adjustable weight
   C. tare weight
   D. vernier weight

6. An osmometer is an instrument used to measure 6.____

   A. osmosis
   B. osmolality
   C. osmotic pressure
   D. osmoles

7. *Which one* of the following methods is *MOST* appropriate for the quantitative measurement of triglyceride? 7.____

   A. Electrophoresis
   B. Gas chromatography
   C. UV spectrophotometry
   D. Atomic absorption

8. When not in immediate use, the electrodes of a pH meter should be 8.____

   A. stored in a refrigerator
   B. kept immersed in distilled water

C. kept immersed in normal saline
D. dried and the fluid emptied from inside the electrode

9. The normal pH of blood is about 7.4. This means that blood is 9.____

A. strongly acidic
B. very slightly acidic
C. strongly alkaline
D. very slightly alkaline

10. Bile is secreted by the 10.____

A. small intestine
B. pancreas
C. gallbladder
D. liver

11. *Which one* of the following solutions has the *LOWEST* pH? 11.____

A. 1N hydrochloric acid
B. 1N acetic acid
C. 1N ammonium hydroxide
D. 1N sodium hydroxide

12. *What* is the molecular weight of oxygen? 12.____

A. 1
B. 8
C. 16
D. 40

13. *Which one* of the following chemicals is *NOT* flammable, and can be used if there is a burning flame in the room? 13.____

A. Amyl alcohol
B. Potassium hydroxide
C. Benzene
D. Xylene

14. If 17.3 gms of copper sulfate are required to make one liter of a solution, *how much* copper sulfate would be needed to make 350 ml of solution? 14.____

A. 1.73 gms
B. 6.06 gms
C. 17.3 gms
D. 35.0 gms

15. A biological substance that increases the rate of a chemical reaction is a(n) 15.____

A. solvent
B. antigen
C. enzyme
D. buffer

16. *Which one* of the following is *NOT* a carbohydrate? 16.____

A. Starch
B. Glucose
C. Glycine
D. Galactose

17. Electrophoresis measures the 17.____

A. migration of proteins
B. ionic strength of a solution
C. solubility product
D. voltage of a solution

18. The purpose of the photocell in a flame photometer is to 18.____

A. remove dust particles
B. filter out the proteins
C. convert light energy to electrical energy
D. multiply the electrical signal

19. Titration of an acid with a base yields a(n) 19.____

A. acid
B. alcohol
C. base
D. salt

20. *What* is the pH of the commonly used buffer, phosphate buffered saline? 20.____

A. 6.5 B. 7.4 C. 8.3 D. 9.2

21. A potential explosive chemical which is used in clinical chemistry is 21.____

A. nitric acid
B. picric acid
C. potassium nitrate
D. sodium nitrate

22. In using an Autoanalyzer, the *PRIMARY* reason for dialysis is to 22.____

A. prevent coagulation
B. prepare a clear solution
C. remove salt
D. remove protein

23. Of the following materials that are commonly added to whole blood, *which one* will have the *LEAST* effect on a calcium assay? 23.____

A. Heparin B. EDTA C. Oxalate D. Fluoride

24. Isotonic saline is 24.____

A. 0.1% NaCl
B. 0.9% NaCl
C. 5% NaCl
D. 9% NaCl

25. *Which* element is used as an internal standard in clinical chemistry? 25.____

A. La B. I^{125} C. Sr D. Li

KEY (CORRECT ANSWERS)

1. A
2. B
3. B
4. D
5. C

6. B
7. C
8. B
9. D
10. D

11. A
12. C
13. B
14. B
15. C

16. C
17. A
18. C
19. D
20. B

21. B
22. D
23. A
24. B
25. D

TEST 2

DIRECTIONS: Each question or incomplete statement is followed by several suggested answers or completions. Select the one that *BEST* answers the question or completes the statement. *PRINT THE LETTER OF THE CORRECT ANSWER IN THE SPACE AT THE RIGHT.*

1. In using micropipettes, the *usual* source of measurement error is caused by 1.____

   A. dirt
   B. hanging drops
   C. poor tips
   D. contamination

2. Enzymes are reported in 2.____

   A. pH units
   B. concentration units
   C. mg/dl units
   D. activity units

3. Assume that a beaker contains 700 ml. of 0.3M NaOH. *HOW much* of a 10M NaOH solution must be added to the solution in the beaker to bring it to 0.5M NaOH? 3.____

   A. 7 ml B. 10 ml C. 14 ml D. 30 ml

4. If one dissolves 25 gms of a solid in a liter, *how much* is present in 100 microliters? 4.____

   A. 2.5 mgms
   B. 25 mgms
   C. 250 micrograms
   D. 250 nanograms

5. Cholesterol does *NOT* exist in the form of a(n) 5.____

   A. hormone B. alcohol C. steroid D. fat

6. Amylase is an enzyme that acts on starch to produce 6.____

   A. alcohol B. sucrose C. amyloid D. glucose

7. *Which* is *NOT* an electrolyte? 7.____

   A. Phosphate
   B. Urea nitrogen
   C. Calcium
   D. icarbonate

8. The protein component found in the greatest concentration in normal human serum is 8.____

   A. hemoglobin B. globulia C. fibrinogen D. albumin

9. *Which one* cannot be used as a substrate for alkaline phosphatase? 9.____

   A. Sodium phosphate
   B. Phenyl phosphate
   C. δ-napthyl phosphate
   D. p-nitrophnyl phosphate

10. Insulin is secreted by the 10.____

    A. pancreas B. liver C. thyroid D. spleen

11. *Which* of the following is *NOT either* a product *or* a reactant in a SGOT assay? 11.____

    A. Alanine
    B. δ-Ketoglutaric acid
    C. Glutamic acid
    D. Oxalocetic acid

12. *Which one* of the following is *MOST* alkaline? 12.____

A. 1N ammonia hydroxide
B. 1N sodium bicarbonate
C. 1N sodium carbonate
D. 1N sodium hydroxide

13. How many more hydrogen ions does a solution of pH3 have compared to a solution of pH5? ______ as many. 13.____

A. One hundred times
B. Two times
C. 1.67 times
D. 1.33 times

14. *Which one* of the following statements *BEST* describes the pH of distilled water? Freshly distilled water is 14.____

A. slightly alkaline because of the CO_2 dissolved in it
B. slightly acid because of the CO_2 dissolved in it
C. neutral
D. neither acid, alkaline, nor neutral

15. The *MOST* effective buffer consists of a 15.____

A. strong acid and a strong base
B. weak acid and a weak base
C. mixture of two salts
D. strong acid and its salt

16. A double beam colorimeter is *better* than a single beam colorimeter because 16.____

A. two measurements can be made at the same time
B. corrections for non-specific absorbances can be done
C. two substances can be determined at the same time
D. corrections for light intensity fluctuations can be made

17. The *advantage* of a bichromatic colorimeter over a monochromatic colorimeter is that 17.____

A. two measurements can be made at the same time
B. corrections for non-specific absorbances can be done
C. two substances can be determined at the same time
D. corrections for light intensity fluctuations can be made

18. If one thickness of a neutral density filter reduces the transmitted light by 50%, *how much* will two thicknesses of the same filter reduce the transmitted light? 18.____

A. 25%
B. 50%
C. 75%
D. 100%

19. If all the controls in the day's run for the assay of glucose come out proportionately high, *which* of the following would *MOST* likely be the cause? A 19.____

A. systematic error due to elevated room temperature
B. random error due to faulty pipetting
C. systematic error due to deterioration of the standards
D. systematic error due to the colorimeter not being set properly

20. *Why* is it important to have *GREATER* precision in sodium assay than for a glucose assay? 20.____

    A. Sodium is a more important clinical component.
    B. There is more sodium in the body.
    C. There is more glucose in the body.
    D. There is less percentage variation in the normal range of sodium.

21. *Which* of the following components is *NOT* found in the usual chart recorder? 21.____

    A. Pen driver
    B. Amplifier
    C. Cathode ray
    D. Chant driver

22. CPK is an enzyme *MAINLY* found in the 22.____

    A. serum
    B. pancreas
    C. liver
    D. muscle

23. The *MOST* effective method of preserving a serum specimen for acid phosphatase assay is to 23.____

    A. refrigerate it
    B. add one drop of 10% Na Citrate per 2 ml
    C. add 50 mg NaF per 2 ml
    D. add one drop of 5% Thymol per 2 ml

24. Bilirubin is a 24.____

    A. hemoglobin metabolite
    B. steroid
    C. bile salt
    D. digestive by-product

25. Thyroxine is a 25.____

    A. hormone
    B. steroid
    C. lipid
    D. protein

KEY (CORRECT ANSWERS)

1. B
2. D
3. C
4. A
5. A
6. D
7. B
8. D
9. A
10. A
11. A
12. C
13. A
14. C
15. B
16. D
17. B
18. C
19. C
20. D
21. C
22. D
23. B
24. A
25. A

HEMATOLOGY

EXAMINATION SECTION
TEST 1

DIRECTIONS: Each question consists of a statement. You are to indicate whether the statement is TRUE (T) or FALSE (F). *PRINT THE LETTER OF THE CORRECT ANSWER IN THE SPACE AT THE RIGHT.*

1. Sickle cell trait and sickle cell anemia are one and the same condition. 1.____
2. A low RBC indicates anemia. 2.____
3. The sedimentation rate is never diagnostic. 3.____
4. It is possible to have an elevated sedimentation rate with a normal plasma protein level. 4.____
5. *Polychromatophilia* and *diffuse basophilia* are the same thing. 5.____
6. The BEST test for making the diagnosis of hemophilia is the clotting time. 6.____
7. In anemia due to vitamin B12 deficiency or folic acid deficiency, the reticulocyte count is low. 7.____
8. Target cells are RARELY found in sickle cell disease. 8.____
9. Jaundice of the obstructive type is NEVER accompanied by increased red cell fragility. 9.____
10. In hemophilia, the partial thromboplastin time is prolonged, but, the bleeding time, the clot retraction time, the platelet count, and the capillary fragility remain normal. 10.____
11. In classical hemophilia, the prothrombin time is prolonged. 11.____
12. The presence of an abnormal hemoglobin is responsible for sickle cell formation. 12.____
13. Thromboplastin is present in tissue extracts. 13.____
14. It is actually BETTER to report a hemoglobin test in percent than in grams. 14.____
15. The bleeding time is USUALLY normal in hemophilia. 15.____
16. A low MCV would be expected in an untreated PA case. 16.____
17. A high PCV indicates anemia. 17.____
18. A marked eosinophilia can occur ONLY in allergic or parasitic conditions. 18.____
19. The presence of large platelets indicates increased (or rapid) platelet production. 19.____
20. Reticulocyte stains include Janus green, Nile blue sulfate, and new methylene blue. 20.____

KEY (CORRECT ANSWERS)

1. F
2. T
3. T
4. T
5. T

6. F
7. T
8. F
9. T
10. T

11. F
12. T
13. T
14. F
15. T

16. F
17. F
18. F
19. T
20. T

TEST 2

DIRECTION: Match the items in Column I with the items in Column II. *PRINT THE LETTER OF THE CORRECT ANSWER IN THE SPACE AT THE RIGHT.*

COLUMN I	COLUMN II	
1. Reticulocyte count	A. No blood preparation required	1.____
2. Sedimentation rate	B. Suspension of patient's cells or of cells from the cord	2.____
3. PCV (hematocrit reading)	C. Diluted blood from patient	3.____
4. Capillary fragility test	D. Patient's plasma	4.____
5. Differential white cell count	E. Smear of patient's blood	5.____
6. Prothrombin time	F. Patient's whole blood	6.____
7. Capillary resistance test	G. Patient's serum	7.____
8. Direct Coombs	H. No blood preparation (or wet films)	8.____
9. Eosinophil count	I. Bone marrow smears	9.____
10. Direct platelet count		10.____
11. Indirect platelet count		11.____
12. Malarial parasites		12.____
13. Bone marrow studies		13.____
14. Hemoglobin determinations		14.____
15. Rh titer		15.____
16. Indirect Coombs		16.____
17. Clotting time		17.____
18. RBC		18.____
19. WBC		19.____
20. Sickle cells		20.____
21. Bleeding time		21.____
22. Clot retraction		22.____
23. Heterophil antibody test		23.____

KEY (CORRECT ANSWERS)

1. E
2. F
3. F
4. A
5. E
6. D
7. A
8. B
9. C
10. C
11. E
12. E
13. I
14. C,F
15. G
16. G
17. A
18. C
19. C
20. H
21. A
22. A
23. G

TEST 3

DIRECTIONS: Match the items in Column I with the items in Column II. *PRINT THE LETTER OF THE CORRECT ANSWER IN THE SPACE AT THE RIGHT.*

COLUMN I	COLUMN II	
1. Typhoid fever	A. Leukocytosis (high total white cell count)	1.____
2. Meningitis	B. Leukopenia (low total white cell count)	2.____
3. Brucellosis		3.____
4. Pneumonia		4.____
5. Influenza		5.____
6. Appendicitis		6.____
7. Measles		7.____
8. Neutropenia		8.____
9. Leukemia		9.____
10. Diphtheria		10.____

KEY (CORRECT ANSWERS)

1.	B	6.	A
2.	A	7.	B
3.	B	8.	B
4.	A	9.	A, B
5.	B	10.	A

HEMATOLOGY EXAMINATION SECTION

TEST 1

DIRECTIONS: Each question or incomplete statement is followed by several suggested answers or completions. Select the one that BEST answers the question or completes the statement. *PRINT THE LETTER OF THE CORRECT ANSWER IN THE SPACE AT THE RIGHT.*

1. Which of the following animal parasites CANNOT be present in a blood smear? 1.____

   A. Plasmodium
   B. Anopheles
   C. Trypanosoma
   D. Schistosoma

2. Pernicious anemia is caused by a deficiency of vitamin 2.____

   A. K
   B. B_{12}
   C. D
   D. A

3. Another vitamin deficiency that is similar to pernicious anemia in that it presents with anemia, macrocytic r.b.c., and megaloblasts in the marrow is ______ deficiency. 3.____

   A. folic acid
   B. vitamin D
   C. vitamin B_2
   D. vitamin K

4. In typhus, brucellosis, tuberculosis, and monocytic leukemia, you would expect the monocytes to be 4.____

   A. increased
   B. decreased
   C. normal in number
   D. either increased or decreased

5. In mumps, whooping cough, and infectious mononucleosis, you would expect the lymphocytes to be 5.____

   A. increased
   B. decreased
   C. normal in number
   D. either increased or decreased

6. A neutrophilic leukocytosis with *shift to the left* occurs in 6.____

   A. radiation sickness
   B. viral hepatitis
   C. leukemia
   D. appendicitis

7. In appendicitis, meningitis, diphtheria, pneumonia, and leukemia, you would expect the total white cell count to be 7.____

   A. increased
   B. decreased
   C. normal
   D. increased or decreased

8. The percent number of monocytes is INCREASED in 8.___
   I. whooping cough
   II. tuberculosis
   III. typhus fever
   IV. hay fever
   The CORRECT answer is:
   A. I, II B. II, III C. III, IV D. I, IV

9. In typhoid fever, influenza, measles, brucellosis, and neutropenia, you would expect the total white cell count to be 9.___
   A. increased B. decreased
   C. normal D. increased or decreased

10. The percent number of lymphocytes is INCREASED in 10.___
    I. whooping cough
    II. tuberculosis
    III. scarlet fever
    IV. infectious mononucleosis
    The CORRECT answer is:
    A. I *only* B. II, III, IV
    C. I, IV D. I, II, III, IV

11. Atypical lymphocytes are seen in the following conditions: 11.___
    A. Toxoplasmosis B. Cytomegalovirus infection
    C. Infectious hepatitis D. All of the above

12. A macrocytosis characteristically occurs in 12.___
    A. sickle cell anemia B. Tay-Sachs disease
    C. lead poisoning D. pernicious anemia

13. With a normal rate of red cell production in a newborn infant, the following percentage of circulating r.b.c. is reticulocytes: 13.___
    A. 0.5 - 1.0% B. 1.0 - 2.0%
    C. 2.0 - 6.0% D. 6.0 - 7.5%

14. In a normal bone marrow smear, you would expect to find the following number of reticulocytes: 14.___
    A. 0 - 1.0% B. 1 - 5.0%
    C. 5 - 15.0% D. 15 - 35.0%

15. In a normal bone marrow smear, you would expect to find the following number of lymphocytes: 15.___
    A. 0 - 3.0% B. 3 - 11.3%
    C. 4 - 16.0% D. 20 - 27.5%

16. In a normal bone marrow smear, you would expect to find the following number of plasma cells: 16.___
    A. 0 - 1.0% B. 1.0 - 1.5%
    C. 1.5 - 2.0% D. 2.0 - 2.5%

17. In a normal bone marrow smear, you would expect to find the following number of normoblasts: 17.____

A. 0 - 5.0%
B. 1 - 2.0%
C. 2 - 5.0%
D. 5 - 20.0%

18. In a normal bone marrow smear, you would expect to find the following number of myeloblasts: 18.____

A. 0 - 5.0%
B. 5 - 10.0%
C. 10 - 15.0%
D. 15 - 20.0%

19. In a normal bone marrow smear, you would expect to find the following number of neutrophilic myelocytes: 19.____

A. 0 - 2.5%
B. 2.5 - 5.0%
C. 5 - 20.0%
D. 20 - 29.8%

20. In a normal bone marrow smear, you would expect to find the following number of neutrophilic metamyelocytes: 20.____

A. 0 - 1.0%
B. 1 - 3.0%
C. 3 - 4.0%
D. 5 - 10.0%

21. In a normal bone marrow smear, you would expect to find the following number of neutrophilic band (stab) cells: 21.____

A. 0 - 2.0%
B. 2 - 5.0%
C. 10 - 15.0%
D. 15 - 35.0%

22. In a normal bone marrow smear, you would expect to find the following number of segmented neutrophils: 22.____

A. 0 - 5.0%
B. 7 - 30.0%
C. 35 - 60.0%
D. 60 - 96.0%

23. A consistently reliable means of differentiating between human and animal blood is the _______ test. 23.____

A. Van Slyke
B. Guaiac
C. Teichmann's
D. Precipitin

24. After ACTH injection, the circulating eosinophil count is normally 24.____

A. increased
B. decreased
C. unaffected
D. either A or B

25. The 0.85% solution of sodium chloride is known as 25.____

A. Helly's fluid
B. Zenker's fluid
C. Bouin's fluid
D. normal saline

KEY (CORRECT ANSWERS)

1. D
2. B
3. A
4. A
5. A

6. D
7. A
8. B
9. B
10. C

11. D
12. D
13. C
14. B
15. C

16. A
17. D
18. A
19. C
20. D

21. D
22. B
23. D
24. B
25. D

TEST 2

DIRECTIONS: Each question or incomplete statement is followed by several suggested answers or completions. Select the one that BEST answers the question or completes the statement. *PRINT THE LETTER OF THE CORRECT ANSWER IN THE SPACE AT THE RIGHT.*

1. Which of the following solutions may be employed as diluting fluids for a red cell count? 1.____

   A. Hayem's solution
   B. 3% acetic acid
   C. Hydrochloric acid
   D. Zenker's fluid

2. The TOTAL ruled area of the counting chamber covers ______ sq.mm. 2.____

   A. 3 B. 9 C. 18 D. 27

3. The dilution range of a red cell pipette is 3.____

   A. 1:10 - 1:100
   B. 1:20 - 1:200
   C. 1:50 - 1:500
   D. 1:100 - 1:1,000

4. The dilution range of a white cell pipette is 4.____

   A. 1:10 - 1:100
   B. 1:20 - 1:200
   C. 1:50 - 1:500
   D. 1:100 - 1:1,000

5. In routing RBC, the red cells are counted under high power in the following number of smallest squares: 5.____

   A. 24 B. 32 C. 64 D. 80

6. An RBC should be replated whenever the greatest variation between *R* squares EXCEEDS ______ cells. 6.____

   A. 5 B. 20 C. 50 D. 75

7. For routine RBC, the blood is diluted 1:200 and, in order to report r.b.c./cu.mm., the number of these cells counted in 80 of the smallest squares may be directly multiplied by 7.____

   A. 50 B. 100 C. 1000 D. 10,000

8. In routine WBC, the white cells are counted under low power in the following number of sq. mm.: 8.____

   A. 1 B. 2 C. 3 D. 4

9. A WBC should be replated whenever the greatest variation between *W* squares EXCEEDS ______ cells. 9.____

   A. 4 B. 6 C. 8 D. 12

10. For routine WBC, the blood is diluted 1:20 and, in order to report w.b.c. per cu. mm., the number of these cells counted within 4 sq. mm. may be directly multiplied by 10.____

    A. 50 B. 100 C. 1,000 D. 10,000

11. Which of the following tests ALWAYS require blood drawn from a vein? 11.____

A. Capillary fragility
B. Lee & White
C. Ivy bleeding time
D. Fonio's thrombocyte count

12. Which of the following tests does NOT call for dilution of blood in a special diluting pipette? 12.____

A. Total erythrocyte count
B. Total leukocyte count
C. Sedimentation rate
D. Circulating eosinophil count

13. Which of the following tests does NOT require the preparation of a blood smear? 13.____

A. Reticulocyte count
B. Sedimentation rate
C. Direct Coombs
D. Mean corpuscular diameter

14. The hemoglobin concentration of blood may be INCREASED in: 14.____

I. Anemia
II. Polycythemia vera
III. Dehydration
IV. Pernicious anemia

The CORRECT answer is:

A. I, IV
B. II,III
C. II, III, IV
D. III, IV

15. The total body hemoglobin is INCREASED in: 15.____

I. Anemia
II. Polycythemia vera
III. Dehydration
IV. Erythremia secondary to severe pulmonary disease or congenital heart disease

The CORRECT answer is:

A. II *only*
B. II, III, IV
C. II, IV
D. I, II

16. In a case of obstructive jaundice, you would expect the erythrocyte fragility to be 16.____

A. increased
B. decreased
C. normal
D. either A or B

17. In a case of hereditary spherocytosis, you would expect the erythrocyte fragility to be 17.____

A. increased
B. decreased
C. normal
D. either A or B

18. In cases of sickle cell anemia, the red cells become sickle-shaped when 18.____

A. oxygen is added to the cells
B. oxygen is removed from the cells
C. cell fragility is increased
D. cell fragility is decreased

19. In disseminated intravascular coagulation, the following coagulation components are frequently depleted: 19.____

A. Platelets
B. Factor VIII
C. Factor II
D. All of the above

20. Hypochromia is seen in 20.____

A. iron deficiency anemia
B. thallasemia
C. the anemia of chronic disease
D. all of the above

21. Heinz bodies occur in r.b.c. in which of the following conditions? 21.____

I. Drug-induced hemolysis
II. Hemolysis associated with the unstable hemoglobins
III. Hemolysis associated with hereditary deficiency of glucose-6-phosphate dehydrogenase
IV. PKT

The CORRECT answer is:

A. II *only*
B. II, III
C. I, II, III
D. I, II, III, IV

22. The counting chamber has the following depth: ______ mm. 22.____

A. 0.05
B. 0.10
C. 0.15
D. 0.20

23. The counting chamber has a depth of 1/10 mm. and a total ruled area which measures 3 mm. on each side. 23.____
Therefore, the counting area of a chamber has a ruled area of 9 sq. mm., a depth of 0.1 mm., and a volume of ______ cu. mm.

A. 0.3
B. 0.9
C. 1.2
D. 1.5

24. Each of the smallest squares of the hemocytometer grating measures ______sq. mm. 24.____

A. 1
B. 1/4
C. 1/40
D. 1/400

25. The so-called *direct method* of thrombocyte enumeration requires a 25.____

A. dilution of blood in a red pipette using a special (such as Rees-Ecker) fluid
B. blood smear
C. both A and B
D. neither A nor B

KEY (CORRECT ANSWERS)

1. A
2. B
3. D
4. A
5. D

6. B
7. D
8. D
9. D
10. A

11. B
12. C
13. B
14. B
15. C

16. B
17. A
18. B
19. D
20. C

21. C
22. B
23. B
24. D
25. A

TEST 3

DIRECTIONS: Each question or incomplete statement is followed by several suggested answers or completions. Select the one that BEST answers the question or completes the statement. *PRINT THE LETTER OF THE CORRECT ANSWER IN THE SPACE AT THE RIGHT.*

1. To remove fresh blood from a lab coat, you would apply 1.____

   A. a 3% hydrogen peroxide solution, then rinse thoroughly with water
   B. methyl alcohol
   C. a 10% solution of sodium carbonate
   D. a solvent such as benzene or chloroform

2. Which of the following achromatic objectives would be an oil immersion objective? N.A. 2.____

   A. 0.35 B. 0.65 C. 0.85 D. 1.25

3. The abnormal variation in shape among r.b.c. is called 3.____

   A. anisocytosis
   B. poikilocytosis
   C. polychromatophilia
   D. spherocytosis

4. The abnormal variation in size among r.b.c. is called 4.____

   A. anisocytosis
   B. poikilocytosis
   C. polychromatophilia
   D. spherocytosis

5. Polychromatophilia is also called 5.____

   A. poikilocytosis
   B. polychromasia
   C. erythroblastosis
   D. neutrophilia

6. *Juveniles* are technically known as 6.____

   A. myelocytes
   B. metamyelocytes
   C. microcytes
   D. segmented cells

7. Which of the following cells is NOT a member of the granulocytic series? 7.____

   A. Basophil
   B. Monocyte
   C. Eosinophil
   D. Neutrophil

8. Which of the following cells is characterized by a number of bluish-black coarse cytoplasmic granules? 8.____

   A. Monoblast
   B. Neutrophil
   C. Eosinophil
   D. Basophil

9. Which of the following cells is characterized by numerous large brilliant red cytoplasmic granules? 9.____

   A. Basophil
   B. Neutrophil
   C. Eosinophil
   D. Monocyte

10. Which of the following cells of the granulocytic series is characterized by a bean- or kidney-shaped nucleus? 10.___

A. Myelocyte
B. Metamyelocyte
C. Basophil
D. Segmented cell

11. Which of the following tests would NOT be included in a routine CBC? ______ count. 11.___

A. Differential leukocyte
B. Total erythrocyte
C. Reticulocyte
D. Total leukocyte

12. ·The test which determines the circulating eosinophils before and four hours after treatment with ACTH is the ______ test. 12.___

A. Widal
B. Lee & White
C. Ascoli
D. Thorn

13. The IMMEDIATE precursor of the thrombocyte is 13.___

A. Promegakaryocyte
B. Megakaryocyte
C. Megakaryoblast
D. Embryoblast

14. With a normal rate of red cell production in adults, the following percentage of circulating r.b.c. are reticulocytes: 14.___

A. 0 - 0.5%
B. 0.5 - 1.0%
C. 1.5 - 2.0%
D. 2.0 - 2.5%

15. The NORMAL adult female values for the red cell count (RBC) are ______ millions/cu. mm. 15.___

A. 2.5 - 3.3
B. 3.4 - 4.2
C. 4.3 - 5.5
D. 5.5 - 6.6

16. The NORMAL range of erythrocyte count (RBC) in adult males is ______ millions/cu. mm. 16.___

A. 3.0 - 4.0
B. 4.0 - 4.5
C. 4.5 - 6.0
D. 6.0 - 8.8

17. The NORMAL range of PCV in adult males is 17.___

A. 33 - 38%
B. 40 - 44%
C. 45 - 49%
D. 50 - 56%

18. The NORMAL range of MCH is 18.___

A. 28-32 micromicrograms
B. 33 - 38%
C. 1.7 - 2.5 microns
D. 80-94 cu. microns

19. The NORMAL range of MCV is 19.___

A. 28-32 micromicrograms
B. 80 - 94 cu. microns
C. 33 - 38%
D. 1.8 - 2.3 microns ·

20. The NORMAL number of grams of hemoglobin in an adult female is ______ plus or minus 2 grams%. 20.___

A. 10
B. 12
C. 14
D. 16

21. The dilution correction factor for ordinary red cell counts (RBC) is 21.____

A. 100 B. 125 C. 150 D. 200

22. Which of the following blood dilutions is employed for routine RBC? 22.____

A. 1:10 B. 1:50 C. 1:100 D. 1:200

23. Which of the following blood dilutions is employed for routine WBC? 23.____

A. 1:10 B. 1:20 C. 1:30 D. 1:100

24. When you draw blood to the 1.0 mark of an RBC pipette and platelet diluting fluid to the 101 mark, you have the following blood dilution: 24.____

A. 1:20 B. 1:50 C. 1:100 D. 1:200

25. When you draw blood to the 1.0 mark of a WBC pipette and white cell diluting fluid to the 11.0 mark, you have the following blood dilution: 25.____

A. 1:10 B. 1:20 C. 1:100 D. 1:200

KEY (CORRECT ANSWERS)

1. A
2. D
3. B
4. A
5. B

6. B
7. B
8. D
9. C
10. B

11. C
12. D
13. B
14. B
15. C

16. C
17. C
18. A
19. B
20. C

21. D
22. D
23. B
24. C
25. A

EXAMINATION SECTION
TEST 1

DIRECTIONS: Each question or incomplete statement is followed by several suggested answers or completions. Select the one that BEST answers the question or completes the statement. *PRINT THE LETTER OF THE CORRECT ANSWER IN THE SPACE AT THE RIGHT.*

1. Which one of the following solutions has the LOWEST pH above neutrality? 1 N _______. 1.____

   A. sodium carbonate
   B. potassium hydroxide
   C. sodium bicarbonate
   D. sodium hydroxide

2. Which one of the following solutions has the HIGHEST pH below neutrality? 1 N _______ acid. 2.____

   A. hydrochloric
   B. acetic
   C. sulfuric
   D. nitric

3. The one of the following body fluids which normally has the LOWEST pH is 3.____

   A. whole blood
   B. cerebrospinal fluid
   C. gastric contents
   D. urine

4. Which pH indicator changes from a colored to a colorless solution when the pH of a solution is decreased from 10 to 5? 4.____

   A. Brom phenol blue
   B. Methyl red
   C. Phenol red
   D. Phenolphthalein

5. The mordant used when preparing a gram stain is 5.____

   A. Gentian violet
   B. alcohol
   C. iodine
   D. safranin

6. Of the following, the LEAST common of the white blood cells in human blood is the 6.____

   A. eosinophil
   B. neutraphil
   C. lymphocyte
   D. basophil

7. Which one of the following compounds is a carbohydrate? 7.____

   A. Albumin
   B. Adenine
   C. Cholesterol
   D. Inulin

8. Which substance commonly added to blood is NOT an anticoagulant? 8.____

   A. Sodium oxalate
   B. Heparin
   C. Ethylenediamine tetraacetate
   D. Sodium fluoride

9. Which substance is miscible with water? 9.____

   A. Alcohol
   B. Chloroform
   C. Toluene
   D. Immersion oil

10. Which substance is NOT a surface-active agent? 10.____

A. EDTA
B. Soap
C. Desoxycholate
D. TRITON X

11. Which sugar is the same as levulose? 11.____

A. Glucose
B. Galactose
C. Fructose
D. Lactose

12. Biochemical reactions that proceed at rates lower than their maximum can be speeded up by all of the following EXCEPT 12.____

A. addition of an enzyme
B. increasing the pH to 11.0
C. increasing the temperature
D. addition of more substrate

13. You are measuring the optical density of a colored solution in a spectrophotometer. You first make a measurement using a tube with a 16-mm diameter. Then, using an adapter, you take another measurement with the solution in a tube that has a 10-mm diameter. The optical density reading of the second tube should be of the first tube. 13.____

A. about two-thirds higher than that
B. the same as that
C. lower than that
D. about one-third higher than that

14. Penicillin G powder has a potency of 1677 units per mg. If a vial of penicillin G contains 1 million units, how many ml of water must be added to the vial to make a solution of penicillin G containing 10,000 micrograms per ml? 14.____

A. 10
B. 60
C. 100
D. 600

15. You are preparing the following: (1) add 28 G of disodium phosphate to 1 liter of water; (2) add 27.6 G of monosodium phosphate to another liter of water; and (3) mix 77 ml of solution (1) with 23 ml of solution (2). The resultant product should be a 15.____

A. buffer solution
B. white precipitate
C. pH indicator
D. lipid solvent

16. You have 10 ml of a solution with a specific gravity of 1.25.
In order to have an amount of distilled water that has the same weight as that solution, you must have how many ml of the distilled water? 16.____

A. 7.5
B. 10
C. 12.5
D. 15

17. Assume that 1 ml of a suspension of bacteria is diluted into 9 ml of saline. One ml of this diluted suspension is again diluted into another 9 ml of saline. This procedure is repeated two more times. Finally, 0.1 ml of the last dilution is spread onto a nutrient agar plate, and the plate is incubated. After allowing for growth, there are 150 bacterial colonies on the plate. The number of bacteria in the original suspension was 17.____

A. 1.5×10^5
B. 1.5×10^6
C. 1.5×10^7
D. 1.5×10^{10}

18. The normal value of an adult male microhematocrit determination is 18.____

A. 17% B. 25% C. 38% D. 47%

19. How many microliters (lambdas) of a 1:250 dilution of erythrocytes must be added to 10 ml of saline to give a 1:50,000 dilution of the erythrocytes? 19.____

A. 20 B. 50 C. 200 D. 5000

20. Assume that a urine sample was measured with a hydrometer, and the value was found to be 1.036. 20.____
Of the following, the MOST likely explanation is that the urine sample

A. was too diluted
B. was taken over a 24-hour period
C. contained too many dissolved substances
D. contained erythrocytes

KEY (CORRECT ANSWERS)

1.	C	11.	C
2.	B	12.	B
3.	C	13.	C
4.	D	14.	B
5.	C	15.	A
6.	D	16.	C
7.	D	17.	C
8.	D	18.	D
9.	A	19.	B
10.	A	20.	C

TEST 2

DIRECTIONS: Each question or incomplete statement is followed by several suggested answers or completions. Select the one that BEST answers the question or completes the statement. *PRINT THE LETTER OF THE CORRECT ANSWER IN THE SPACE AT THE RIGHT.*

1. A 1 N solution of a compound with two replaceable hydrogens should be prepared by adding one gram molecular weight of the compound to _______ ml of solute. 1.____

   A. 100 B. 500 C. 1000 D. 2000

2. The amount of solids in 1 liter of urine may be estimated by multiplying the last two figures of the specific gravity of the urine by 2.6.
   If a given sample of urine has a specific gravity of 1.018, how many grams of solids are there in 500 ml of the solution? 2.____

   A. 9.0 B. 13.0 C. 23.4 D. 46.8

3. Thirty-seven degrees centigrade MOST closely approximates which one of the following temperatures? 3.____

   A. Temperature at which water boils
   B. Normal body temperature
   C. Normal refrigerator temperature
   D. Temperature at which water freezes

4. The procedure in which a blood smear from a finger is stained with Wright's stain, examined under a microscope, and the number of each type of leukocyte is counted is known as a 4.____

   A. GTT
   B. 2 hr pp
   C. hematocrit
   D. differential count

5. The term *target cell* refers to a 5.____

   A. red blood cell
   B. white blood cell
   C. heart muscle cell
   D. beta cell of the pancreas

6. The solution which should NOT be used in an emergency to extinguish a small paper fire is 6.____

   A. benzene
   B. 0.1 N NaOH
   C. dilute HCl
   D. phosphate buffer

7. Which one of the following parasitic diseases would be the MOST likely to cause changes in the blood? 7.____

   A. Amoebiasis
   B. Tapeworm
   C. Malaria
   D. Trichomonas

8. Cross-matching of blood will test for *all* of the following blood types EXCEPT type 8.____

   A. A B. B C.) D. Rh

9. Hematomas may sometimes develop after collecting blood from the arm vein for *all* of the following reasons EXCEPT failure to 9.____

A. use a needle that is large enough
B. have the needle completely in the vein
C. release the tourniquet before withdrawing the needle
D. apply finger pressure to the wound for sufficient time

10. Certain unheated sera, when mixed with incompatible blood cells, will destroy the cells. Heating the sera at 56° C for 30 minutes prevents this reaction. 10.____
This cellular destruction is called

A. isoagglutination
B. Rh hemolysis
C. isohemolysis
D. false agglutination

11. The anti-sera used for testing blood groupings must agglutinate Type A cells in a dilution of AT LEAST 11.____

A. 1:10 B. 1:100 C. 1:128 D. 1:512

12. Which blood typing system does NOT test for the Rh factor? 12.____

A. Wiener
B. Lewis
C. Fisher-Race
D. Rosenfield

13. A phenylhydrazine test is used to identify which one of the following types of compounds? 13.____

A. Sugars
B. Hormones
C. Blood gases
D. Urinary salts

14. Which procedure is essential for the determination of acid phosphatase, but is NOT used to determine alkaline phosphatase? 14.____

A. Incubating the reaction mixture at a temperature of 37° C
B. Using a spectrophotometer
C. Adding merthiolate for sterility
D. Keeping the specimen cold at all times

15. Which sugar that might be found in the urine does NOT give a positive Benedict's or Clinitest reaction? 15.____

A. Sucrose B. Fructose C. Ribose D. Galactose

16. Which one of the following findings in a 24-hour urine sample would be considered ABNORMAL? 16.____

A. Glucose
B. pH - 6.2
C. Specific gravity - 1.021
D. Volume - 2700 ml

17. How should a protein-free filtrate of blood be prepared? By 17.____

   A. using only whole blood
   B. adding acid to serum
   C. allowing the blood to clot
   D. inactivating prothrombin

18. When you collect blood by use of the finger-puncture method, you should discard the first drop of blood because it 18.____

   A. is contaminated with skin bacteria
   B. is diluted with tissue matter and fluid
   C. has a higher white cell count
   D. is diluted with skin moisture

19. A blood smear from a finger stained with Wright's stain shows erythrocytes in *stacked chips* arrangement. 19.____
This cell arrangement is called

   A. agglutination
   B. rouleaux formation
   C. Hargrave's cells
   D. hyaline casts

20. When a tube of heparinized blood is centrifuged, a layer of white blood cells forms above the erythrocytes. This reaction occurs because 20.____

   A. white cells are motile and red cells are not
   B. white cells are heavier than red cells
   C. red cells are larger than white cells
   D. red cells are heavier than white cells

KEY (CORRECT ANSWERS)

1.	B	11.	C
2.	C	12.	B
3.	B	13.	A
4.	D	14.	D
5.	A	15.	A
6.	A	16.	D
7.	C	17.	B
8.	D	18.	B
9.	A	19.	B
10.	C	20.	D

EXAMINATION SECTION
TEST 1

DIRECTIONS: Each question or incomplete statement is followed by several suggested answers or completions. Select the one that BEST answers the question or completes the statement. *PRINT THE LETTER OF THE CORRECT ANSWER IN THE SPACE AT THE RIGHT.*

1. According to psychoanalytic theory, the part of the personality which is in closest contact with reality is the 1.____

   A. id B. superego
   C. libido D. ego

2. An individual who gives socially acceptable reasons for his behavior, either verbally, by thought, or conduct, is adjusting through the use of 2.____

   A. rationalization B. sublimation
   C. retrogression D. displacement

3. Of the following statements, the MOST nearly correct one regarding the rate of mental growth is that 3.____

   A. there is a deceleration of the rate of growth with age
   B. there is an increase in the rate of growth with age
   C. mental growth is constant throughout the period of childhood
   D. mental growth is constant during adulthood

4. In early childhood, the individual tends to pattern himself on or to identify himself MOST generally with 4.____

   A. glamorous or romantic figures
   B. age contemporaries
   C. characters in movies or on TV
   D. parents or parent substitutes

5. With respect to physical growth, superior children as compared with children of average intelligence are 5.____

   A. slightly inferior B. above average
   C. slightly superior D. markedly inferior

6. A candidate in an examination says, "I passed the written and the performance tests, but they failed me in the interview." The mechanism of personality defense which he is employing is 6.____

   A. compensation B. sublimation
   C. identification D. projection

7. The psychological forces or needs that influence human behavior are labeled 7.____

   A. extrasensory B. generalized
   C. intrinsic D. extrinsic

8. Reactions of nail biting, grimacing, clawing, spitting, etc. in a fourth-grade child are usually considered symptomatic evidence of 8.____

   A. low intelligence B. psychological conflict
   C. hypothyroidism D. nervousness

9. The greatest "social distance" in boy-girl relationships has been found to be during the ages 9.____

   A. 13 to 17 years B. 9 to 13 years
   C. 5 to 9 years D. 2 to 5 years

10. According to available findings, the effect of deprivation of affection on intellectual development is MOST likely to appear in a curtailment of the 10.____

   A. speed of learning even when the task is rather simple
   B. ability to memorize new material
   C. ability to retain material, once it has been learned
   D. ability to conceptualize

11. Of the following, the one which would MOST likely indicate faulty emotional development in a girl of six is 11.____

   A. striving for perfection in all her work
   B. stronger liking for music than other school work
   C. little interest in doll play
   D. reluctance to engage in competitive sports

12. When a six-year-old child violates the standards of conduct of the group, the teacher should 12.____

   A. criticize him in the presence of the group
   B. accept his behavior as the expression of a deep need
   C. support him in order to alleviate his guilt feelings
   D. discourage his behavior by showing why it is wrong

13. A shy child is MOST likely to be fairly well adjusted if he has 13.____

   A. clearly defined interests
   B. marked intellectual ability
   C. obvious physical handicaps
   D. outstanding artistic talent

14. A kindergarten child shows habitual reluctance to undertake a new activity. This is BEST interpreted as evidence of 14.____

   A. an inability to cope with adult authority
   B. a general attitude of insecurity
   C. a specific fear conditioned in infancy
   D. a persevering and independent attitude

15. For a four-year-old child, the events of the present are 15.____

   A. less vivid than those of the past
   B. less vivid than those of the future
   C. more vivid than those of the past or future
   D. as vivid as those of the past or future

16. The "ideal self" represents what an individual 16.____

A. believes he ought to be
B. believes others ought to be
C. knows he can be
D. knows he cannot be

17. Girls generally prefer groups of girls and boys prefer groups of boys during 17.____

A. early childhood
B. latency
C. pre-adolescence
D. adolescence

18. The rate and pattern of early motor development are largely determined by 18.____

A. experience
B. learning
C. maturation
D. training

19. Which of the following books describes how parents and other adults can help youngsters overcome problems of an urban environment? 19.____

A. YOUR ADOLESCENT, L. K. and Mary Frank
B. STUDIES IN ADOLESCENCE, Robert E. Grinder
C. IN DEFENSE OF YOUTH, by Earl C. Kelley
D. THE AMERICAN TEENAGER, by H.H. Remmers and D.H. Radler

20. When a person has gained some insight into his own emotional behavior, usually following resolution of an acute conflict, we often describe him as having increased his range of 20.____

A. emotional repression
B. affective mobility
C. understanding
D. clinical synapses

21. Sibling rivalry is the term used to describe the competitive feeling between two or more individuals who 21.____

A. are in the same school grade
B. are children of the same parents
C. have similar goals of achievement
D. are in the same chronological age group

22. The mental mechanism of minimizing one's own faults and deficiencies by criticizing and blaming others is known as 22.____

A. compensation
B. rationalization
C. transference
D. projection

23. Etiology is concerned primarily with 23.____

A. symptomology
B. racial origin
C. causation
D. language facility

24. Syndrome is BEST defined as a 24.____

A. form of obsession in which the subject sees himself as someone else
B. form of neurosis in which the subject constantly compares himself with others
C. cardiac condition which has no apparent organic basis
D. constellation of symptoms which characteristically occur together in a specific ailment

25. Girls tend to be superior to boys of the same age in 25.___

A. linguistic fluency
B. speed of reaction time
C. arithmetical reasoning
D. most forms of perception

26. Of the following, a major recreational activity common to both 10- and 15-year-old boys and girls is 26.___

A. going to the movies
B. riding a bicycle
C. watching athletic sports
D. social dancing

27. In general, juvenile fiction comprises the major part of the reading choices of 27.___

A. girls between 9 and 13
B. boys of all ages
C. girls of all ages
D. boys between 12 and 16

28. The behavior of the typical adolescent is BEST described as characteristically 28.___

A. stubborn and willful, showing disregard for strictures of family and society
B. inconsistent, alternating between childish and adult reactions
C. irresponsible, exhibiting lack of judgment and poor taste
D. individualistic, reflecting indifference to approval from parents and peers

29. Of the following observed behavior symptoms, the one which may BEST be described as "regression" is the pupil's 29.___

A. use of infantile speech and verbal expressions
B. thrusting aside of present desires in order to avoid conflict in a direct solution of a problem
C. attempt to dominate every situation in which he finds himself
D. evasion of possible failure by selecting an easier goal

30. UNDERSTANDING GROUP BEHAVIOR OF BOYS AND GIRLS was written by 30.___

A. Helen H. Jennings
B. Ruth Cunningham
C. Jane Waters
D. Alice V. Crow

31. When we compare young children and adolescents with respect to the relative effectiveness of distributed and concentrated practice as a learning technique, we find that 31.___

A. young children learn better by distributed practice; adolescents by concentrated practice
B. young children learn better by concentrated practice; adolescents by distributed practice
C. both young children and adolescents learn better by concentrated practice
D. both young children and adolescents learn better by distributed practice

32. Research has demonstrated that there is an increase in racial prejudice during adolescence. Of the following, the factor that contributes MOST significantly to this increase is 32.___

A. dislike for deviants from norms of social groups
B. influence of parental opinion
C. segregation of groups in school and community
D. fear of economic pressure from minority groups

33. Of the following teachers, the one MOST liked by the largest number of junior high school pupils is the one who 33.____

A. sets easily attainable standards
B. demonstrates a high level of intellectual competence
C. maintains an impersonal, objective attitude
D. is sympathetic

34. Of the following, the behavior which would be considered MOST indicative of potential or actual maladjustment in a junior high school boy is 34.____

A. treating his classmates to sodas in an attempt to buy their votes in a school election
B. spending his entire allowance each week on science fiction paperbacks
C. finding fault with the work of his classmates
D. failing to take care of school property

35. The proportion of TREATED juvenile delinquents who exhibit subsequent histories of failure to adjust to society is about 35.____

A. 5% B. 25% C. 45% D. 65%

36. Current evidence and thinking on the causative factors in juvenile delinquency support the view that 36.____

A. social factors are more basic than psychological factor
B. psychological factors are more basic than social factor
C. psychological factors and social factors are of about equal importance
D. physiological factors are more important than either social or psychological factors

37. Studies involving the relative mental abilities of delinquent and non-delinquent children have generally 37.____

A. shown that there are no significant differences between them
B. shown that delinquent children are slightly but significantly brighter than non-delinquents
C. shown that non-delinquent children are somewhat brighter than delinquent children
D. been about evenly divided some finding the delinquent children brighter, others finding mental superiority for non-delinquents

38. Separation of the infant from his mother can be a traumatic experience. The amount of emotional damage to the infant and the consequent effects on his personality depend MAINLY on the 38.____

A. quality and consistency of the substitute mothering he receives
B. reasons for and duration of the separation
C. kind of preparation for separation the infant receives
D. degree of the mother's acceptance of the placement

39. Research studies of language development in young children have shown that 39.____

A. the multiple mothering of children in a large family delays language development
B. language delay in otherwise normal children is usually related to inadequate language stimulation
C. language delay is always associated with slow motor development
D. children are usually slow in learning to talk when more than one language is spoken in the home

40. The two MOST important influences on the cultural development of a seven-year-old child are the 40.____

A. home and peer group
B. school and peer group
C. home and school
D. home and church

41. In our culture, a child gains his sense of identity MAINLY from 41.____

A. knowledge about and experience with his parents and extended family
B. association with members of his own ethnic group
C. a study of the historical and ethnic factors in this culture
D. association with his peers

42. Of the following, the MOST important influence on the personality development of a child during the first year is the 42.____

A. family as a whole
B. mother
C. way his siblings react to him
D. relationship between the parents

43. Of the following, the term which is generally applied to the situation in which an infant in foster care has insufficient interaction with a substitute mother is 43.____

A. maternal rejection
B. mothering complex
C. maternal deprivation
D. interaction deficiency

44. The normal four-year-old child should be expected to 44.____

A. cut her meat with a knife
B. bathe herself without help
C. care for herself at the toilet
D. tell time to the nearest quarter hour

45. It is usually not a good idea to take a child under the age of five to a movie that may frighten him MAINLY because young children cannot 45.____

A. appreciate a cultural experience
B. behave themselves in a movie theater
C. distinguish clearly between real life and make believe
D. see movies without acting out what they see

46. The average five-year-old child spends the MAJOR part of his play time 46.____

    A. playing by himself
    B. watching other children play
    C. playing cooperatively with other children
    D. playing competitive games involving teams

47. A children's counselor faced with a question about sex from a six-year-old child in her group should 47.____

    A. tell the child she is too young to understand such things
    B. give the child as honest and simple an answer as possible
    C. realize that an older child must have told the six-year-old to ask that question
    D. answer the question in such a way as to discourage the child from asking any more questions about sex

48. Most studies of children's fears indicate that fears of the supernatural are MOST common among the 48.____

    A. pre-schoolers
    B. latency-age group
    C. pre-adolescents
    D. adolescents

49. The boy who trips on the leg of a chair and then accuses the chair is using the mechanism of 49.____

    A. rationalization
    B. regression
    C. daydreaming
    D. projection

50. Mild amounts of emotion, such as anxiety, irritation, and apprehension, tend to have which of the following influences on learning and performance? 50.____

    A. Integrative
    B. Mildly disintegrative
    C. Disruptive
    D. Relatively little influence

KEY (CORRECT ANSWERS)

1. D	11. A	21. B	31. D	41. A
2. A	12. D	22. D	32. A	42. B
3. A	13. A	23. C	33. D	43. C
4. D	14. B	24. D	34. C	44. C
5. C	15. C	25. A	35. B	45. C
6. D	16. A	26. A	36. B	46. C
7. C	17. B	27. A	37. C	47. B
8. B	18. C	28. B	38. A	48. B
9. B	19. C	29. A	39. B	49. D
10. D	20. B	30. B	40. C	50. A

TEST 2

DIRECTIONS: Each question or incomplete statement is followed by several suggested answers or completions. Select the one that BEST answers the question or completes the statement. *PRINT THE LETTER OF THE CORRECT ANSWER IN THE SPACE AT THE RIGHT.*

1. The process by which children take to themselves the values, the thinking, and the social behavior of their parents is known as 1.____

   A. projection
   B. identification
   C. denigration
   D. sublimation
   E. imitation

2. An understanding of the family relationships of a youngster who presents a problem of under-achievement 2.____

   A. is worthwhile but not essential
   B. is important but not within the province of the teacher
   C. may reveal factors that have an important bearing on his problem
   D. is unlikely to be related to the difficulties the young person has with his school work
   E. is important but not within the province of the guidance counselor

3. Which of the following is the MOST correct statement concerning puberty and physical maturity? 3.____

   A. Boys and girls who experience early puberty will achieve physical maturity and cease growing later than will the late maturers.
   B. Boys and girls who experience early puberty will achieve physical maturity and cease growing sooner than will the late maturers.
   C. Boys and girls who experience early puberty will achieve physical maturity and cease growing at approximately the same time as the late maturers.
   D. Boys and girls who experience early puberty will achieve physical maturity and cease growing in any standard pattern, together with the late maturers.
   E. None of the above.

4. The MOST prominent difficulties of the middle years of childhood revolve around 4.____

   A. relations with peer groups
   B. parent-child relationships
   C. schooling and the ability to learn
   D. physical development
   E. emotional and spiritual development

5. The MOST accurate statement concerning anxiety, of the following, is that anxiety is 5.____

   A. needed for the socialization process
   B. not needed for the socialization process
   C. less produced by "mental" punishment than by physical punishment
   D. of negligible effect in producing neurosis
   E. neutralized by feelings of guilt and inadequacy

6. Most studies of children's fears indicate that fears of the supernatural are MOST common among the 6.____

A. early childhood group
B. latency-age group
C. pre-teen group
D. adolescents
E. early childhood group and adolescents as contrasted with the pre-teen and latency-age groups

7. The boy who trips on the leg of a chair and then accuses the chair is using the mechanism of 7.____

A. rationalization
B. regression
C. sublimation
D. projection
E. delusion

8. Mild amounts of emotion, such as anxiety, irritation, and apprehension, tend to have which of the following influences on learning and performance? 8.____

A. Integrative
B. Mildly disintegrative
C. Disruptive
D. Integrative and segregative
E. Disruptive and disintegrative

9. The "ideal self" represents what an individual 9.____

A. believes he ought to be
B. believes others ought to be
C. knows he can be
D. knows others can be
E. believes he ought to be and can be

10. Girls generally prefer groups of girls AND boys prefer groups of boys during 10.____

A. early childhood
B. latency
C. pre-adolescence
D. adolescence
E. early childhood and pre-adolescence

11. The rate and pattern of early motor development are largely determined by 11.____

A. experience
B. learning
C. maturation
D. training
E. practice

12. Changes in cognitive behavior between childhood and adolescence are in the direction of greater 12.____

A. understanding of abstractions
B. reliance on concrete realities
C. dependence on vicarious experiences
D. emphasis on intuition
E. collection of scattered peripheral details

13. Gesell refers to the child's development between the ages of six and ten as 13.____

A. an ever-widening spiral
B. a task phase
C. a latency period
D. a transitional interval
E. an imitative stage

14. A defense mechanism defined as the adoption of an attitude opposite to one that precedes anxiety is 14.____

A. sophistry
B. reaction formation
C. fantasy
D. verification
E. rationalization

15. Experiments with the reactions of varying age groups to snakes indicated that, in general, the greatest fear was exhibited by 15.____

A. infants
B. primary pupils
C. latency-age children
D. adolescents
E. E. adults

16. As children get older, the differences in ability between the bright and the dull tend to 16.____

A. become smaller
B. become larger
C. remain about the same
D. vary in no set pattern
E. become larger, level off, and then become smaller

17. Which one of the following descriptions is characteristic of the actively-rejected home? 17.____

A. Parents show highly emotional attitude, warmth without understanding.
B. Parents tend to use severe punishment only if irritated.
C. Parents restrict child's independence with many rules and requirements.
D. Child is expected to make his own decisions, although advice is unavailable.
E. Parents are jealous of, and in active competition with, their children.

18. Homesickness is an example of which type of adjustment mechanism? 18.____

A. Guilt
B. Identification
C. Reaction
D. Sublimation
E. Regression

19. Children below the age of 10 when asked to write on "The person I would like to be" most frequently want to vie with 19.____

A. peers
B. older siblings
C. parents
D. real or imaginary heroes
E. teachers

20. When a child strikes out at a person who did not provoke the anger, the child is exhibiting 20.____

A. depression
B. retrogression
C. compensation
D. displaced aggression
E. projection

21. Which of the following statements describes the effect upon intellectually gifted children of early school entrance and acceleration? 21.____

    A. It serves to delay their social development.
    B. It produces underachievers.
    C. It creates emotional problems.
    D. It leads to favorable and valuable results.
    E. It substantially affects the development of motor skills.

22. The psychological forces or needs that influence human behavior are labeled 22.____

    A. extrasensory
    B. extrinsic
    C. intrinsic
    D. generalized
    E. contingent

23. Reactions of nail biting, grimacing, clawing, spitting, etc. in a fourth-grade child are usually considered symptomatic evidence of 23.____

    A. anxiety
    B. dementia
    C. low intelligence
    D. hypothyroidism
    E. psychological conflict

24. An individual who gives socially acceptable reasons for his behavior, either verbally, by thought, or conduct, is adjusting through the use of 24.____

    A. rationalization
    B. displacement
    C. sublimation
    D. retrogression
    E. projection

25. Of the following statements, the MOST NEARLY correct one regarding the rate of mental growth is that 25.____

    A. there is a deceleration of the rate of growth with age
    B. mental growth is constant during adulthood
    C. mental growth is constant throughout the period of childhood
    D. there is an increase in the rate of growth with age
    E. the rate of mental growth increases and decreases in a standard pattern

26. In early childhood, the individual tends to pattern himself on or to identify himself MOST generally with 26.____

    A. glamorous or romantic figures
    B. age contemporaries
    C. characters in movies or on TV
    D. parents or parent substitutes
    E. older siblings

27. With respect to physical growth, mentally superior children as compared with children of average intelligence are 27.____

    A. markedly inferior
    B. slightly inferior
    C. slightly superior
    D. markedly superior
    E. about average

28. A candidate in an examination says, "I passed the written and the performance tests, but they failed me in the interview." The mechanism of personality defense which he is employing is 28.____

A. compensation
B. sublimation
C. identification
D. projection
E. rationalization

29. The psychologist whose name is MOST often associated with the theory that the experience of birth has a profound influence on personality development and that an individual who has a slow, prolonged birth is likely to have a personality which fights, struggles and plunges is 29.____

A. Horney
B. Freud
C. Sullivan
D. Rank
E. McDougall

30. Two different studies have suggested that children who will probably have lower I.Q.'s are those who have been reared in 30.____

A. institutions
B. broken homes
C. foster homes
D. upper class homes
E. lower class homes

31. Studies of twins reared together indicate that the correlation coefficients of intelligence tests scores for identical twins lie in the range of 31.____

A. .40-.55
B. .65-.74
C. .75-.79
D. .80-.90
E. .90-1.00

32. As a means of changing the current behavior pattern of an adolescent, which of the following forces will generally prove to be MOST potent? Disapproval of the behavior pattern by 32.____

A. the adolescent's parents
B. an adult he admires
C. a group of his peers
D. his classroom teacher
E. older siblings

33. If the results of studies of boys' clubs are applicable to the school situation, one may expect the greatest amount of aggressive behavior to be noted in classes where the classroom climate may be described as 33.____

A. permissive
B. laissez-faire
C. democratic
D. autocratic
E. unstructured

34. Of the following, the LEAST effective way of dealing with children's fears is 34.____

A. explaining and reassuring
B. helping the child to face the feared situation
C. simply ignoring the child's fears
D. setting examples of fearlessness
E. removing the cause of fear from the child's environment

35. The age at which individuals cease to grow in intellectual ability is 35.____

A. 13 years
B. 16 years
C. 21 years
D. 35 years
E. probably none of these

36. The theory that physical compensation for a feeling of physical or social inferiority is responsible for the development of a psychoneurosis is attributed to 36.____

A. Adler
B. Horney
C. Freud
D. Sullivan
E. Jung

37. Which of the following terms refers to the maintenance of stability in the physiological functioning of the organism? 37.____

A. functional autonomy
B. canalization
C. homeostasis
D. maturation
E. physiological integration

38. Which of the following authors would you be LEAST likely to recommend for information about child care? 38.____

A. Sidonie Gruenberg
B. Jean Piaget
C. Ernest Harms
D. Benjamin Spock
E. Arnold Gesell

39. All of the following statements are generally TRUE of children of elementary school age EXCEPT 39.____

A. girls mature approximately one year earlier than do boys
B. girls have poorer health than boys
C. girls excel in body balance and fine hand coordination
D. girls excel in school achievement
E. girls tend to get their second set of teeth earlier than boys

40. The teacher of a sixth-grade class is likely to find all of the following characteristics among children of this growth level EXCEPT that they 40.____

A. are influenced very little by what their peers do
B. are beginning to rebel against adult domination
C. are at a receptive stage for indoctrination of all sorts
D. enjoy giving assistance to younger children in the lower grades
E. are beginning to show more discrimination in the selection of possessions and in the care of them

KEY (CORRECT ANSWERS)

1.	B	11.	C	21.	D	31.	D
2.	C	12.	A	22.	C	32.	C
3.	B	13.	A	23.	E	33.	D
4.	C	14.	B	24.	A	34.	C
5.	A	15.	E	25.	A	35.	E
6.	B	16.	B	26.	D	36.	A
7.	D	17.	C	27.	C	37.	C
8.	A	18.	E	28.	D	38.	B
9.	A	19.	C	29.	D	39.	B
10.	B	20.	D	30.	A	40.	A

EXAMINATION SECTION
TEST 1

DIRECTIONS: Each question or incomplete statement is followed by several suggested answers or completions. Select the one that BEST answers the question or completes the statement. *PRINT THE LETTER OF THE CORRECT ANSWER IN THE SPACE AT THE RIGHT.*

1. Epilepsy is MAINLY associated with 1.____

   A. brain injury
   B. migraine
   C. dysrhythmia
   D. aggressivity

2. A disturbance of language perception and expression is called 2.____

   A. aphasia
   B. amnesia
   C. amentia
   D. alexia

3. Alcoholism is MOST commonly connected with 3.____

   A. dysrhythmia
   B. neurosis
   C. psychopathy
   D. overt homosexuality

4. The polygraph is MOST useful for diagnosing 4.____

   A. epilepsy
   B. aggressivity
   C. deception
   D. brain damage

5. The electroencephalogram is MOST useful for diagnosing 5.____

   A. brain tumor
   B. epilepsy
   C. brain injury
   D. mental deficiency

6. Shock therapy was recommended for 6.____

   A. paranoid schizophrenics
   B. depressed psychotics
   C. severe psychoneurotics
   D. psychopaths

7. Prefrontal lobotomy had been recommended for 7.____

   A. aggressive psychotics
   B. apathetic psychotics
   C. paranoid psychotics
   D. psychopaths

8. Most authorities believe that mental deficiency is ______ hereditary. 8.____

   A. never
   B. always
   C. sometimes
   D. rarely

9. Recent experiments utilizing glutamic acid in an attempt to raise the intellectual level of retarded children have resulted in 9.____

   A. inconclusive findings
   B. a marked temporary rise in intellectual level
   C. a marked permanent rise in intellectual level
   D. a slight temporary decline in intellectual level

10. An individual's Rorschach protocol may be MOST profitably interpreted in the light of his 10.____

    A. behavior while being tested
    B. case history
    C. other test results
    D. presenting problems

11. If a child is mentally retarded, his academic potential can be explained MOST readily to his parent in terms of the status of other children 11.____

A. in his class
B. of similar CA
C. of similar MA
D. of similar IQ

12. It is MOST probable that a school-age child characterized, on the basis of psychological tests, as a mental defective might, in fact, be 12.____

A. epileptic
B. deaf
C. mute
D. schizophrenic

13. The classroom behavior MOST characteristic of the brain injured child includes 13.____

A. distractibility, hyperactivity, and lack of inhibition
B. listlessness, withdrawal, and compulsiveness
C. aggressiveness, fearfulness, and egocentrism
D. perseveration, fatigue, and apathy

14. A child's MOST rapid rate of mental growth generally occurs 14.____

A. during the first few months of life
B. between the ages of 3-6
C. between the ages of 6-12
D. during early adolescence

15. A psychopath may be distinguished by the fact that he commits antisocial acts 15.____

A. consistently
B. without customary reaction to guilt
C. without awareness of what he is doing
D. violently

16. Of the following techniques, the one which is considered to be characteristic of non-directive or client-centered therapy is 16.____

A. encouraging transference
B. reflection of feeling
C. free association
D. permissive questioning

17. Psychoanalytic writers consider the MOST important aspect of an analyst's training to be his 17.____

A. training in psychoanalytic concepts
B. training in medicine
C. training in analysis
D. general psychological training

18. In the transference situation, it is MOST probable that there will be ______ feeling(s) between analyst and patient. 18.____

A. positive
B. negative
C. neutral
D. positive and negative

19. The sequelae of encephalitis 19.____

    A. are now preventable in virtually every case of the disease
    B. may become evident long after an acute attack of the disease
    C. respond readily to treatment when detected
    D. are physical and emotional but rarely mental

20. The mental mechanism most strongly EMPHASIZED in psychoanalytic formulations of schizophrenia is 20.____

    A. repression
    B. conversion
    C. projection
    D. regression

21. Paranoia differs from the paranoid type of schizophrenia in 21.____

    A. the occurrence of delusions in one and not the other
    B. the fact that the paranoid patient does not act on the basis of his delusions
    C. the amount of *psychopathic tainting* in the family history
    D. that the delusions are more systematized

22. According to the Freudian psychoanalysts, the personality changes in general paresis are due to 22.____

    A. oedipus complex
    B. infantile sex urges
    C. sublimations
    D. changes in narcissism

23. A patient who touched his chin when asked to touch his nose would be MOST likely to be suffering from 23.____

    A. motor apraxia
    B. motor ataxia
    C. sensory apraxia
    D. agnosia

24. Shock treatment for schizophrenia, especially by the use of metrazol, was introduced at first because of the theory that 24.____

    A. shock arouses special physiological defense mechanisms by way of the *alarm reaction*
    B. shock stimulates the autonomic nervous sytem and thus facilitates homeostasis
    C. convulsions protect epileptics against developing schizophrenic symptoms
    D. shock as a form of punishment gratifies the patient's masochistic tendencies

25. From his survey of experimental evidence on the effect of infant care on later personality, Orlansky was led to the conclusion that such factors as breastfeeding and toilet-training 25.____

    A. are of no significance for later personality
    B. are significant determiners of personality
    C. are relevant to personality only insofar as they indicate the mother's attitude, which is the effective factor
    D. may help determine personality but constitutional and post-infantile factors should receive major emphasis

KEY (CORRECT ANSWERS)

1. C
2. A
3. B
4. C
5. B
6. B
7. A
8. C
9. A
10. B
11. C
12. D
13. A
14. A
15. B
16. B
17. C
18. D
19. B
20. D
21. D
22. D
23. A
24. C
25. D

TEST 2

DIRECTIONS: Each question or incomplete statement is followed by several suggested answers or completions. Select the one that BEST answers the question or completes the statement. *PRINT THE LETTER OF THE CORRECT ANSWER IN THE SPACE AT THE RIGHT.*

1. A part of the nervous system NOT known to have any connection with emotional behavior is referred to as the 1.____

   A. parasympathetic nervous system
   B. basal ganglia
   C. frontal lobes of cerebral cortex
   D. temporal lobes of cerebral cortex

2. A phobia is ______ anxiety. 2.____

   A. less specific than
   B. more specific than
   C. synonymous with an
   D. less acute than

3. The division of the autonomic nervous system that coordinates bodily changes in fear and anger is 3.____

   A. sacral
   B. sympathetic
   C. emergency
   D. cranial

4. The effect of familiarity in the case of inter-racial attitudes is 4.____

   A. dependent upon the nature of the contact
   B. a tendency to breed contempt
   C. greater understanding and acceptance
   D. of little importance one way or the other

5. Negativism is MOST typical of children at the age of ______ year(s). 5.____

   A. one
   B. three
   C. six
   D. nine

6. Children's groups about the age of two typically show 6.____

   A. much cooperation
   B. sex segregation
   C. parallel activity
   D. none of the above

7. In which of the following functions does development depend MOST completely upon maturation? 7.____

   A. Roller skating
   B. Swimming
   C. Singing
   D. Walking

8. In the first months of an infant's life, the baby's reflex responses are 8.____

   A. almost the only reactions the baby shows
   B. virtually absent from behavior
   C. more accurate than later in life
   D. less conspicuous than generalized mass reactions

9. Play and reading interests of boys and girls will be found to be most DIFFERENT at the age of _______ years. 9.____

A. three B. six C. twelve D. eighteen

10. The unsociability often reported for very bright children is MOST likely to be due to 10.____

A. their biological makeup
B. their complete absorption in intellectual pursuits
C. their lack of personal attractiveness
D. the absence of suitable companions

11. If we measure a number of individuals upon a variety of complex mental functions, we will find that the different functions show _______ relationship. 11.____

A. a negative
B. no
C. a fairly high degree of positive
D. practically a perfect positive

12. Of the following general statements about deterioration in mental patients, which is the MOST questionable at present? 12.____

A. More recently acquired forms of reaction are lost before those formed earlier in life.
B. Generalization and abstraction in psychoses is qualitatively the same as that in the young child.
C. Deterioration in many cases regarded as hopeless appears to be reversible.
D. The responses of a deteriorated person show generally a definite patterning which tends to mask his defects.

13. Concerning the course of intellectual deterioration in the mental disorders, it is CORRECT to state that 13.____

A. defect in the ability to generalize is more characteristic of schizophrenia than of other psychotic states
B. concept formation deteriorates more slowly in schizophrenia than in senile psychosis
C. decreased speed and persistence in mental activity are characteristic of epilepsy
D. senile patients suffer more impairment in the recall of long past events than in recent memory

14. According to mental test comparisons of cooperative patients in the various disease groups, the group which shows the LEAST intellectual impairment is 14.____

A. paranoid schizophrenia B. psychopathic personality
C. hebephrenic schizophrenia D. hysteria

15. Schizophrenic speech is BEST characterized by 15.____

A. loose, approximate use of words and reaction to superficial similarities among ideas and objects
B. loose, approximate use of words and failure to make use of similarities or analogies

C. unusual amount of stammering and reaction to superficial similarities among ideas and objects
D. unusual amount of stammering and failure to make use of similarities or analogies

16. It is the central, distinguishing feature of the depressive phase of manic-depressive psychosis that the patient 16.____

A. is keenly aware of lacking a motive for existence
B. attaches his depression to some irrelevant or imaginary cause
C. is excessively disturbed over some recent trouble
D. is overactive, restless, and even agitated

17. In which of the following abilities do dull and gifted children tend to differ most markedly? 17.____

A. Arithmetical computation
B. Drawing
C. Reading comprehension
D. Spelling

18. The schizophrenic patient is said to exhibit loss of affect.
This amounts to 18.____

A. decreased attention to one's personal feeling tone
B. lack of emotional reaction toward abstract ideas
C. increased affectivity to ideas and decreased affectivity concerning persons and events
D. increased affectiveness in environment but less to abstractions

19. Ability to establish a conditioned response in the eyelid has been found to be a point of differentiation between 19.____

A. idiopathic epilepsy and hysterical seizures
B. malingering and traumatic neurosis
C. senile dementia and cerebral arteriosclerosis
D. hysterical and organic blindness

20. The MAIN distinction between normal grief and reactive neurosis is in the 20.____

A. feelings of inadequacy and unreality
B. lack of basis in real occurrence
C. duration and intensity of the emotional display
D. intellectual retardation

21. Kretschmer's dysplastic type applies to those with 21.____

A. compact, round, fleshy habitus
B. strong, solid, muscular build
C. slender bodies, long bones, little muscular strength
D. conspicuous disharmony due to abnormal functioning of the endocrine glands

22. Which of the following is NOT characteristic of anxiety neurosis? 22.____

    A. Increase of irritable tension
    B. Vague somatic complaints
    C. Hypersensitivity to external stimuli
    D. Temporary muscular paralysis of the limbs

23. Involutional melancholia is usually characterized by a 23.____

    A. marked motor agitation
    B. motor depression
    C. flight of ideas
    D. loss of affect

24. From our knowledge about hallucinatory phenomena, it can be stated reliably that 24.____

    A. hallucinations occur in association with a dreamlike state
    B. hallucinations and imagery are similar processes differing only in intensity
    C. mescal-induced hallucinations are not similar to schizophrenic hallucinations
    D. organized hallucinations can be produced by direct stimulation of the brain surface

25. Which of the following is NOT a form of epilepsy? 25.____

    A. Grand mal
    B. Pyknolepsy
    C. Jacksonian
    D. Parkinsonian

KEY (CORRECT ANSWERS)

1. B
2. B
3. D
4. A
5. B

6. C
7. D
8. D
9. C
10. D

11. C
12. B
13. A
14. A
15. A

16. A
17. C
18. C
19. D
20. C

21. D
22. D
23. A
24. D
25. D

EXAMINATION SECTION
TEST 1

DIRECTIONS: Each question or incomplete statement is followed by several suggested answers or completions. Select the one that BEST answers the question or completes the statement. *PRINT THE LETTER OF THE CORRECT ANSWER IN THE SPACE AT THE RIGHT.*

1. Because studies of learning show that events occurring close together in time are easier to associate than those occurring at widely different times, parents should PROBABLY avoid ______ punishment. 1.____

   A. corporal
   B. mild
   C. consistent
   D. inescapable
   E. delay of

2. According to Abraham Maslow's hierarchy of needs, which of the following statements is TRUE? 2.____

   A. Individuals may have peak experiences when meeting physiological needs.
   B. Self-actualization will always precede the meeting of needs for esteem.
   C. There are cultural differences in the rate at which individuals attain self-actualization.
   D. Women are more likely to reach self-actualization than men are.
   E. Physiological needs must be met before an individual achieves self-actualization.

3. A teenager would MOST probably draw on which of the following to recall her tenth birthday party? 3.____

   A. Episodic memory
   B. Semantic memory
   C. Echoic memory
   D. Eidetic imagery
   E. State-dependent learning

4. Leadership, job satisfaction, and employee motivation are all studied in ______ psychology. 4.____

   A. human factors
   B. industrial-organizational
   C. community
   D. counseling
   E. experimental

5. According to the ethical guidelines set by the American Psychological Association (APA), of the following, it is TRUE that psychological research in which animals are used as subjects 5.____

   A. must not involve the use of surgical procedures
   B. is no longer permitted by the APA without special authorization
   C. should conform to all APA ethical guidelines for animal research
   D. must be limited to investigations that use correlational procedures
   E. may not be conducted by psychologists who do not have a license

6. Which of the following is INCORRECTLY matched with the hormone that it secretes? 6.____

A. Thyroid gland - thyroxine
B. Adrenal gland - epinephrine
C. Pituitary gland - prolactin
D. Pancreas - insulin
E. Ovary - testosterone

7. Hunger and eating are PRIMARILY regulated by which of the following? 7.____

A. Androgens
B. Estrogens
C. The hypothalamus
D. The kidneys
E. The medulla oblongata

8. Elena is presented with a list of 20 numbers. When asked to recall this list, she remembers more numbers from the beginning than from the end of the list. 8.____
This phenomenon demonstrates which of the following types of effect?

A. Mnemonic
B. Primacy
C. Recency
D. Secondary
E. Clustering

9. A prototype is BEST defined as 9.____

A. an example of habituation
B. an example of bottom-up processing
C. the equivalent of feature abstraction
D. the hypothetical *most typical* instance of a category
E. an essential element of category membership

10. Theories of motivation that assert the existence of biological motives to maintain the body in a steady state are called 10.____

A. mechanistic
B. homeostatic
C. reductionistic
D. genetic
E. instinctual

11. According to attribution theory, Pablo is MOST likely to attribute his high score on a difficult exam to 11.____

A. good luck
B. his intelligence
C. his instructor's teaching ability
D. the low level of difficulty of the exam
E. his classmates' inadequate preparation for the exam

12. In which of the following types of research are the same children tested periodically at different points in their development? 12.____

A. Clinical case study
B. Between subjects
C. Cross-sectional
D. Ethnographic
E. Longitudinal

13. The occipital lobes contain the 13.____

A. primary visual cortex
B. prefrontal cortex
C. somatosensory cortex

D. pons
E. sensory and motor connections to other brain regions

14. Eleanor Gibson and her colleagues have used the visual cliff to measure an infant's ability to perceive 14.____

A. patterns
B. depth
C. size constancy
D. shape constancy
E. different hues

15. The MOST well-adjusted and socially competent children tend to come from homes where parents employ which of the following parental styles? 15.____

A. Minimal supervision
B. Authoritarian
C. Authoritative
D. Indulgent
E. Permissive

16. Which of the following approaches to psychology emphasizes observable responses over inner experiences when accounting for behavior? 16.____

A. Behaviorist
B. Cognitive
C. Existentialist
D. Psychodynamic
E. Structuralist

17. Carla tutors other students because she likes to be helpful, whereas Jane tutors classmates strictly for pay. Their behaviors demonstrate the difference between 17.____

A. primary and secondary drives
B. instinctive and derived drives
C. appetitive and aversive motivation
D. intrinsic and extrinsic motivation
E. positive and negative reinforcement

18. The view that human emotions are universal has been supported by studies of 18.____

A. facial expressions
B. body language
C. linguistic structures
D. hedonic relevance
E. biological symmetry

19. Dopamine, norepinephrine, and acetylcholine are all 19.____

A. hormones excreted by the endocrine glands
B. secretions of the exocrine glands
C. drugs used in the therapeutic treatment of memory disorders
D. enzymes involved with the degradation of interneuron signals
E. neurotransmitters that excite or inhibit a neural signal across a synapse

20. The cognitive theory of depression states that depression results from 20.____

A. anger directed toward the self and significant others
B. an excess of certain neurotransmitters in the brain
C. failure in adult love relationships
D. maladaptive interpretations of life events
E. oral fixations from disturbed mother-infant relationships

21. All of the following infant behaviors are usually considered by developmental psychologists to be reflexes EXCEPT 21.____

A. rooting
B. reaching
C. sucking
D. grasping
E. crying

22. The MOST common form of color blindness is related to deficiencies in the 22.____

A. blue-yellow system
B. red-green system
C. process of visual summation
D. bipolar cells
E. secretion of rhodopsin

23. A person is asked to listen to a series of tones presented in pairs, and asked to say whether the tones in each pair are the same or different in pitch. 23.____
In this situation, the experimenter is MOST likely measuring the individual's

A. sound localization ability
B. dichotic listening ability
C. difference threshold
D. echoic memory
E. attention span

24. A survey shows that children who have encyclopedias in their homes earn better grades in school than children whose homes lack encyclopedias. The researcher concludes that having encyclopedias at home improves grades. 24.____
This conclusion is erroneous PRIMARILY because the researcher has incorrectly

A. failed to allow for experimeter bias
B. identified the independent variable
C. identified the dependent variable
D. inferred correlation from causation
E. inferred causation from correlation

25. The release of those with mental disorders from mental hospitals for the purpose of treating them in their home communities is called 25.____

A. deinstitutionalization
B. milieu therapy
C. primary prevention
D. secondary prevention
E. noncrisis intervention

KEY (CORRECT ANSWERS)

1. E
2. E
3. A
4. B
5. C
6. E
7. C
8. B
9. D
10. B
11. B
12. E
13. A
14. B
15. C
16. A
17. D
18. A
19. E
20. D
21. A
22. B
23. C
24. E
25. A

TEST 2

DIRECTIONS: Each question or incomplete statement is followed by several suggested answers or completions. Select the one that BEST answers the question or completes the statement. *PRINT THE LETTER OF THE CORRECT ANSWER IN THE SPACE AT THE RIGHT.*

1. The painful experience associated with termination of the use of an addictive substance is known as 1.____
   A. discontinuance
   B. tolerance
   C. withdrawal
   D. forced independence
   E. transduction

2. When parents refuse to accept several psychologists' diagnosis of a child's mental illness, they are using which of the following defense mechanisms? 2.____
   A. Denial
   B. Displacement
   C. Projection
   D. Rationalization
   E. Regression

3. After several trials during which a dog is given a certain kind of food at the same time that a specific tone is sounded, there is evidence of conditioning if the dog salivates when ______ presented______. 3.____
   A. the tone is; only
   B. the food is; only
   C. the food and tone are; together
   D. a different tone is; with the food
   E. a different kind of food is; without a tone

4. A complex pattern of organized, unlearned behavior that is species-specific is called a(n) 4.____
   A. drive
   B. need
   C. motive
   D. emotion
   E. instinct

5. Of the following, the firing of neurons would be CORRECTLY described as a(n) 5.____
   A. protoplasmic transfer of ions
   B. finely graded response
   C. all-or-none response
   D. osmotic process
   E. symbiotic function

6. Distrust of others is symptomatic of 6.____
   A. mania
   B. dementia
   C. catatonia
   D. paranoia
   E. hebephrenia

7. Sigmund Freud believed that dream analysis was a useful device for 7.____
   A. decreasing repression
   B. sublimating the id
   C. strengthening the superego
   D. displacing instinctual forces
   E. gaining insight into unconscious motives

8. When rehearsal of incoming information is prevented, which of the following will MOST likely occur? 8.____

   A. The information will remain indefinitely in short-term memory.
   B. There will be no transfer of the information to long-term memory.
   C. The sensory register will stop processing the information.
   D. Retrieval of the information from long-term memory will be easier.
   E. Information already in long-term memory will be integrated with the incoming information.

9. Which of the following behavior-therapy techniques is normally used to reduce fear of heights? 9.____

   A. Time-out
   B. Punishment
   C. Discrimination learning
   D. Token economy
   E. Systematic desensitization

10. Painkilling substances produced by the brain are known as 10.____

    A. cortisols B. endorphins C. glucocorticoids
    D. pheromones E. hormones

11. Receptors that are especially important for helping a person maintain balance are located in the 11.____

    A. gyrus cinguli B. inner ear C. tendons
    D. ossicles E. ligaments

12. In terms of the effect on the central nervous system, alcohol is MOST accurately classified as which of the following types of drug? 12.____

    A. Depressant B. Narcotic C. Psychoactive
    D. Stimulant E. Hallucinogen

13. Research findings in the area of interpersonal attraction indicate that individuals are MOST likely to be attracted to others who are 13.____

    A. critical of them
    B. similar to them in attitudes and values
    C. like their parents
    D. willing to do favors for them
    E. indulgent of their failings

14. On a fishing trip, Ed realizes that he has mistakenly packed the sewing box instead of the tackle box. He wants to fish but returns home because he does not have any line or hooks.
    Ed's failure to realize that sewing thread can be used as fishing line and that a bent needle can be used as a hook is an example of 14.____

    A. poor problem representation
    B. cognitive accommodation
    C. backward masking

D. functional fixedness
E. proactive interference

15. Of the following, the response MOST likely acquired through classical conditioning would be the 15.____

A. startled response of a baby the first time the baby hears thunder
B. child's fear of dogs after he has been bitten by a dog
C. cry of pain expressed by a man whose hand has been cut on a piece of broken glass
D. uncontrollable blinking of a woman who has just gotten dust in her eye
E. salivation of a dog that is halfway through a bowl of its favorite food

16. If a man who is a heavy smoker is given an electric shock every time he takes a puff on a cigarette, which of the following behavior-modification techniques is being used? 16.____

A. Systematic desensitization
B. Modeling
C. Aversive conditioning
D. Homogeneous reinforcement
E. Interlocking reinforcement

17. The failure of bystanders to give victims of automobile accidents needed assistance is sometimes explained as an instance of 17.____

A. group polarization
B. deindividuation
C. situational attribution
D. diffusion of responsibility
E. mere exposure effect

Questions 18-19.

DIRECTIONS: Questions 18 and 19 are to be answered on the basis of the situation described below.

In an experiment designed to determine whether watching violent scenes on television increases the frequency of aggressive behavior in children, one group of subjects saw a nonviolent cartoon and another group saw a violent cartoon. In the play period that followed the viewing of the cartoons, researchers observed the two groups of children together and counted instances of aggressive behavior.

18. The control group in the experiment is the group that 18.____

A. the researchers thought would be most aggressive
B. performed the larger number of aggressive acts
C. performed the smaller number of aggressive acts
D. watched the violent cartoon
E. watched the nonviolent cartoon

19. The dependent variable in the experiment is the 19.____

A. amount of aggressive behavior exhibited by the children
B. amount of time that each child spent interacting with the other children

C. group in which each child was originally placed
D. violent cartoon
E. nonviolent cartoon

20. Which of the following is MOST characteristic of individuals with chronic schizophrenia? 20.____

A. Extreme mood swings
B. Disordered thinking
C. Profound sadness
D. Unaccountable loss of body function
E. Loss of memory

21. Activation of the sympathetic branch of the autonomic nervous system results in a(n) _______ in _______. 21.____

A. increase; salivation
B. increase; digestion
C. increase; respiratory rate
D. decrease; heart rate
E. decrease; pupil dilation

22. The terms *modeling* and *imitation* are MOST closely associated with which of the following? 22.____

A. Classical conditioning
B. Gestalt theory
C. Hypothesis testing
D. Operant conditioning
E. Social learning theory

23. In a famous series of experiments conducted by Harry Harlow, infant monkeys were separated from their mothers at birth. The infants were then given two surrogate mothers (a terrycloth *mother* and a wire *mother*), each of which alternately had a nursing bottle that provided food to the infants. 23.____
The experimental results showed that in frightening situations, the infant monkeys

A. were more likely to become aggressive toward the wire mother than toward the terrycloth mother
B. failed to seek out either of the mothers because of their lack of experience in seeking contact comfort
C. preferred the wire mother, even when the terrycloth mother had the nursing bottle
D. preferred the terrycloth mother, even when the wire mother had the nursing bottle
E. would run and cling to whichever mother had the nursing bottle

24. According to Sigmund Freud, a child's early experience in coping with external demands leads to the development of the 24.____

A. unconscious
B. preconscious
C. Oedipus complex
D. id
E. ego

25. According to Albert Bandura, people who believe that their efforts will be successful and that they are in control of events have a high level of 25.____

A. insight
B. self-efficacy
C. social responsibility
D. reciprocal determinism
E. self-monitoring skill

KEY (CORRECT ANSWERS)

1. C
2. A
3. A
4. E
5. C
6. D
7. E
8. B
9. E
10. B
11. B
12. A
13. B
14. D
15. B
16. C
17. D
18. E
19. A
20. B
21. C
22. E
23. D
24. E
25. B

TEST 3

DIRECTIONS: Each question or incomplete statement is followed by several suggested answers or completions. Select the one that BEST answers the question or completes the statement. *PRINT THE LETTER OF THE CORRECT ANSWER IN THE SPACE AT THE RIGHT.*

1. Which of the following has been MOST effective in the treatment of schizophrenia? 1.____

   A. Administration of L-dopa
   B. Prefrontal lobotomy
   C. Psychoanalytic therapy
   D. Drug therapy that blocks neurotransmitter sites
   E. Drug therapy that increases the activity of limbic system neurons

2. Which of the following allows the examination of living brain tissue visually without performing surgery? 2.____

   A. Computerized axial tomography
   B. Stereotaxic examination
   C. Retrograde degeneration
   D. Biofeedback
   E. Ablation

3. The change in the curvature of the lens that enables the eye to focus on objects at various distances is called 3.____

   A. accommodation B. adaptation C. conduction
   D. convergence E. consonance

4. The hypothesis that intelligence is in part inherited is BEST supported by the fact that the IQ correlation for 4.____

   A. pairs of twins reared together is greater than the correlation for pairs of twins reared apart
   B. pairs of identical twins is greater than for pairs of fraternal twins
   C. pairs of fraternal twins is greater than the correlation for other pairs of siblings
   D. adopted children and their adoptive parents is greater than zero
   E. adopted children and their adoptive parents is greater than the correlation for the same children and their biological parents

5. The technique of strengthening behavior by reinforcing successive approximations is called 5.____

   A. positive reinforcement B. negative reinforcement
   C. distributed practice D. modeling
   E. shaping

6. According to Jean Piaget, which is the EARLIEST stage at which a child is capable of using simple logic to think about objects and events? 6.____

   A. Sensorimotor B. Preoperational
   C. Symbolic D. Concrete operational
   E. Formal operational

7. Bipolar disorders are MOST effectively treated with a combination of tricyclic antidepressants and 7.____

   A. acetaminophen
   B. antianxiety drugs
   C. beta-blockers
   D. amphetamines
   E. lithium carbonate

8. The tendency of most people to identify a three-sided figure as a triangle, even when one of its sides is incomplete, is the result of a perceptual process known as 8.____

   A. closure
   B. proximity
   C. similarity
   D. feature analysis
   E. shape constancy

9. According to Carl Rogers, the role of the therapist in person-centered psychotherapy is to 9.____

   A. accept the client unconditionally so that the client's own desire for mental health and positive growth will flourish
   B. express warmth and empathy and suppress negative feelings that arise in the relationship with the client
   C. use a didactic approach to teach the client to correct maladaptive behavior
   D. establish behavior-change programs to alter the problematic behavior that is often learned in early childhood
   E. define ideal characteristics of mental health for the client and to encourage the client to incorporate these elements in his or her personality

10. One criticism of Sigmund Freud's psychosexual theory of development is that it 10.____

    A. emphasizes developmental changes in the oral and anal stages
    B. views adult disorders as adjustments to the environment
    C. views fear of loss as a motivating drive
    D. is based on empirically unverifiable constructs
    E. is based on ethnographic studies

11. For MOST people, which of the following is an activity based in the right hemisphere of the brain? 11.____

    A. Muscular control of the right hand
    B. Simple spatial reasoning
    C. Arithmetic reasoning
    D. Language comprehension
    E. Speech

12. Which of the following are the stages in Hans Selye's general adaptation syndrome? 12.____

    A. Appraisal, stress response, coping
    B. Shock, anger, self-control
    C. Anxiety, fighting, adapting
    D. Alarm, resistance, exhaustion
    E. Attack, flight, defense

13. Of the following situations, the defense mechanism of reaction formation is BEST exemplified when a(n) 13.____

A. college student speaks sharply to her roommate after quarreling with her professor about her grades
B. woman who is unaware of her anger toward her friend expresses affection for that friend
C. runner forgets the name of the opponent who just defeated her in an event for which she held the record
D. man who dislikes his supervisor believes that his supervisor dislikes him
E. elderly man lights up a cigarette just after learning that he has been cured of a respiratory ailment

14. The reticular activating system 14.____

A. is the major system in the brain for controlling emotions
B. functions primarily in the control of motor responses
C. regulates levels of arousal
D. regulates body temperature
E. controls the uptake of pituitary hormones

15. Which of the following types of test is designed to measure an individual's knowledge of a subject? 15.____

A. Achievement
B. Attitude
C. Aptitude
D. Projective
E. Interest inventory

16. A word or part of a word that is in itself meaningful, but that cannot be broken into smaller meaningful units, is called a 16.____

A. grapheme
B. morpheme
C. phoneme
D. performative
E. holophrase

17. Which of the following studies has had the MOST profound impact on ethical issues in psychological research? 17.____

A. Stanley Milgram's study of obedience
B. Solomon Asch's study of conformity
C. Daryl Bem's study of self-perception
D. William McGuire's study of self-concept
E. Leon Festinger's study of cognitive dissonance

18. Behaviorally oriented therapists seek to modify a client's behavior by 18.____

A. repressing the client's deviant thoughts
B. relating past events to the client's current behavior
C. removing the underlying causes of the client's behavioral problems
D. explaining the significance of the client's dreams
E. changing the contingencies of reinforcement for the client

19. If Carmelita stares at a red spot for one minute and then shifts her gaze to a white piece of paper, she is likely to experience an afterimage that is 19.____

A. green
B. red
C. blue
D. violet
E. black

20. The place in the retina where the optic nerve exits to the brain is called the 20.____

A. lens
B. sclera
C. fovea
D. blind spot
E. aqueous humor

21. Responses extinguish fastest when they are learned through which type of reinforcement schedule? 21.____

A. Continuous
B. Negative
C. Variable-interval
D. Variable-ratio
E. Fixed-interval

22. According to Benjamin Whorf's linguistic relativity hypothesis, which of the following is TRUE? 22.____

A. Individuals have a natural predisposition to learn language.
B. Individuals learn positive instances of concepts faster than they learn negative instances.
C. Children learn their first language from their relatives and their peer group.
D. Different languages predispose those individuals who speak them to think about the world in different ways.
E. Children learn quantifying words such as *more* and *further* sooner than they do absolutes such as *every* and *all.*

23. In their discussions of the process of development, the advocates of nature in the nature-nurture controversy emphasize which of the following? 23.____

A. Socialization
B. Cognition
C. Maturation
D. Experience
E. Information processing

24. Which of the following is an example of metacognition? 24.____

A. Memorizing 100 words in a foreign language
B. Recognizing the faces of people after meeting them once
C. Solving a complex problem in a slow, deliberate way
D. Understanding the role of various parts of the brain in memory
E. Knowing the effectiveness of different strategies for learning statistical formulas

25. The debate over whether development occurs gradually, without discernible shifts, or through a series of distinct stages is termed ______ vs. ______. 25.____

A. nature; nurture
B. developmental; cognitive
C. cross-sectional; longitudinal
D. continuity; discontinuity
E. maturation; learning

KEY (CORRECT ANSWERS)

1. D
2. A
3. A
4. B
5. E
6. D
7. E
8. A
9. A
10. D
11. B
12. D
13. B
14. C
15. A
16. B
17. A
18. E
19. A
20. D
21. A
22. D
23. C
24. E
25. D

TEST 4

DIRECTIONS: Each question or incomplete statement is followed by several suggested answers or completions. Select the one that BEST answers the question or completes the statement. *PRINT THE LETTER OF THE CORRECT ANSWER IN THE SPACE AT THE RIGHT.*

1. Lawrence Kohlberg's theory of moral reasoning is BEST described by which of the following? 1.____

   A. Personal conscience is innate and all human beings develop it at the same rate.
   B. By adulthood, all people judge moral issues in terms of self-chosen principles.
   C. Ethical principles are defined by ideals of reciprocity and human equality in individualistic societies, but by ideals of law and order in collectivistic societies.
   D. Children grow up with morals similar to those of their parents.
   E. Children progress from a morality based on punishment and reward to one defined by convention, and ultimately to one defined by abstract ethical principles.

2. The intelligence quotient (IQ) has traditionally been based on the relationship between an individual's mental age and his or her 2.____

   A. stage of cognitive development
   B. level of physiological development
   C. reading ability
   D. chronological age
   E. quantitative aptitude

3. In Ivan Pavlov's experiments in classical conditioning, the dog's salivation was a(n) 3.____

   A. unconditioned stimulus *only*
   B. unconditioned response *only*
   C. conditioned response *only*
   D. unconditioned and a conditioned stimulus
   E. unconditioned and a conditioned response

4. Which of the following is a characteristic common to all individuals with a narcissistic personality disorder? 4.____

   A. A domineering attitude toward others
   B. An unwarranted sense of self-importance
   C. Restricted ability to express warmth and affection
   D. Inability to form social relationships
   E. Oversensitivity to rejection or possible humiliation

5. Hypnosis has been found useful in the treatment of 5.____

   A. pain B. autism C. dementia
   D. paranoia E. schizophrenia

6. In a normal distribution of test scores, the percentage of scores that fall at or below the mean score is 6.____

   A. 17.5 B. 25 C. 50 D. 66.6 E. 95

7. Persistent repetitive thoughts that cannot be controlled are known as 7.____

A. compulsions B. obsessions C. phobias
D. delusions E. sublimations

8. Of the following statements, it is TRUE that behaviorism 8.____

A. was formulated to account for cognitive development
B. is rooted in Sigmund Freud's view of the importance of early experiences
C. focuses on the development of thought processes and knowledge
D. holds that development is largely a product of learning
E. emphasizes the dominance of heredity over environment

9. Individuals diagnosed as having personality disorders 9.____

A. are typically afraid to leave their homes
B. are consistently psychotic in their cognition and affect
C. may function reasonably well in society
D. experience symptoms characterized by sudden onset and short duration
E. develop their problems as a result of drug abuse

10. The mean will be higher than the median in any distribution that 10.____

A. is symmetrical
B. is not normal
C. is positively skewed
D. represents measures for a random sample
E. represents measures for a biased sample

11. Which of the following is usually cited as a characteristic of autistic children? 11.____

A. Minor developmental delays in academic achievement
B. Above-average performance on tests of creativity
C. Severely impaired interpersonal communication
D. Tendency to seek younger playmates
E. Paranoia comparable with that experienced in schizophrenia

12. The goal of rational-emotive therapy is to help clients 12.____

A. focus on the significance of childhood events for current feelings of self-worth
B. correct self-defeating thoughts about their lives
C. avoid putting themselves in risky situations
D. practice relaxation techniques and autohypnosis to reduce anxiety
E. use introspection to alleviate their feelings of self-doubt

13. A person with sight in only one eye lacks which of the following visual cues for seeing in depth? 13.____

A. Retinal disparity B. Linear perspective
C. Motion parallax D. Relative size
E. Texture gradient

14. Multiple personality disorder is a type of 14.____

A. dissociative disorder
B. schizophrenia
C. dementia praecox
D. bipolar disorder
E. manic-depressive psychosis

15. The intensity at which a sound becomes audible for a given individual is known as the individual's 15.____

A. contrast sensitivity
B. absolute threshold
C. response threshold
D. critical frequency
E. just noticeable difference

16. A teacher asks students to think of as many uses for a brick as possible. By listing 50 uses, most of which the class finds new and unusual, Susan is displaying 16.____

A. computational learning
B. paired-associate learning
C. hypothetical thinking
D. divergent thinking
E. convergent thinking

17. The PRIMARY effect of the myelin sheath is to 17.____

A. increase the velocity of conduction of the action potential along the axon
B. increase the velocity of conduction of the action potential across the synapse
C. facilitate the incoming stimulus signals at sensory receptors
D. reduce the amount of unused neurotransmitter in the synaptic cleft
E. protect the terminal buttons of the neuron from destruction by enzymes

18. Which of the following was TRUE of Solomon Asch's experiments on conformity? 18.____

A. People conformed if they knew and respected the authority figure present.
B. An increase from 7 to 12 confederates increased conformity by experimental subjects.
C. Experimental subjects conformed less frequently when their judgments were made known to the group.
D. About 99% of the judgments made by the experimental subjects were wrong.
E. If the confederates' judgments were not unanimous, the degree of conformity by experimental subjects decreased.

19. Which of the following concepts was advanced by social psychologists to help explain why people who are part of a crowd sometimes commit aggressive, antisocial acts that they would not commit if they were alone? 19.____

A. Groupthink
B. Cognitive dissonance
C. Social facilitation
D. Deindividuation
E. Catharsis

20. A somatoform disorder is BEST described as an illness that 20.____

A. results from inadequate parenting in childhood
B. occurs when defense mechanisms are used inappropriately
C. is psychological in nature with no physical symptoms
D. is physical in nature with no psychological symptoms
E. is physical in nature and caused by psychological factors

21. It is widely known in Jerry's social circle that he is the most stubborn and inflexible member of the group. Yet Jerry complains that all his friends are opinionated and rigid. Jerry's complaints are MOST clearly a sign of 21.____

A. displacement
B. repression
C. projection
D. reaction formation
E. rationalization

22. Which of the following is a genetic disorder that results in a deficiency of a liver enzyme which, if not treated soon after birth, may eventually lead to profound mental retardation? 22.____

A. Down syndrome
B. Tay-Sachs disease
C. Fetal alcohol syndrome
D. Toxoplasmosis
E. Phenylketonuria (PKU)

23. Electroconvulsive therapy has been MOST successful in the treatment of 23.____

A. phobias
B. schizophrenia
C. psychogenic amnesia
D. multiple personality
E. clinical depression

24. Of the following, MOST useful in understanding an employer's interpretation of an employee's poor performance would be ______ theory. 24.____

A. Cannon's
B. the reinforcement
C. the attribution
D. the arousal
E. the cognitive dissonance

25. Of the following, a MAJOR change in perspective in the field of developmental psychology over the past twenty-five years is a 25.____

A. shift from an emphasis on childhood and adolescence to an interest in development over the life span
B. shift from a cognitive to a psychoanalytic interpretation of developmental phenomena
C. shift in research focus from cognitive to personality development
D. decrease in interest in the physiological factors affecting growth and development
E. decrease in interest in the study of the cognitive components of intellect

KEY (CORRECT ANSWERS)

1. E
2. D
3. E
4. B
5. A

6. C
7. B
8. D
9. C
10. C

11. C
12. B
13. A
14. A
15. B

16. D
17. A
18. E
19. D
20. E

21. C
22. E
23. E
24. C
25. A

Basic Fundamentals of Anatomy and Physiology

CONTENTS

Basic Fundamentals of Anatomy and Physiology

SECTION A—BODY STRUCTURE AND PHYSIOLOGY

1. Introduction. Operating room personnel must know how organs and systems normally work if they are to understand what is happening during surgical procedures. It is well to think in terms of the functions and of the physiology of the body parts while trying to understand anatomy. Avoid a tendency to think in terms of the anatomical structure on which an operation is being performed. The physiological considerations are also helpful in planning operative setups.

2. Planes, Surfaces, Quadrants, and Positions. The importance of planes, surfaces, quadrants, and positions, as illustrated in figures 1 through 4, cannot be overemphasized. The ability to identify the different positions, as well as place patients in them, is an everyday requirement. Planes are necessary in understanding body motion and direction. Figures 2 and 3 show how body areas are used to describe operative sites. The surgeon often refers to the surface area or the abdominal quadrant through which the incision is made.

3. Body Cavities. The body is divided into two main cavities which are readily identified by looking at a midsagittal section of the body, as illustrated in figure 3–5. These are:

a. *The ventral cavity* which encompasses the thoracic cavity, diaphragm, and peritoneal cavity.

b. *The dorsal cavity* which encompasses the cranial and spinal cavities.

4. Cells. A cell is the structural unit of organic life. Each cell contains a nucleus, cytoplasm, and a cell wall, as illustrated in figure 6. Cells differ in size, shape, chemical composition, and special function within the body. They possess the ability to absorb food and secrete waste, grow in size, reproduce, be irritated, and move.

5. Tissue. When a great number of similar cells are combined, they become visible to the naked eye and in this form are referred to as tissue. Figure 7 shows examples of several types of cells and the manner in which they arrange themselves into the *four main kinds of tissue: epithelial, connective, muscle,* and *nerve tissue*. Table 1 shows some of the body areas in which the different types of tissue are located and the function in each location.

6. Membranes. Membranes are the coverings and linings of the body organs and surfaces. The membranes are actually composed of thin sheets of tissue (usually epithelial and connective), which have been so compounded that they are able to *provide protection, absorb moisture, secrete body fluids, regulate heat, eliminate waste, and receive sensory stimulation.* These functions are performed through *cutaneous, synovial, serous,* or *mucous membranes.*

SECTION B—THE SKELETAL SYSTEM

7. Function of the Skeletal System. The skeletal system is the bony framework of the body. It supports the body in an upright position, protects vital organs, and affords attachment for tendons, muscles, and ligaments. It provides the leverage which, by muscular contraction, permits body movements. Blood cells (red blood cells) are formed in the marrow of bones, and bones act as reservoirs for calcium and other minerals.

8. Bones. Bones consist of a hard, outer shell called compact bone and a spongy, porous center called cancellous bone. The center of long bones is called the medullary canal and contains bone marrow. This is the manufacturing center for red blood cells. At the end of long bones is a smooth, glossy tissue which forms the joint surfaces. The surfaces articulate with, fit into, or move in contact with, similar surfaces of other bones. Bone is covered with a thin membrane called periosteum, which is important in the nourishment of bones. It contains nerves and blood vessels and is essential for bone growth. The periosteum, as well as other parts of the bone, are shown in figure 8.

a. If a bone is closely examined, one can see many projections and depressions. The terms listed below are commonly used to describe these areas:

(1) Condyle—a rounded process at the articular (joint) end of a bone.

(2) Crest—a prominent ridge.

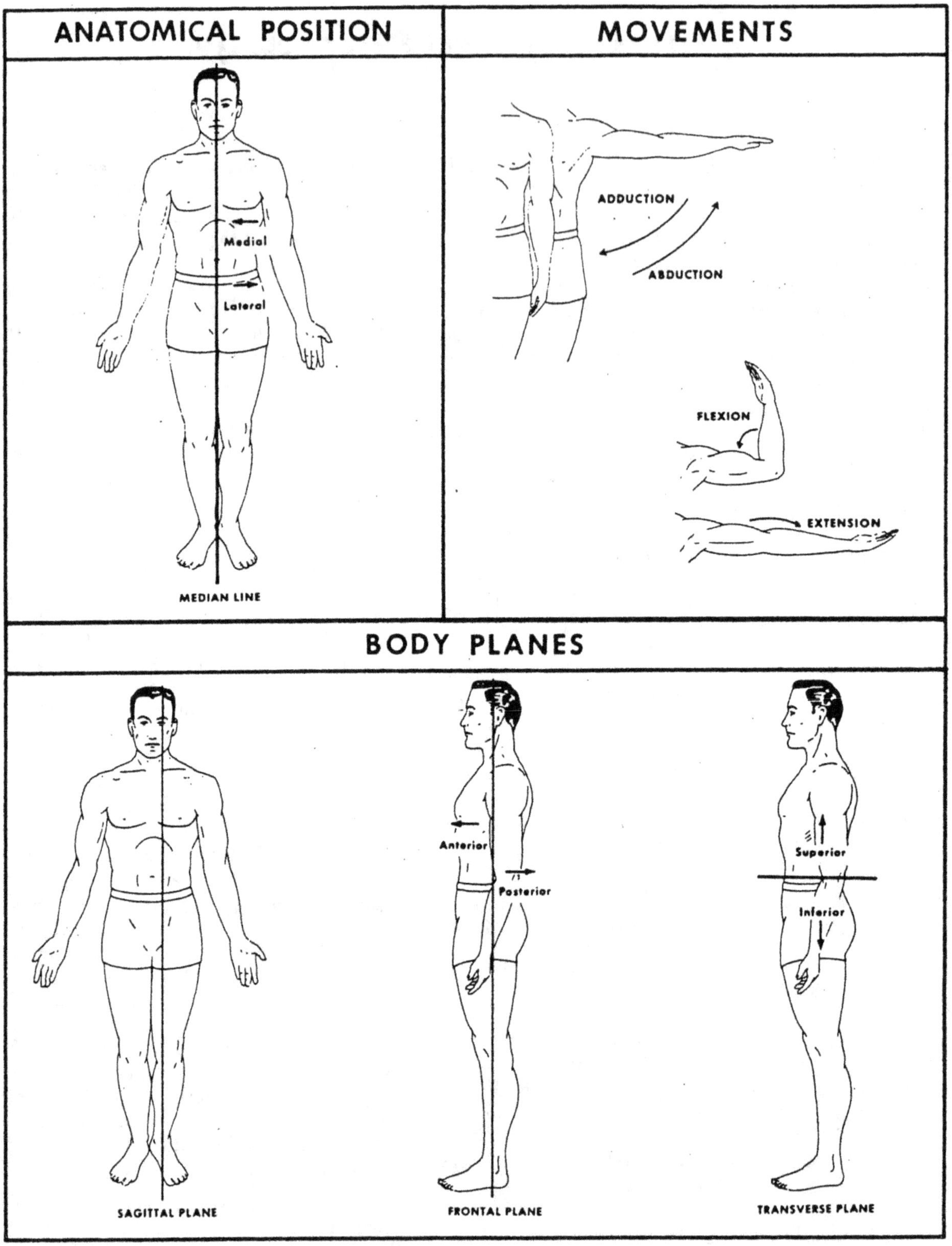

Figure 1. Body Planes and Movements.

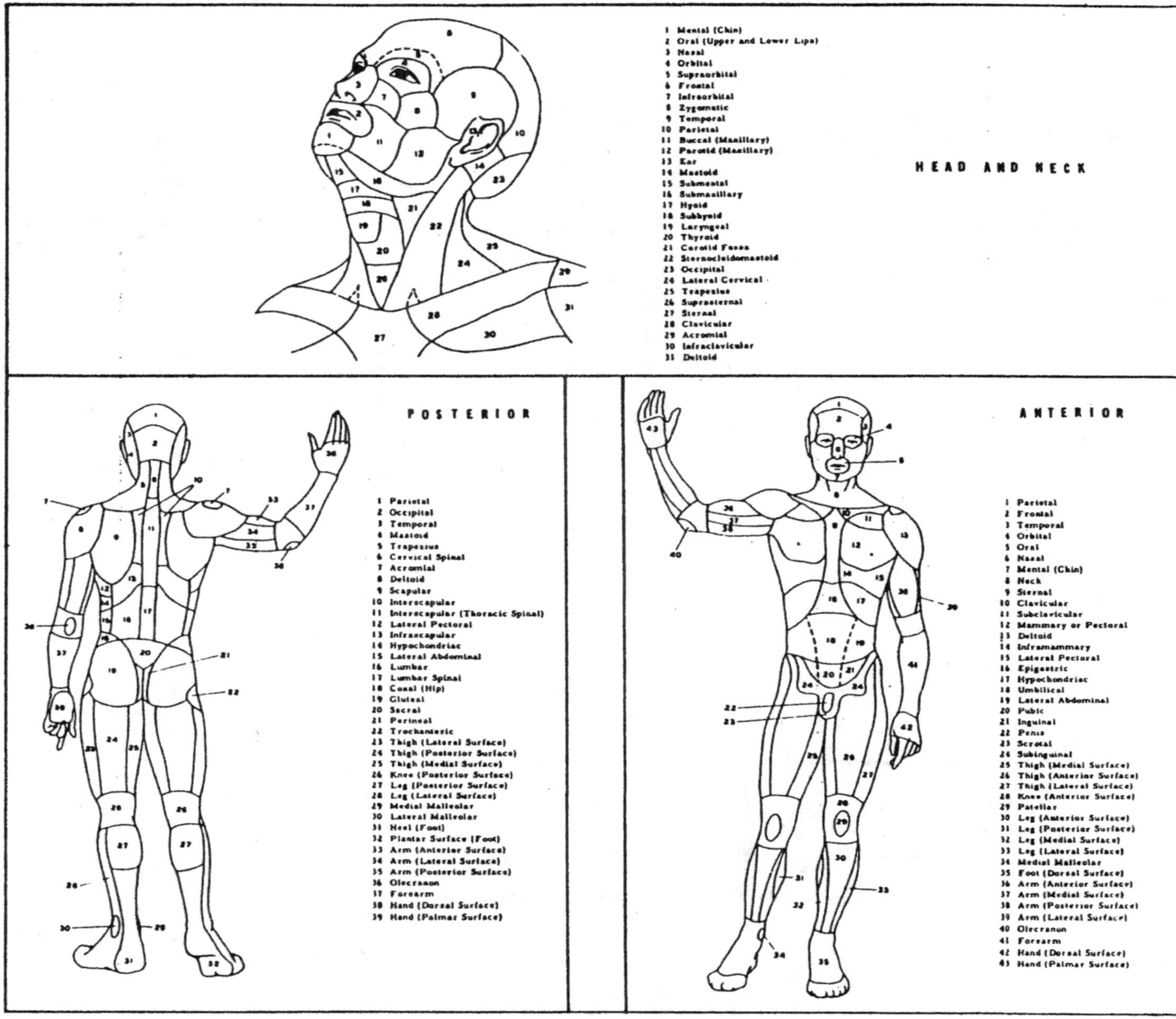

Figure 2. Body Surfaces.

1. Epigastric
2. Upper right quadrant
3. Upper left quadrant
4. Right lateral or lumbar
5. Umbilical
6. Left lateral or lumbar
7. Lower right quadrant (right inguinal)
8. Pubic (hypogastric)
9. Lower left quadrant (left inguinal)

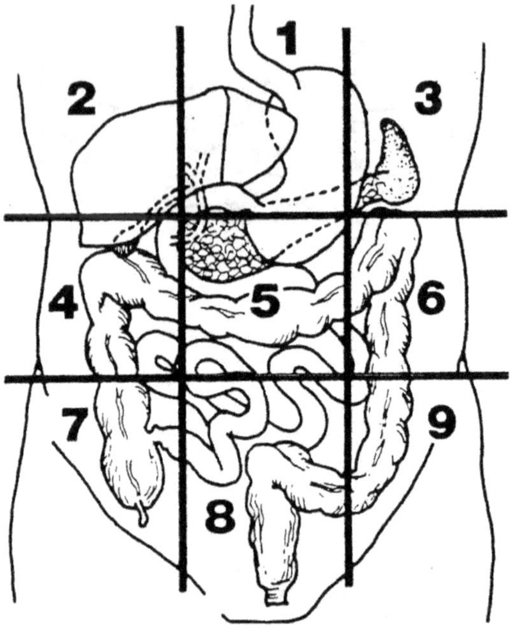

Figure - 3. Anatomic Regions of the Abdomen.

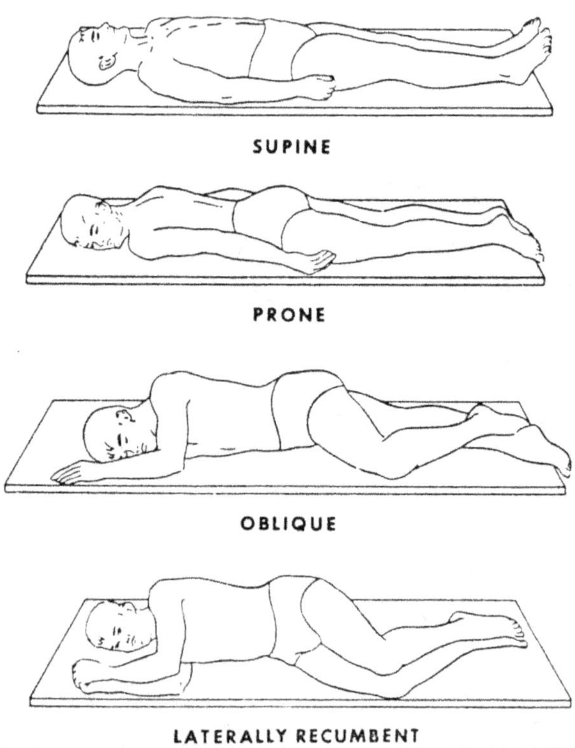

Figure 4. Body Positions.

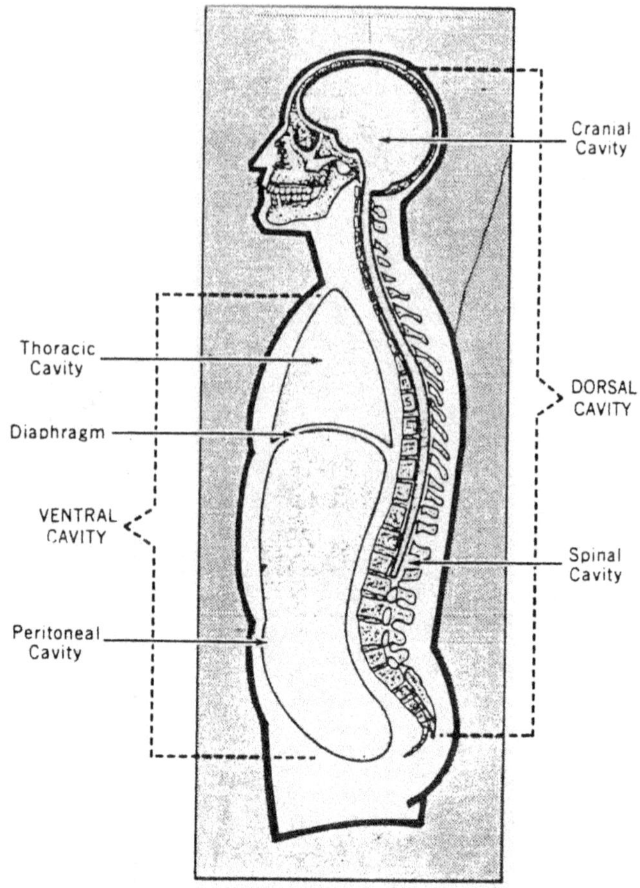

Figure 5. Diagram of Body Cavities as Seen in Midsagittal Section.

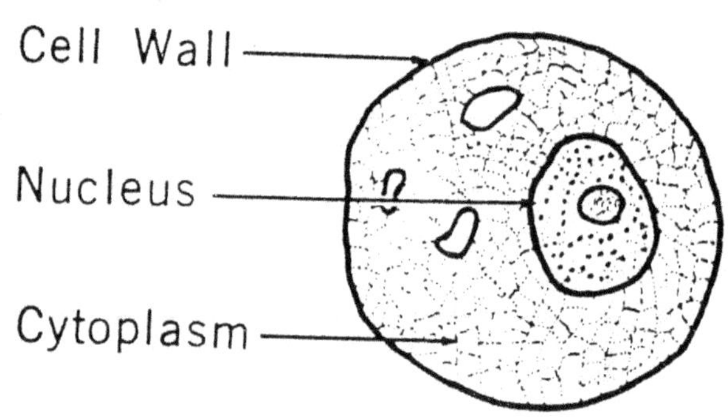

Figure 6. Structure of a Cell.

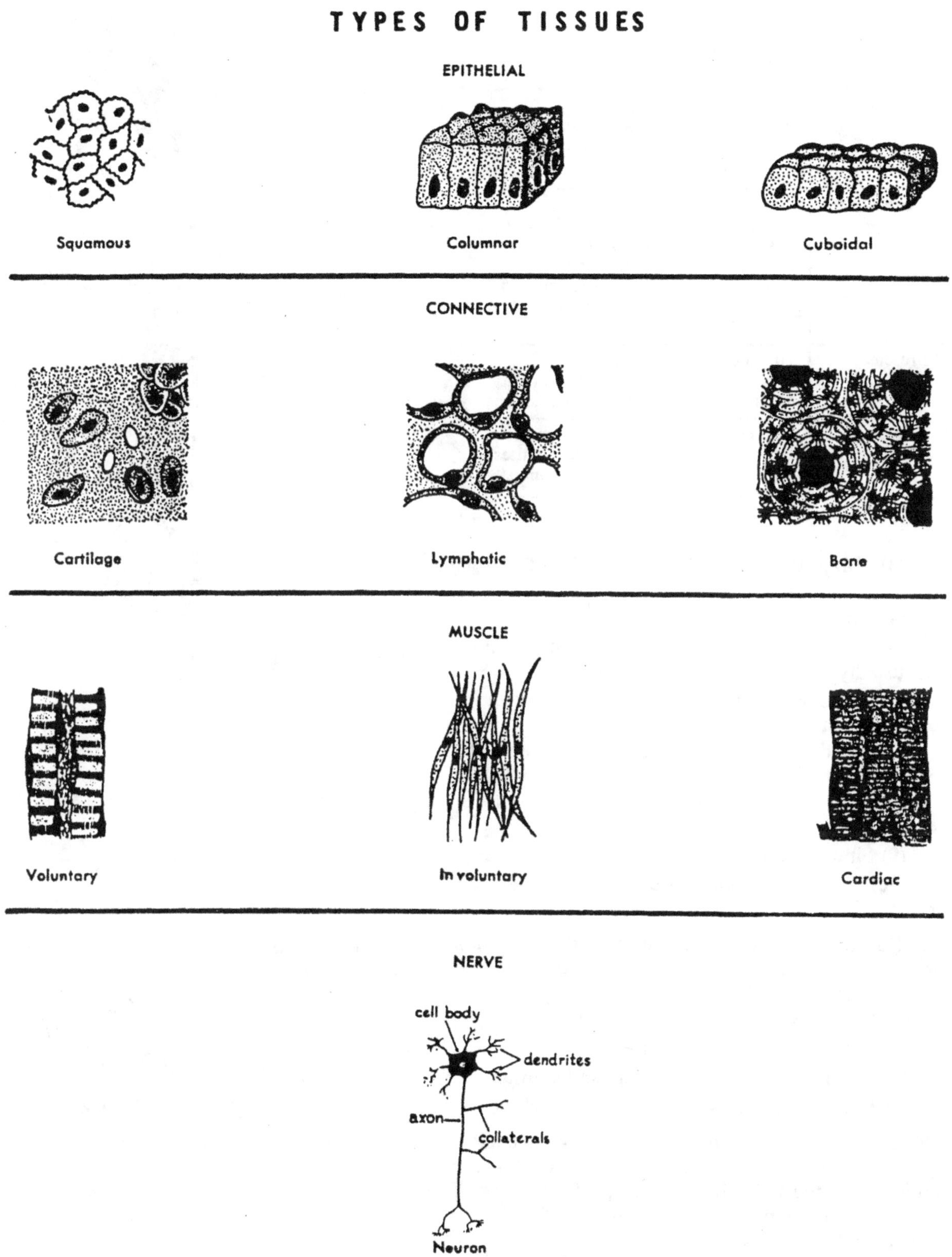

Figure 7. Body Cells and Tissues.

Table 1. Body Tissue.

Body Tissue

Type of Tissue	*Where Located*	*Purpose*
1. Epithelial	Skin Lining of passageways and cavities	Protection Absorption Secretion
2. Connective	Between organs and tissue Walls of vessels Skeleton Blood	Support Elasticity Insulation Protection Transportation of nutrients and waste
3. Muscle	Attached to bones Walls of organs Heart wall	Movement Support, elasticity Heart contractions
4. Nerve	Nerves Brain Spinal cord	Receive stimuli Conduct impulses Effect responses

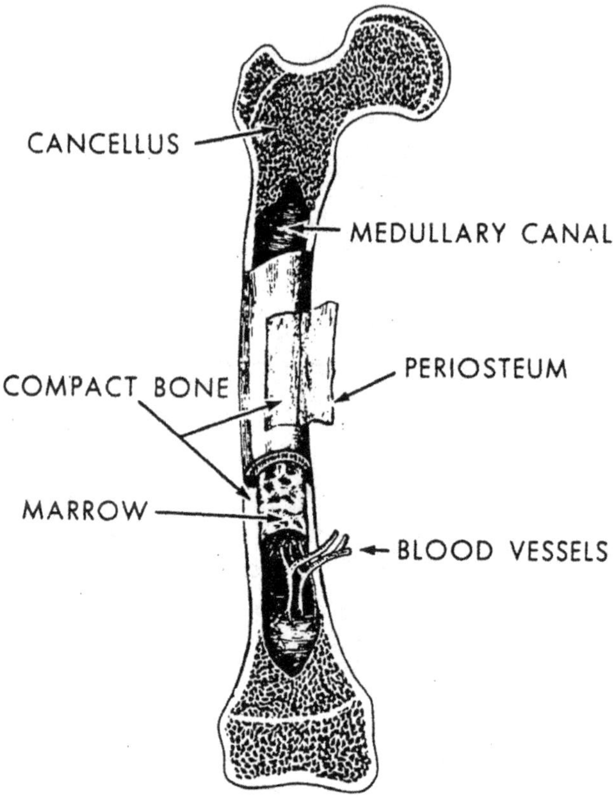

Figure 8. A Long Bone.

(3) Diaphysis—the shaft or body of a long bone.

(4) Epiphysis—the end of a long bone.

(5) Fontanelle—an unossified, membranous area usually found in the infant cranium.

(6) Foramen—a hole in a bone for passage of vessels or nerves.

(7) Head—the enlarged portion at the end of a bone.

(8) Process—a general term for any bony prominence.

(9) Sinus—a cavity in a bone.

(10) Spine or spinous process—a slender projection.

b. Bones are classified according to their location and shape. Examples of bones classified according to their shape are as follows:

(1) Long Bones—femur and humerus.

(2) Short Bones—wrists and ankles.

(3) Flat Bones—skull, shoulder, and sternum.

(4) Irregular Bones—mandible and vertebrae.

9. The Skull. The skull is the framework enclosing the brain. It is divided into two parts—the cranium and the face. It is made-up of 22 bones, 8 forming the cranium and 14 forming the face. The cranial bones support and protect the brain and are very firmly united to each other. The junctions of these bones along their edges are called sutures. Cranial bones include one frontal, one occipital, one sphenoid, one ethmoid, two parietal, and two temporal. These bones, along with the facial bones, are shown in figures 9 and 3–10.

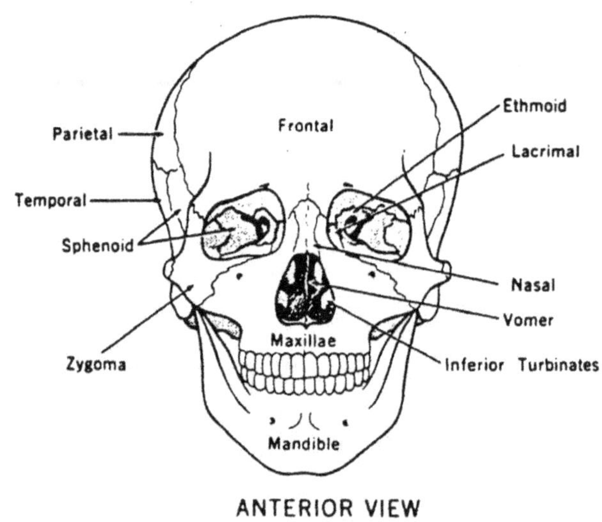

Figure 9. Anterior View of the Skull.

10. The Vertebral Column. The vertebral column consists of 24 movable or true vertebrae, the sacrum, and the coccyx. It is divided into five regions: cervical (neck), thoracic (chest), lumbar (lower back), and the sacral and coccygeal (both in the pelvis). The vertebral column (with its different regions) is shown in figure 11.

a. *Functions of the Vertebrae.* The vertebrae are designed to support and provide motion for the body and extremities, and to serve as a bony protection for the spinal cord, from which nerves arise. A typical vertebra consists of an anterior portion or body and a posterior portion or arch. The body of the vertebra provides support not only for the spinal cord but for other organs of the body as well. Many of the main muscles are also attached to the body of the vertebrae. The various surfaces and processes enable the vertebrae to move upon one another.

b. *Intervertebral Disks.* Between the vertebrae are intervertebral disks. They act as shock absorbers for the vertebral column. They contain an elastic, pulpy substance called nucleus pulposus. A rupture of one of these disks, especially those between the fourth and fifth lumbars, and the fifth lumbar and the sacrum, is a fairly common occurrence. It is termed "herniated nucleus pulposus" (HNP).

c. *Lamina.* The lamina is part of the vertebral arch connected to the pedicles of the vertebra. The laminae are identified in figure 11.

11. The Thorax. The thorax is a cone-shaped, bony cage formed by the 12 thoracic vertebrae, the ribs that terminate anteriorly in articulating cartilages, and the sternum. It houses the heart and lungs. The ribs are curved, flat bones that form most of the posterior and anterior structure and all of the lateral structure of the bony thorax. There are 12 ribs on each side of the thorax, extending from the first through the twelfth thoracic vertebrae. Ribs are identified by number and by the side of the body on which they are located. The first seven pairs are considered true ribs because they are attached to the thoracic vertebrae and to the sternum. The remaining five pairs are considered false ribs because they do not articulate directly with the sternum. The ribs from one to seven become progressively larger; after the seventh rib, they become progressively smaller. The sternum, commonly called the breastbone, is long and flat and is located at the midanterior part of the thoracic cage. It protects the heart, lungs, and greater vessels. The sternum consists of three portions: the manubrium, the body, and the xiphoid process. The entire bony thorax is shown in figure 12.

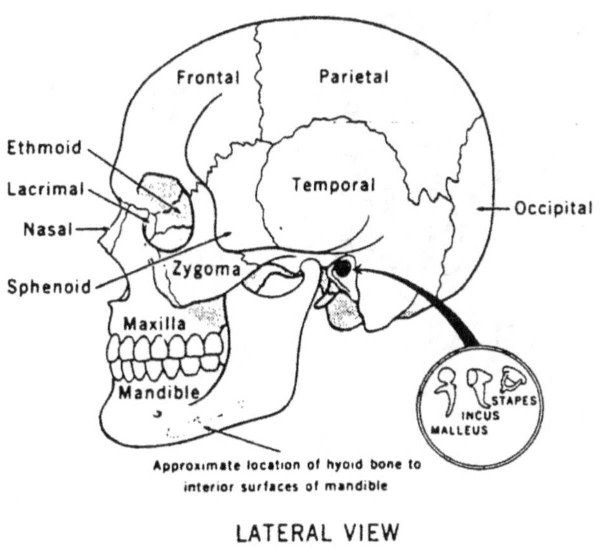

Figure 10. Lateral View of the Skull.

12. The Upper Extremities. Each upper extremity, shown in figure 13, consists of the clavicle, shoulder, arm, forearm, wrist, and hand.

a. *The Clavicle.* The clavicle, or collarbone, forms the anterior part of the shoulder girdle. It lies in a horizontal position just above the first rib. It is attached to the scapula and the sternum. Because of its anterior location, it is often fractured as a result of a fall.

b. *The Scapula.* The scapula (shoulder bone) is a triangular-shaped bone lying in the upper part of the back. It forms the posterior portion of the shoulder girdle and a part of the shoulder joint.

c. *The Humerus.* The humerus is the bone of the upper arm and is classified as a long bone. It articulates with the shoulder girdle to form the shoulder joint and the bones of the forearm to form the elbow joint.

d. *The Forearm.* The bones of the forearm are called the ulna and the radius. From an anatomical position, the radius is on the lateral or thumb side with the ulna on the medial or little finger side. The ulna and radius articulate at their proximal ends with the humerus and at their distal ends with some of the carpal bones.

e. *The Wrist and Hand.* The wrist and hand are made up of 27 separate bones. The wrist contains eight small bones called carpals. The hand consists of 5 metacarpal bones and 14 phalanges. The metacarpal bones are numbered one to five to correspond to the five fingers. The phalanges are the small bones of the fingers and thumb.

13. The Lower Extremities. The bones that make up the lower extremities are the innominate

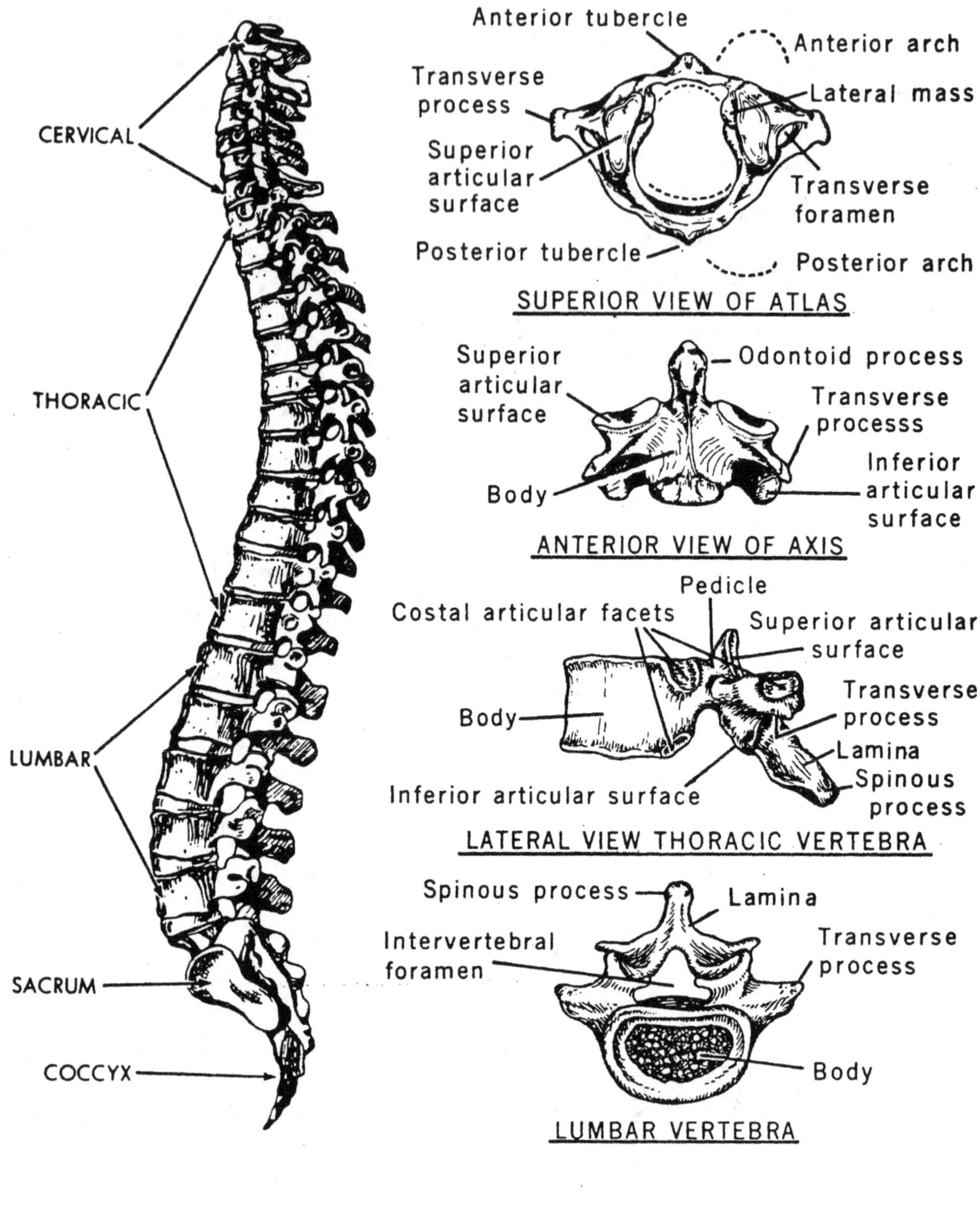

Figure 11. Vertebral Column.

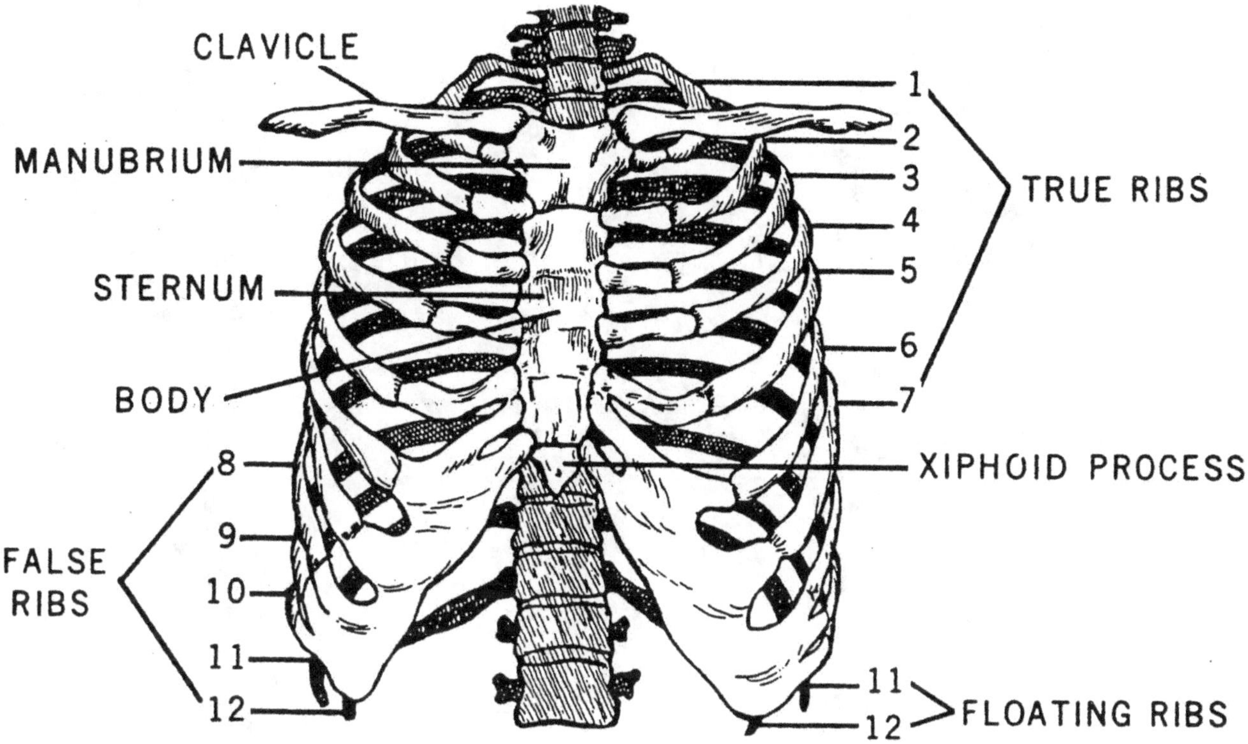

Figure 12. Bony Thorax, Anterior Aspects.

(hipbone), femur, patella, tibia and fibula, tarsals, metatarsals, and the phalanges. Each of these bones is shown in figure 14.

a. *The Pelvic Girdle.* The two hipbones, together with the sacrum and coccyx posteriorly, form the pelvic girdle. This girdle forms a deep basin, which protects the organs of the lower abdomen, the bladder, lower bowel, and reproductive organs.

b. *The Femur.* The femur, or thigh bone, is the longest bone in the body. The proximal end is rounded and has a head that fits into the acetabulum. It also has a neck, the part of the femur most frequently fractured.

c. *The Lower Leg.* The bones of the lower leg are the tibia and fibula. The tibia is the inner and larger bone; it articulates with the femur and the head of the fibula at the top and the talus at the bottom. The fibula is the outer and smaller bone. The fibula is most often fractured, but a fracture of the tibia is generally more serious.

d. *The Ankle and Foot.* The bones of the foot are similar in structure and arrangement to those of the hand. They include the 7 tarsals, 5 metatarsals, and 5 phalanges. The tarsals form the anklebones, and the metatarsals form the sole and instep of the foot. The phalanges form the toes.

14. Joints. The place of union between two or more bones of the skeleton is a joint. Because of the way the bones are attached, the body position can be changed, and hundreds of motions are possible. Figure 15 illustrates range of motion, as used in exercises and orthopedic positions.

a. *Anatomy.* The joints are lined with a membrane that secretes a fluid called synovial fluid. This fluid serves as a lubricant and keeps the joint working smoothly. Cartilage plates cover the ends of the bones and provide a smooth surface for rotation in freely movable joints. When the bones meet to form a joint, they require assistance to stay in place. This is the responsibility of the ligaments. The bursae are sacs filled with a viscid fluid and located between the ends of bones to act as a cushion. They are also found between muscle and bone or between tendons.

b. *Types of Joints.* Joints are of three different types: immovable, slightly movable, and freely movable. Figure 16 illustrates each of these types of joints.

(1) *Immovable.* In immovable joints, the surfaces of the bones are almost in direct contact and are fastened together with a thin layer of intervening fibrous tissue or cartilage. An example of this type of joint is the joining of the bones of the skull.

(2) *Slightly Movable.* In slightly movable joints, the bony surfaces are connected by broad, flattened disks of fibrocartilage or by a fibrous ligament between the bones. Examples of this type of joint

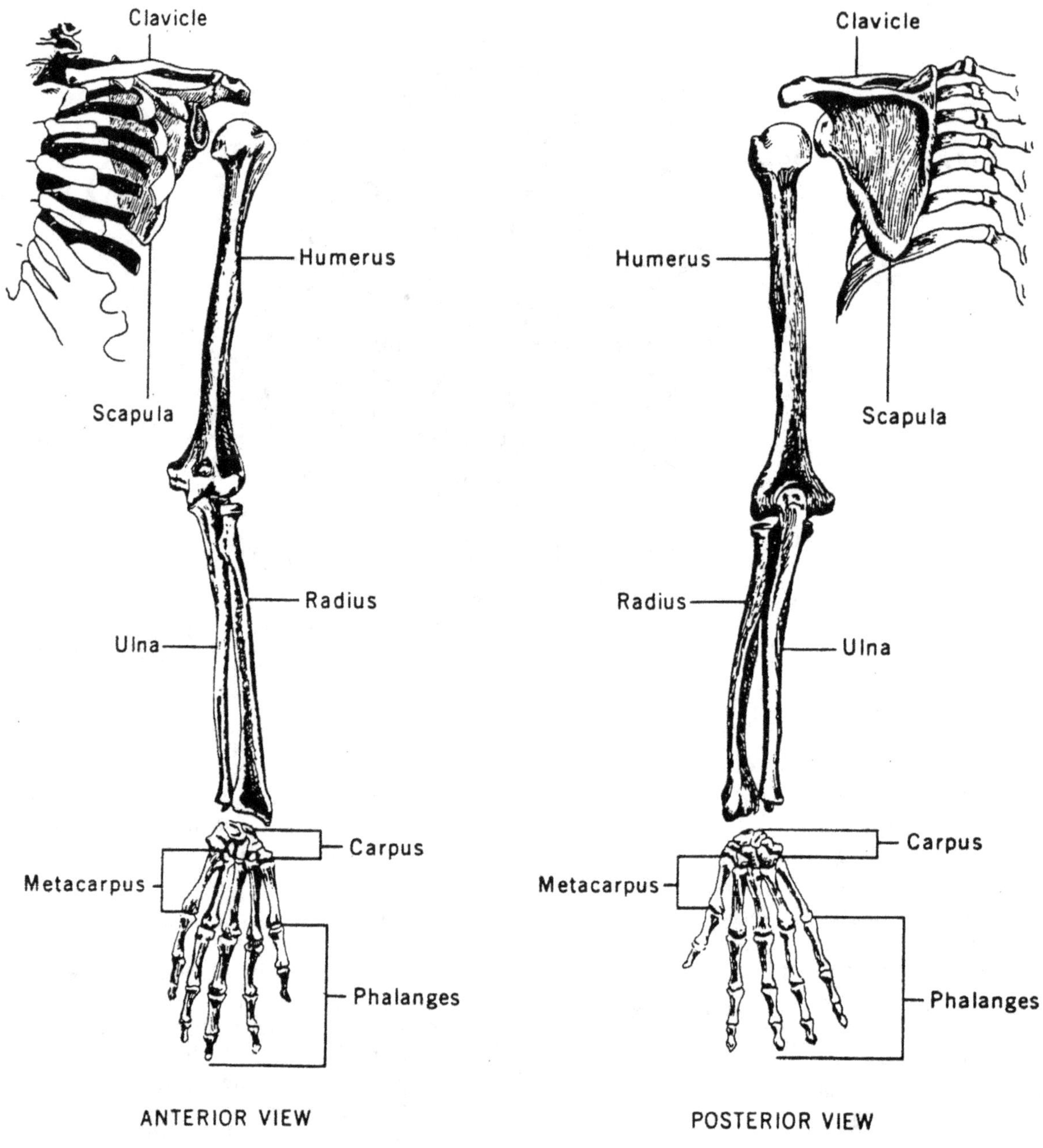

Figure 13. Upper Extremities.

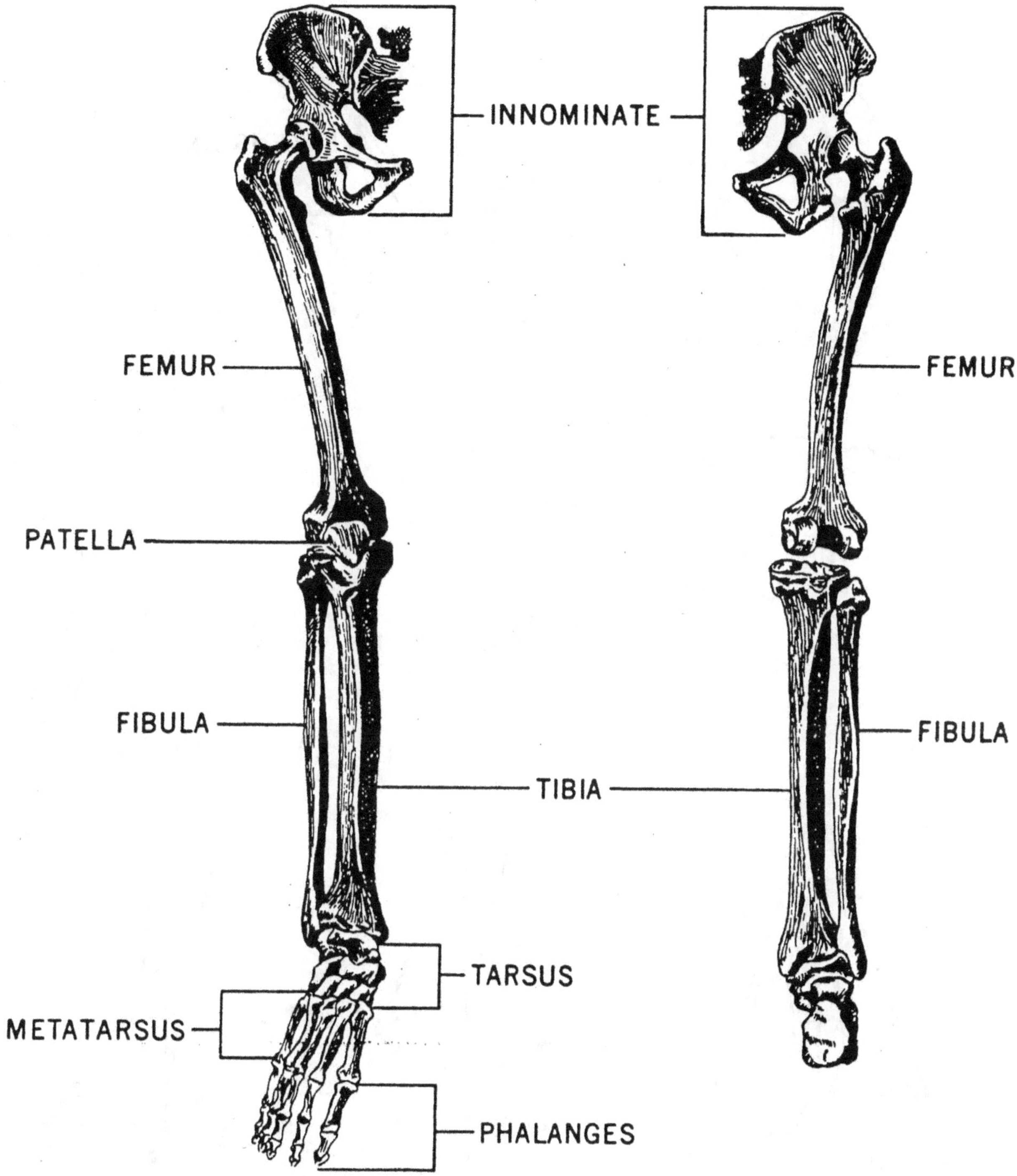

Figure 14. Lower Extremities.

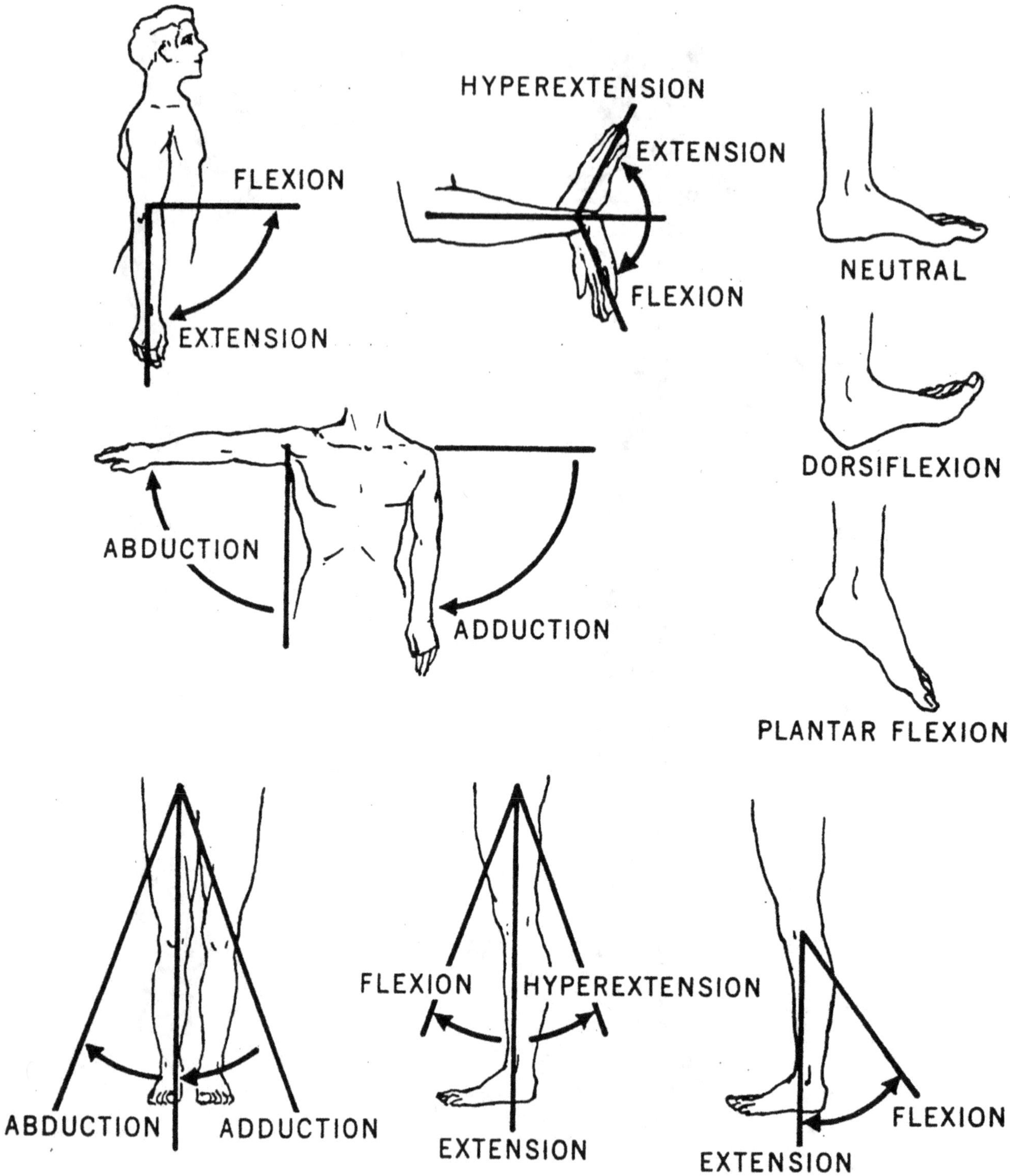

Figure 15. Range of Motion.

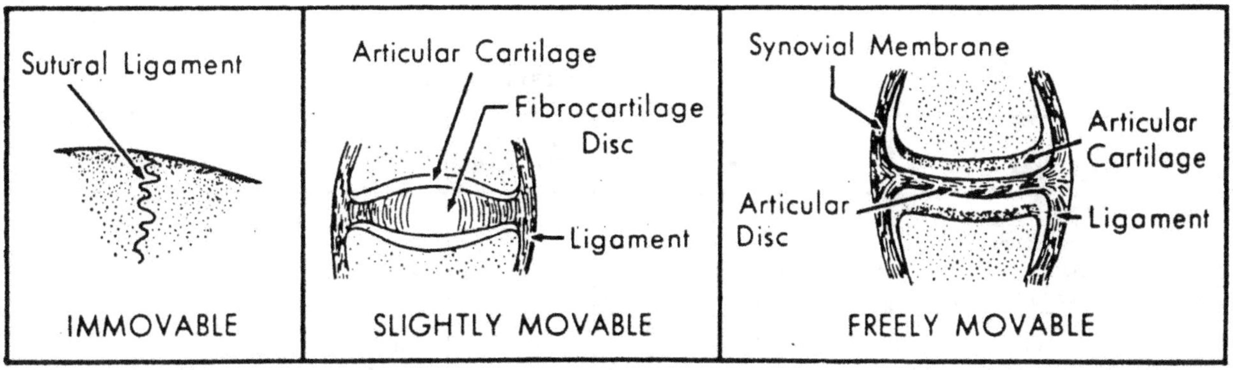

Figure 16. Types of Joints.

are the articulations of the bones of the vertebrae and the symphysis pubis.

(3) *Freely Movable.* Freely movable joints are the most numerous in the body and have a more complex arrangement. The surface of each bone is covered with articular cartilage. The bones are connected by ligaments that pass from one to the other on all sides of the joint, thus forming a capsule. This articular capsule is made up of two layers of tissue. The outer layer is fibrous tissue; the inner layer is the synovial membrane and secretes synovial or lubricating fluid. Some joints are divided completely or incompletely by a disk that is continuous with the articular capsule. Movable joints are classified according to the types of motion permitted by their structures. Some of the main types are:

(a) Hinge joints, such as the elbow and knee.

(b) Ball-and-socket joints, in which the round head of one bone fits into a cuplike cavity of another, such as the shoulder and hip.

(c) Gliding joints, where the surfaces of adjacent bones glide upon each other, such as those of the wrist and ankle.

(d) Pivot (or rotary) joints, where one bone pivots or rotates about another that is stationary, such as the axis about the atlas.

(e) Condyloid joints, in which an oval head of one bone fits into a shallow depression of another, as the carpal bones fit into the finger bones.

15. Overview of the Skeletal System. The skeletal system includes some 206 bones and numerous ligaments and cartilages which make up the joints that attach the bones together. Table 2 lists all of the bones along with their location and body area.

SECTION C—THE MUSCULAR SYSTEM

16. Functions of the Muscular System. The muscular system is important not only because muscular contraction results in movement, locomotion, and maintenance of erect posture, but also because it is involved in such essential bodily functions as pumping the blood around the body and in respiration and digestion.

17. Voluntary and Involuntary Muscles. Muscle is a tissue composed of a number of fibers held together by connective tissue and enclosed in a fibrous sheath called fascia. Muscles are characterized by their ability to contract and, thereby, to move the various parts of the body. All motion of the body, whether conscious or unconscious, is due to action of the muscles. All muscle is normally in a state of partial tension at all times and, therefore, is said to have tone or tonus. The tendency to contract is present throughout life so that if a muscle is cut, the two ends pull apart just as do the cut ends of a stretched rubber band. The muscle tissues of the body vary in shape and structure according to the functions they perform. They are divided into two main groups—voluntary muscles and involuntary muscles.

a. *Voluntary Muscles.* A muscle that is under conscious control is a voluntary muscle. All the muscles attached to the skeleton are of the voluntary type. Groups of muscle bundles held together by fascia make up the individual muscle, each of which is named according to its location, action, or other distinguishing feature. Each skeletal muscle is made up of three main parts—the origin, the belly, and the insertion. The origin is the point where the muscle is anchored, and it usually consists of a short tendon attached to the bone. The belly is the largest part of the body and is made up of many fibers. The insertion is the point on which the action of the muscle is applied, resulting in motion. Here the muscle is attached to a bone by a tendon. Tendons are nonelastic, dense, fibrous tissue. They unite with the periosteum of bones to form secure attachments for the muscles.

b. *Involuntary Muscles.* A muscle whose nerve

Table 2. Skeletal Bones.

SKELETAL BONES

Body Area	*Bone*	*Number in the body*	*Location*
Axial Skeleton (80 bones)			
1. Skull (29 bones)			
a. Cranium (8 bones)	1. Frontal	1	Forehead
	2. Occipital	1	Base of skull
	3. Sphenoid	1	Across midportion of cranial floor
	4. Ethmoid	1	Front of cranial floor
	5. Parietal	2	Bulging two top portions of skull
	6. Temporal	2	Lower two sides, anterior and superior to ears.
b. Face (14 bones)	1. Nasal	2	Bridge of nose
	2. Mandible	1	Lower jaw
	3. Vomer	1	Lower part of nasal system
	4. Maxilla	2	Upper jaw
	5. Zygomatic	2	Cheek bones
	6. Lacrimal	2	Lateral to nasal bones
	7. Inferior turbinates	2	Inner surface of nasal side wall
	8. Palatine	2	Roof of mouth
c. Ear (6 bones)	1. Malleus (hammer)	2	Hammer-shaped bone in middle ear
	2. Incus (anvil)	2	Anvil-shaped bone in middle ear
	3. Stapes (stirrups)	2	Stirrup-shaped bone in middle ear
d. Tongue	1. Hyoid	1	In throat, at root of tongue
2. Chest (25 bones)	1. True ribs	7 pairs	Attached to sternum
	2. False ribs	5 pairs	3 upper pairs attached to cartilage. 2 lower pairs are floating.
	3. Sternum	1	Breast bone
3. Spine (26 bones)	1. Cervical vertebrae	7	First 7 vertebrae (neck)
	2. Thoracic vertebrae	12	Next 12 vertebrae (chest area)
	3. Lumbar vertebrae	5	Next 5 vertebrae (small of back)
	4. Sacrum	1	Lower end of spine (contains 5 fused bones)
	5. Coccyx	1	Remains of a tail (contains 4 fused bones)
Appendicular Skeleton (126 bones)			
1. Upper Extremities (64 bones)	1. Clavicle	2	Collar bone
	2. Scapula	2	Shoulder blade
	3. Humerus	2	Upper arm
	4. Radius	2	Forearm, thumb side
	5. Ulna	2	Forearm, little finger side
	6. Carpals	16	Wrist bones
	7. Metacarpals	10	Palm of hands
	8. Phalanges	28	Fingers and thumbs
2. Lower Extremities (62 bones)	1. Innominate bone	2	Hip or pelvis
	2. Femur	2	Thigh
	3. Patella	2	Knee cap
	4. Tibia	2	Shin
	5. Fibula	2	Calf side of lower leg
	6. Tarsal	14	Ankle
	7. Metatarsal	10	Foot
	8. Phalanges	28	Toes

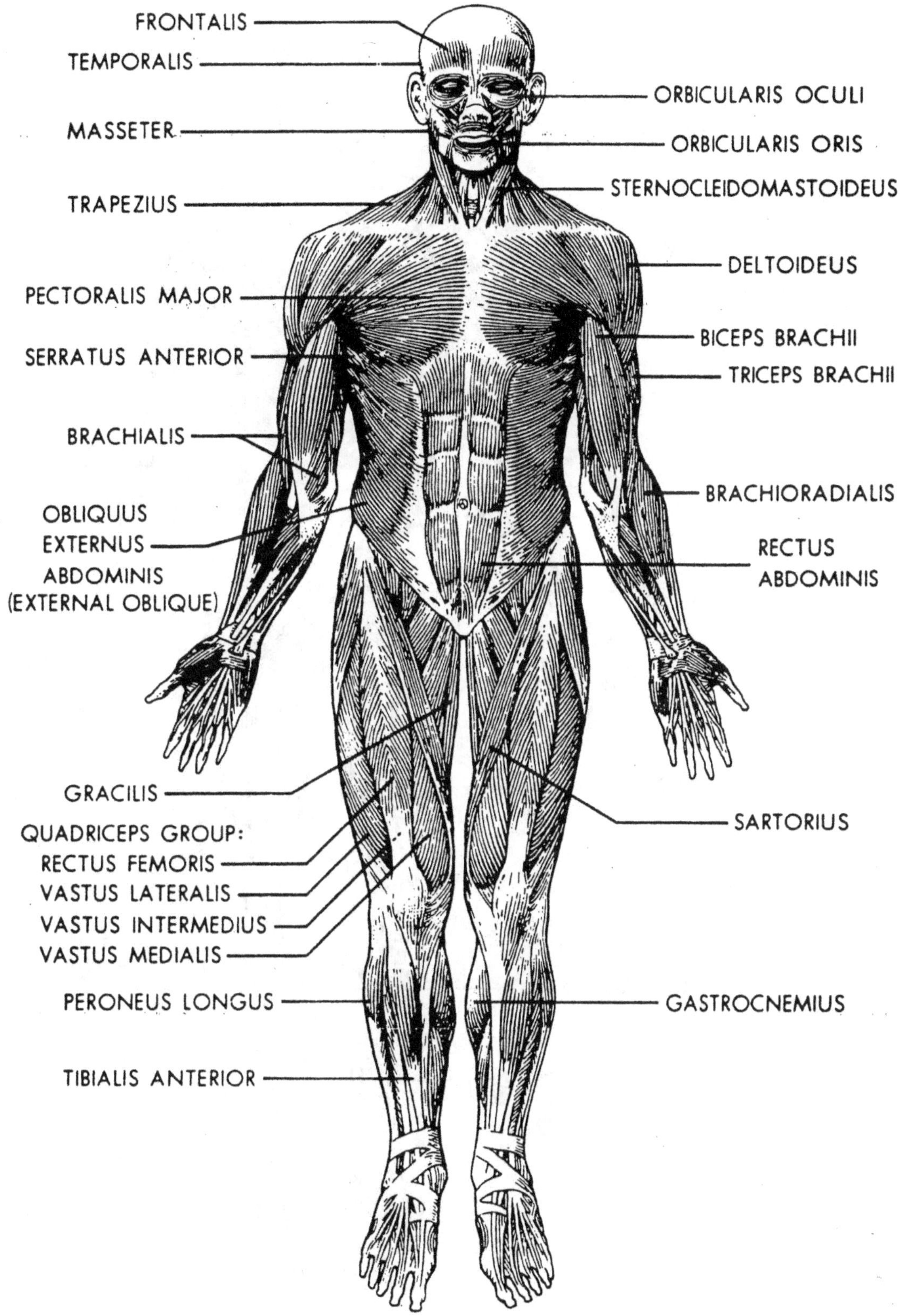

Figure 17. Anterior Superficial Muscles.

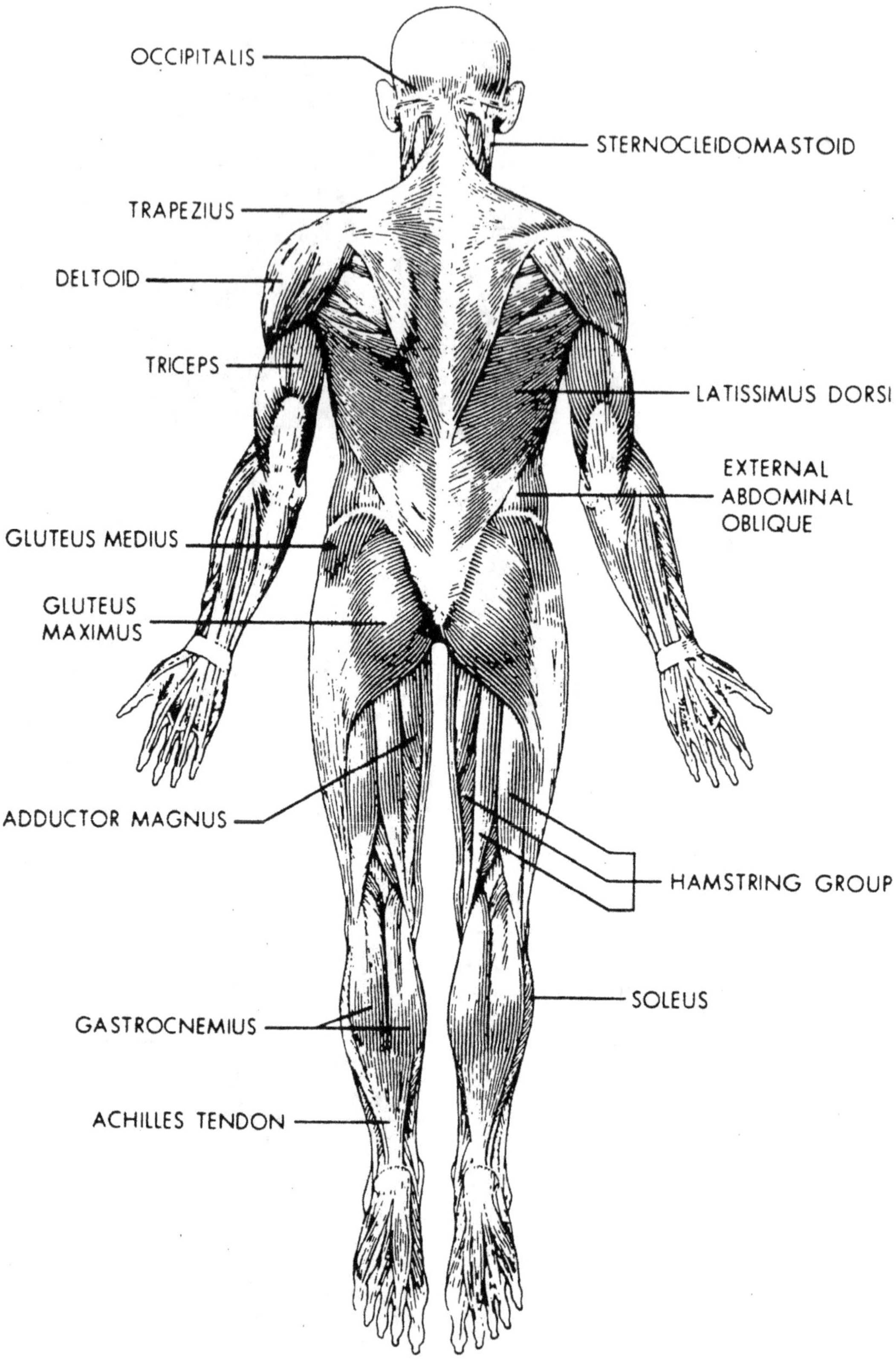

Figure 18. Posterior Superficial Muscles.

supply comes from the autonomic nervous system (the part of our nervous system over which we have no direct control) is an involuntary muscle. These muscles are found in the walls of the blood vessels, in the intestinal tract, and in the glands. Their action is well illustrated in the intestinal tract, where they push food along by rhythmic contractions (peristalsis). A special kind of involuntary muscle is the cardiac muscle. Its structure is quite different from that of any other muscle.

18. Muscles of the Upper and Lower Extremities. The major muscles and muscle groups are illustrated in figures 17 and 18.

a. *Upper Extremities.* The major muscles of the upper extremities consist of the deltoid, the biceps brachii, and the triceps brachii. The first of these, the deltoid, fits as a "cap" over the shoulder and occupies the superolateral portion of the shoulder prominence. It is widely used for injections. The biceps brachii is a large spindle-shaped muscle forming the major portion of the bulge on the anterior surface of the upper arm. The triceps brachii occupies the posterior surface of the arm.

b. *Lower Extremities.* The lower extremities have several major muscles: the gluteus maximus, the quadriceps, the hamstrings, and the gastrocnemius. The first of these, the gluteus maximus, is the large, fleshy muscle forming the prominence of the buttocks. The quadriceps are a four-headed group of muscles forming the anterior portion of the thigh. The hamstrings are three muscles located on the posterior thigh. The gastrocnemius is the large, superficial muscle forming the major portion of the calf of the leg. It is inserted into the heel bone by the Achilles tendon, the largest tendon in the body.

19. The Abdominal Muscles. There are several different abdominal muscles forming broad, thin layers that support the internal organs. These muscles also assist in breathing, in flexing the thorax on the pelvis, and in flexing and rotating the spine.

20. The Back Muscles. The muscles of the back are large and broad. They are attached to the vertebrae and keep the trunk in an erect position, permitting it to bend and turn. These movements occur mainly in the cervical lumbar regions. Some of the major muscle groups, as well as their location and function, are explained in table 3.

Table 3. Location and Purpose of Major Muscle Groups.

Location	*Muscle*	*Purpose*
Head	Occipito frontalis Orbicularis oculi Orbicularis oris Masseter	Raises eyebrows Closes eye Closes lips Closes jaw
Neck	Sternocleidomastoid	Flexes head
Shoulder	Deltoid Trapezius	Abducts upper arm Raises shoulder; extends head
Chest	Pectoralis major	Flexes and adducts anteriorly the upper arm
Abdomen	External abdominal oblique Rectus abdominus Inguinal ligament	Compresses abdomen; flexes trunk Compresses abdomen; flexes trunk Insertion area for external oblique
Back	Latissimus dorsi	Extends upper arm and adducts it posteriorly
Arm	Biceps brachii Triceps brachii Flexors Extensors	Flexes lower arm Extends lower arm Flexes hand Extends hand
Thigh	Gluteus Maximus Adductor group Sartorius Quadriceps femoris Hamstring group	Extends and abducts thigh Adducts and flexes thigh Adducts, flexes and "crosses" lower leg Extends leg; flexes thigh Flexes lower leg
Lower Leg	Gastrocnemius (Achilles tendon) Extensors Soleus	Flexes leg; extends foot Extends toes Extends foot

21. Muscle Tone. Muscles are never completely relaxed; they are always in a state of partial contraction. This state is referred to as *muscle tone*, and it involves a complicated chemical process by which glucose is broken down into lactic acid and energy. This process is more active when the muscle is being consciously contracted, extended, or irritated. Even though muscle tone is advantageous for normal body functions, it can become a problem to the surgeons who would, for example, like to have the abdominal muscles relaxed when they explore a peritoneal cavity. The elasticity which allows flexion of the fingers can also cause a severed tendon to retract deep into surrounding tissue, thus necessitating a probing search on the part of a surgeon who is trying to repair the injury. In the case of needed abdominal relaxation, it may sometimes be necessary to inject muscle-relaxing drugs before deep abdominal surgery can be performed. Figure 19 illustrates the number of muscle layers the surgeon must contend with in his approach to the abdominal cavity.

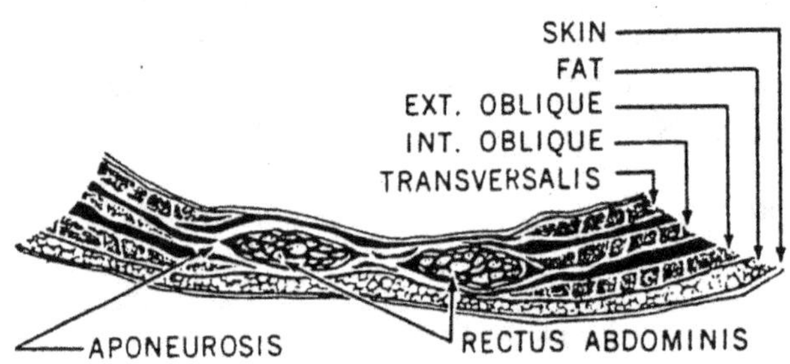

Figure 19. Cross Section of Abdominal Muscle Layers.

SECTION D—THE NERVOUS SYSTEM

22. Function of the Nervous System. The nervous system is the means by which the human body is integrated and enabled to function as a whole. The nervous system is the stimulus-response mechanism that coordinates and regulates all body activity. It is responsible for all the processes that make up the adjustment to both internal and external environment. It is the most highly organized system in the body. The nervous system may be considered as an intricate communications system that transmits impulses from different parts of the body to the brain, and from the brain to organs and structures that react to impulses.

23. Divisions of the Nervous System. The nervous system is both *voluntary* and *involuntary* and is composed of the brain, spinal cord, nerves, and ganglia. It is also divided into a *central nervous system* (CNS) and a *peripheral nervous system* (PNS). The peripheral nervous system also includes the autonomic nervous system, which is self-controlling and is formed from the many nerves that innervate the internal organs, glands, and blood vessels. Table 4 shows the divisions of the CNS and the PNS.

24. Neurons. The basic structural unit of the nervous system is the neuron or nerve cell. Each neuron contains a cell body and cell processes called dendrites and axons. Dendrites carry impulses away from the cell body. A typical nerve cell is shown in figure 7.

Table 4. Divisions of the Nervous System.

DIVISIONS OF THE NERVOUS SYSTEM

Central Nervous System (CNS)	*Peripheral Nervous System (Craniospinal Division)*
Brain: Cerebrum Cerebellum Midbrain Pons Medulla Oblongata	Cranial Nerves and their Functions: 1. Olfactory (smell) 2. Optic (vision) 3. Oculomotor (eye movement and pupil size) 4. Trochlear (eye movement) 5. Trifacial (sensations in face and head, chewing) 6. Abducens (abduction of eye) 7. Facial (facial expressions and taste) 8. Auditory (hearing and equilibrium) 9. Glossopharyngeal (taste and swallowing) 10. Vagus (various sensations and movements in heart, intestines, etc.) 11. Spinal accessory (head and shoulder movement) 12. Hypoglossal (tongue movements)
Spinal Cord	Spinal Nerves and Areas Innervated: 8 cervical (shoulder, neck, head, chest) 12 thoracic (shoulder, chest, arm, hand) 5 lumbar (back, hip, thigh, genitalia) 5 sacral (rectum, buttocks, leg, foot) 1 coccygeal (skin in coccyx area)

25. Afferent and Efferent Neurons. There are two types of neurons—*afferent, which is receptive or sensory,* and *efferent, which is effective or motor.* Afferent neurons carry impulses from the periphery (body) toward the spine and brain. Efferent neurons carry impulses from the brain and spine to the periphery. The bodies of afferent neurons are located in ganglia, just outside the spinal cord. *A ganglion is a group or mass of neurons* that serve as a center of nervous impulses.

26. Nerves. A nerve is a cordlike structure that transmits impulses from one part of the body to another. A nerve has many fibers that are closely associated but have independent functions. A nerve may consist of sensory fibers only, motor fibers only, or a combination of both.

27. The Central Nervous System. The central nervous system is composed of the brain and spinal cord and is contained or located inside the cranial cavity and in the vertebral canal. Figure 20 illustrates the environment of the brain and spinal cord in midsagittal section. The brain, shown in figure 21, receives and interprets impulses and sends out responses.

a. The *cerebrum* (or forebrain) is the largest part of the brain and is divided into right and left halves called hemispheres. Each hemisphere is divided into specialized lobes. named after the cranial bones to which they join. Each of these lobes is a specialized, functional area. The frontal lobe is a motor area; the parietal lobe is a sensory area; the occipital lobe is the center of vision; and the temporal lobe is the center of hearing.

b. The cerebrum presents a wrinkled appearance, characterized by many ridges and convolutions. The outer layer of the cerebrum, called the cortex, is made up of gray matter containing nerve cells. It governs all conscious functions. The interior of the cerebrum is white and contains bundles of axons and nerve tracts. Its functions include accumulation and storage of knowledge, or memory, and the interpretation of sensations.

c. The *cerebellum* is the second largest part of the brain and is located in the lower posterior part of the cranial cavity, beneath the cerebrum. Its primary functions are concerned with the coordination of muscular movements and body balance or equilibrium.

d. The *brain stem* consists of three functional parts: the midbrain, the pons, and the medulla oblongata. The *midbrain* is a small structure containing nuclei for reflex control. The *pons* makes up the middle part of the brain stem and serves as a bridge to connect the brain stem to the cerebellum. It also serves as a place for the exit of cranial nerves and helps to regulate respiration. The *medulla oblongata* is the part of the brain that connects with the spinal cord. It is the location of such vital control centers as respiration, heartbeat, and blood pressure. In addition, many reflex actions such as sneezing, coughing, and peristaltic movement are also controlled by the medulla.

e. The *spinal cord* is the main nerve trunk for the body. It is like a large telephone cable, able to carry hundreds of messages at the same time. It is located inside the vertebral column, extending from the brain to the lower region of the back. The spinal cord is the means by which impulses from the brain reach the periphery of the body, and also the way by which impulses from the periphery reach the brain. The spinal cord contains 31 pairs of spinal nerves, with both sensory and motor fibers, that lead from the cord to all parts of the body.

f. The brain and spinal cord are covered with three layers of special membranes called *meninges.* They serve as protective covering for brain and spinal cord. The space between the middle and inner layers contains cerebrospinal fluid, a clear, watery solution similar to blood plasma. It circulates over the entire surface of the brain and spinal cord and provides a protective cushion as well as a source of nourishment for these structures. The cerebrospinal fluid is continuously being formed by a plexus (network or mass) of blood vessels in the brain, and as it is formed, a like amount is continuously reabsorbed.

28. The Peripheral Nervous System. The peripheral nervous system is made up of 12 pairs of cranial nerves and 31 pairs of spinal nerves stemming from the brain and spinal cord, respectively. These nerves carry both voluntary and involuntary impulses. The cranial nerves are sensory, motor, or mixed.

29. The Autonomic Nervous System. The autonomic nervous system, as shown in figure 22, belongs to the peripheral nervous system and is functional rather than organic. It is formed from the many nerves that innervate the internal organs, glands, and blood vessels. Its action, as the name implies, is automatic. The autonomic nervous system enables the body to maintain an internal environment suitable for all vital body processes. It is further divided into a *sympathetic* and a *parasympathetic* system. These two systems act in opposition to each other. For example, the sympathetic system stimulates nerves which cause acceleration of the heartbeat and a rise in blood pressure. The parasympathetic system acts to slow the heart and lower the blood pressure. By acting in opposition, the two opposing functions tend to keep the body in delicate balance.

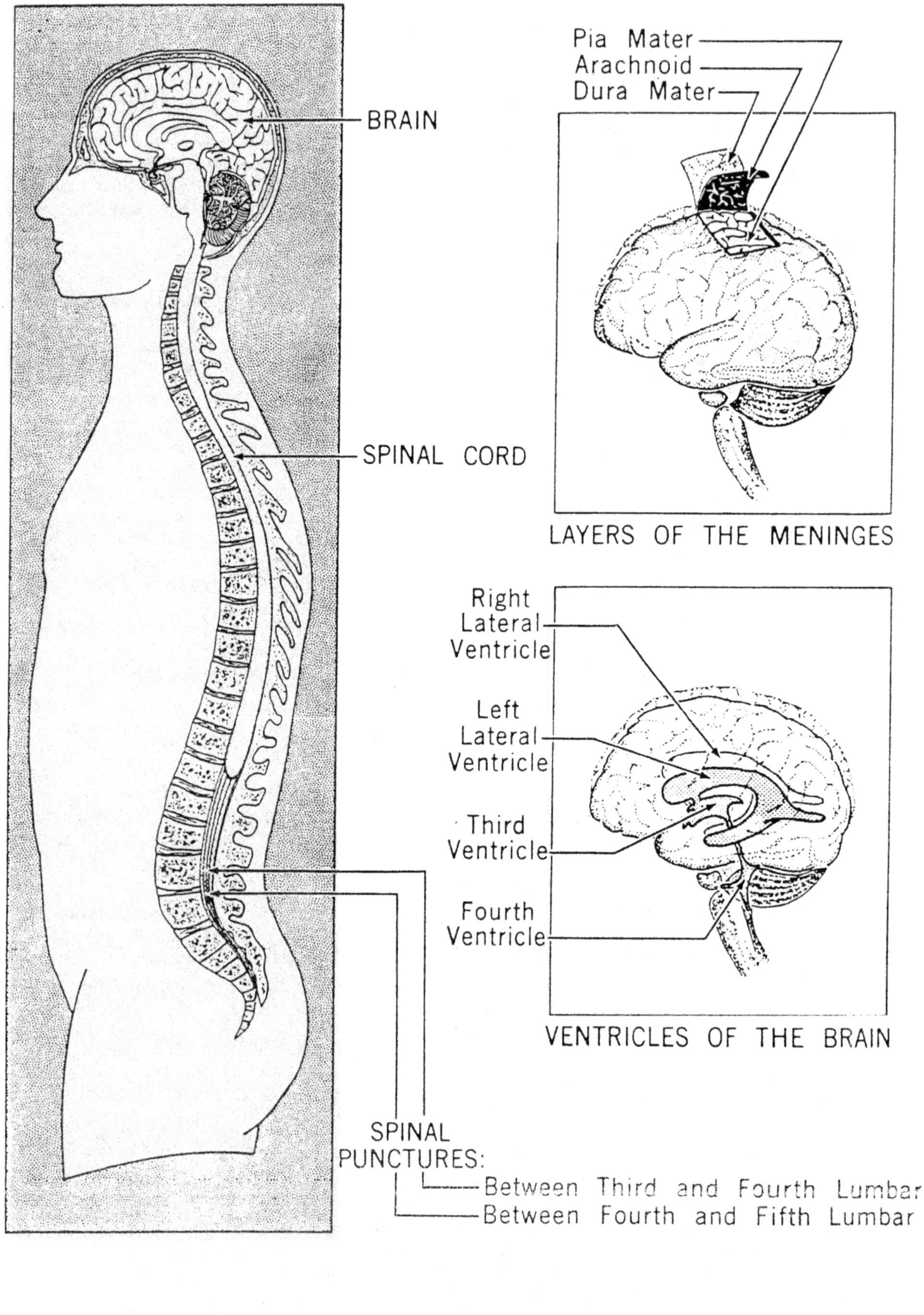

Figure 20. Environment of the Brain and Spinal Cord in Midsagittal Section.

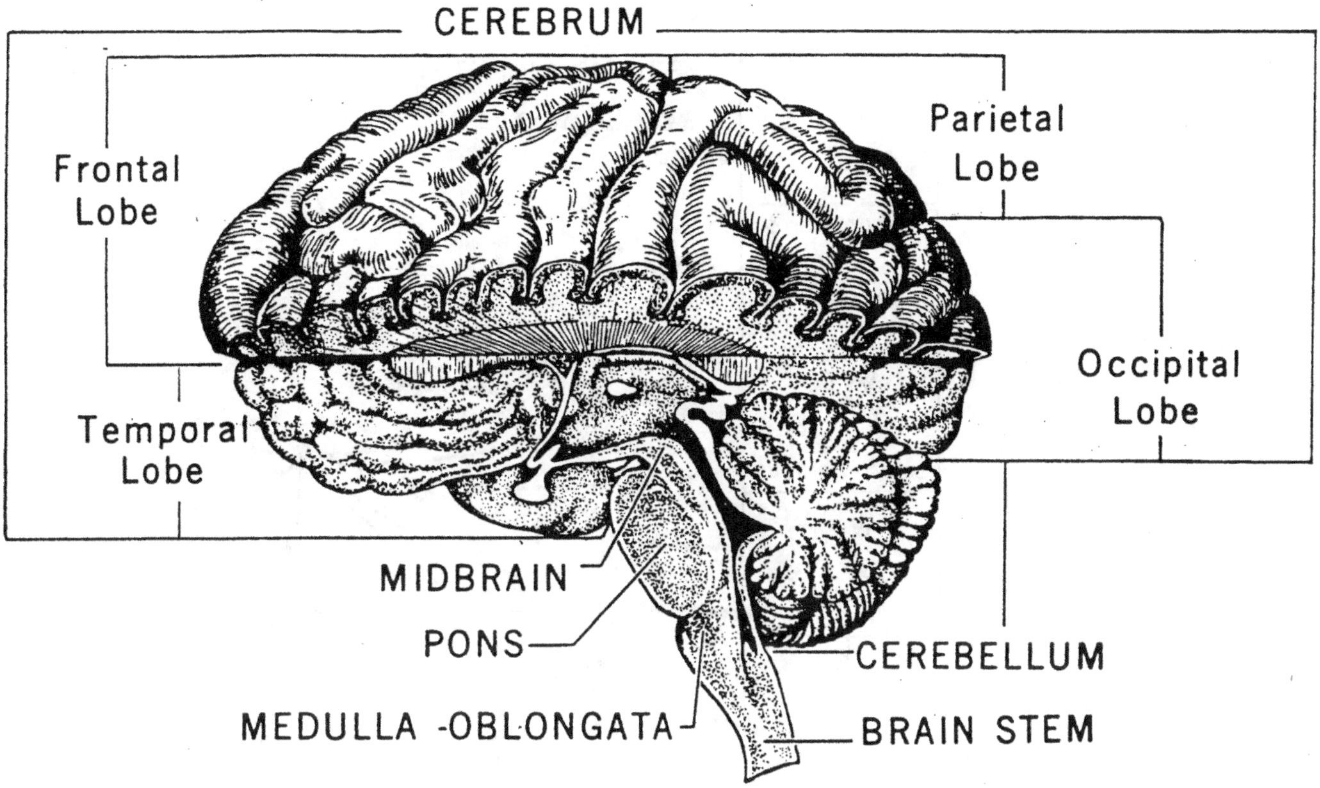

Figure 21. The Brain.

30. The Major Nerve Branches. The major nerve branches are illustrated in figure 23. Each of these branches continues to diverge into numerous fine threads which carry on a communication process throughout the body. It is these fine nerves that conduct local anesthetic agents into the tissues surrounding small operative areas.

31. Sensory Neurons. Sensory neurons carry the impulses into the posterior portion of the cord. They may synapse (connect) with motor neurons at this level, or the cord may act as a cable and transmit the information to the brain for interpretation. Then the responsive impulse is passed down through the anterior portion of the cord, and motor neurons deliver it to the muscle or organ that will react.

a. Sensations which originate in the skin include heat, cold, pain, touch, and pressure. The receptors for each of these are not evenly distributed throughout the body, and for this reason sensitivity to the different stimuli may vary from one part of the body to another.

b. The *eye* is a highly specialized sense organ. It is contained in a cone-shaped, bony cavity called the *orbit*. When reflected light rays enter through the *cornea*, shown in figure 24, they are quickly controlled by the shutter action of the *iris* which allows different sizes of *lens* openings. The *ciliary muscle* adjusts the shape of the lens so that light rays are focused to the rear of the eye on the *retina*. From here, the *optic nerve* sends the impression to the brain, and an interpretation is made. Work in the area of the eye must always be concerned with the delicate nature of eye tissue, and with the measures which will protect the patient from pain or injury.

c. *Hearing* also involves an interpretation by the central nervous system. Sound waves are transferred through the three portions of the ear as illustrated in figure 25. The *outer ear* picks up these sound waves and passes them along a canal or *auditory meatus* until they strike the *tympanic membrane* (ear drum). The vibration produced at this point is transmitted through the middle ear by three small bones, which are shaped like a *hammer* (malleus), an *anvil* (incus), and a *stirrup* (stapes). The eustachian tube, which reaches from the middle ear to the nasopharynx, allows for equalization of air pressure between this area and the outside, but unhappily, it may also serve as a source of infection to the middle ear. At the junction between the middle and inner ear, the vibrations are picked up by a membrane called the *oval window* and are

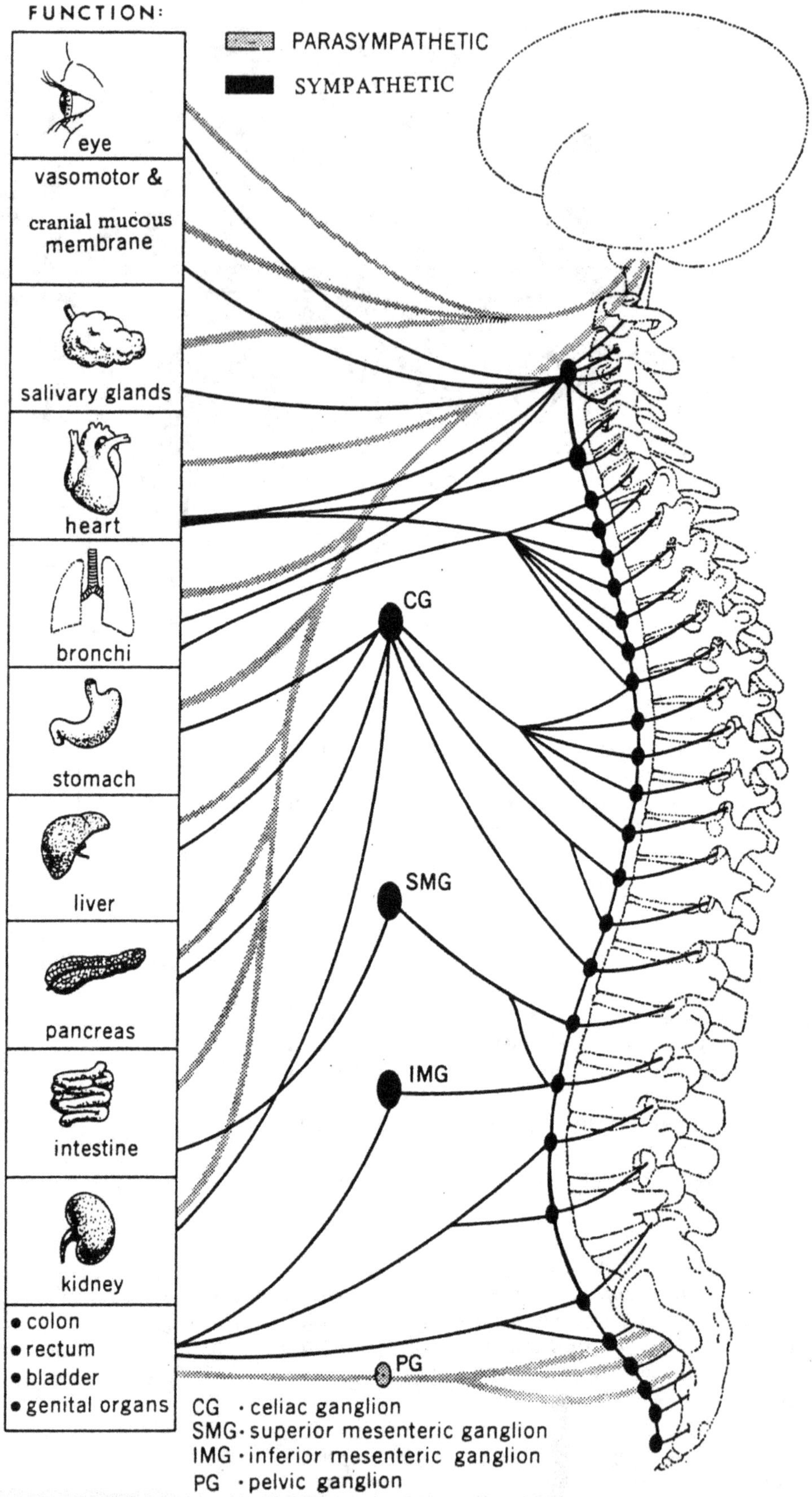

Figure 22. Diagram of the Autonomic Nervous System.

transferred through a fluid medium along the *cochlea*. The auditory (eighth cranial) nerve is stimulated by way of tiny hair cells (*organs of Corti*) which project into this fluid. The impulse is then carried to the auditory area of the brain, and hearing occurs. In addition to the cochlea, the inner ear also contains the semicircular canals. The fibers of the eighth cranial nerve, which controls equilibrium, reach into this organ and pick up messages which inform us of the position of our head. (In other words, this is where dizziness originates.)

d. The last two sensory organs, those of *smell* and *taste*, are closely allied. The nasal cavity contains the receptors of the *olfactory* (first cranial) nerve, and drawing air into the nose stimulates these nerve fibers. There are many kinds of smell receptors, and they fatigue easily as evidenced by how rapidly we become accustomed to any specific type of odor. *There are only four types of taste buds*, capable of stimulation by sweet, sour, bitter, or salty substances. The other flavors which we experience result from a combination of taste and smell.

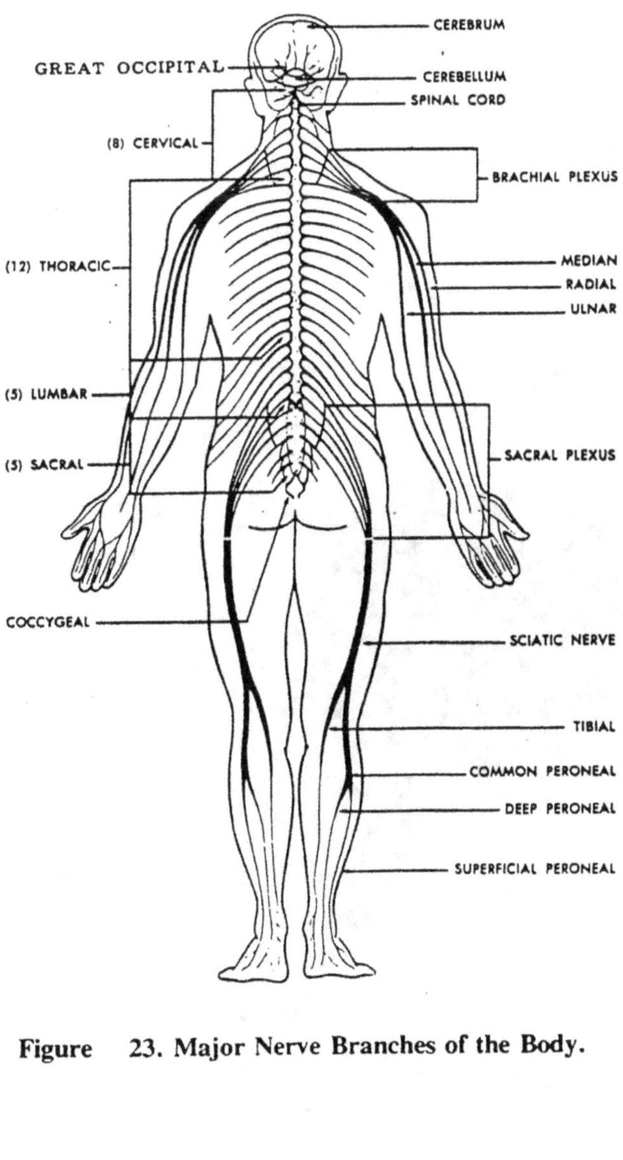

Figure 23. Major Nerve Branches of the Body.

SECTION E—THE CIRCULATORY SYSTEM

32. Functions of the Circulatory System. The circulatory system includes all structures concerned with the transportation and distribution of body fluids. It includes a *cardiovascular system* and a *lymphatic system*. These systems are vital to all other body systems and functions. The cardiovascular system consists of the heart, arteries, arterioles, veins, venules, and capillaries. The lymphatic system is made up of lymph capillaries, lymph vessels, and lymph ducts.

33. The Heart. Figure 26 illustrates the layers of the heart muscle, the four chambers, the valves dividing these chambers, and the manner in which major blood vessels lead into and out of the chambers. Coronary vessels nourish the heart muscle, and branches of the autonomic nervous system supply the impulses that cause the chambers to contract. One of the most common phenomenon associated with heart contractions is the *pulse*. The speed with which the heart contracts produces the *pulse rate*, and the force that blood exerts against the vessel walls with each contraction is *blood pressure*.

34. Circulation. The heart forces blood that has been freshly oxygenated by the lungs through *arterial* vessels, as illustrated in figure 27, to the *capillaries* that feed the cells of the body. *Veins*, shown in figure 28, then return the waste materials from the body cells to the heart, and the process is repeated.

35. Subdivisions of Blood. The two main subdivisions of blood are its *plasma* (liquid portion) and *formed elements*. Facts concerning this group of elements are contained in table 5, and the constituents of plasma are outlined in table 6. There are also certain elements which, by their presence or absence, determine *blood group* and *Rh factor*. The four blood groups are O, A, B, and AB. The Rh factor is indicated as negative (−) or positive (+). Both the blood group and Rh factor are important when a blood transfusion is to be given to a patient. If the blood of the donor and recipient are not compatible, severe reactions may occur which could endanger the life of the recipient.

36. The Lymphatic System. The lymphatic system, illustrated in figure 29, is discussed along with the circulatory system because the two systems

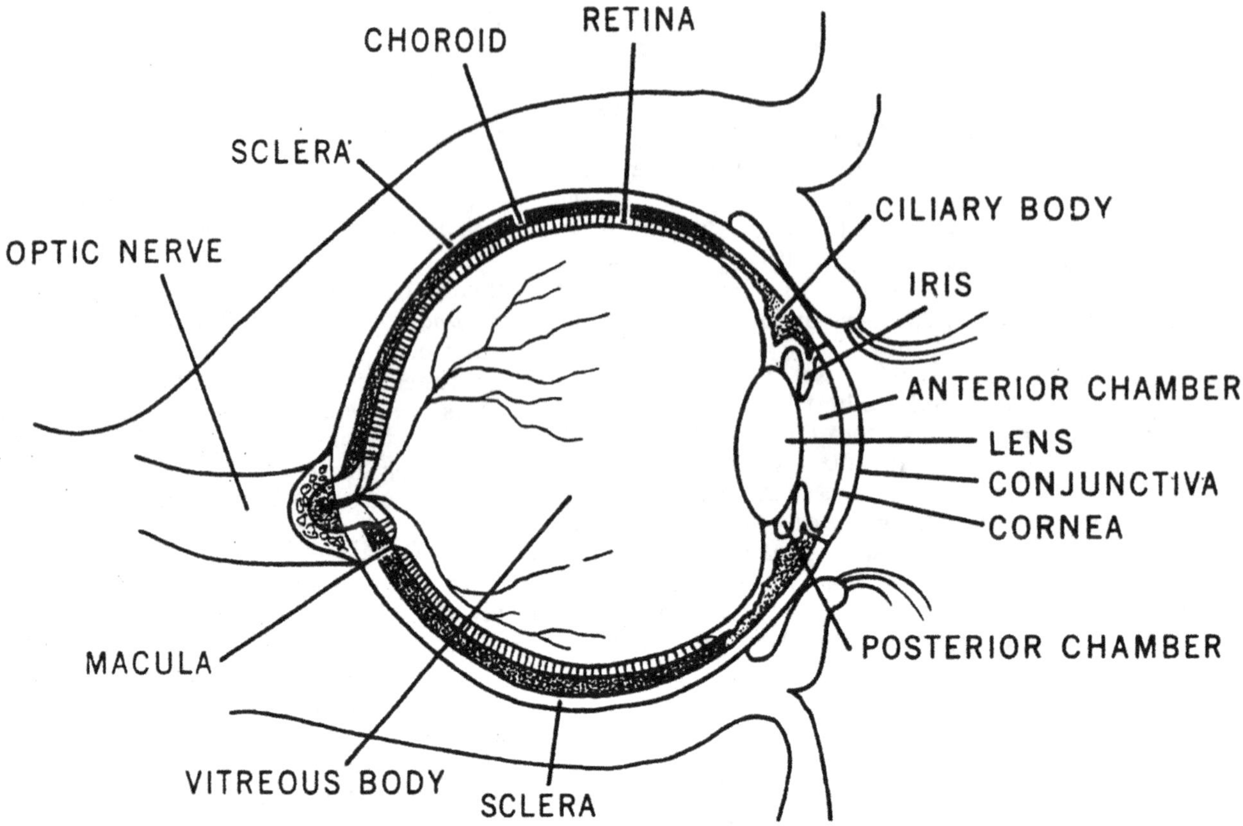

Figure 24. The Eye.

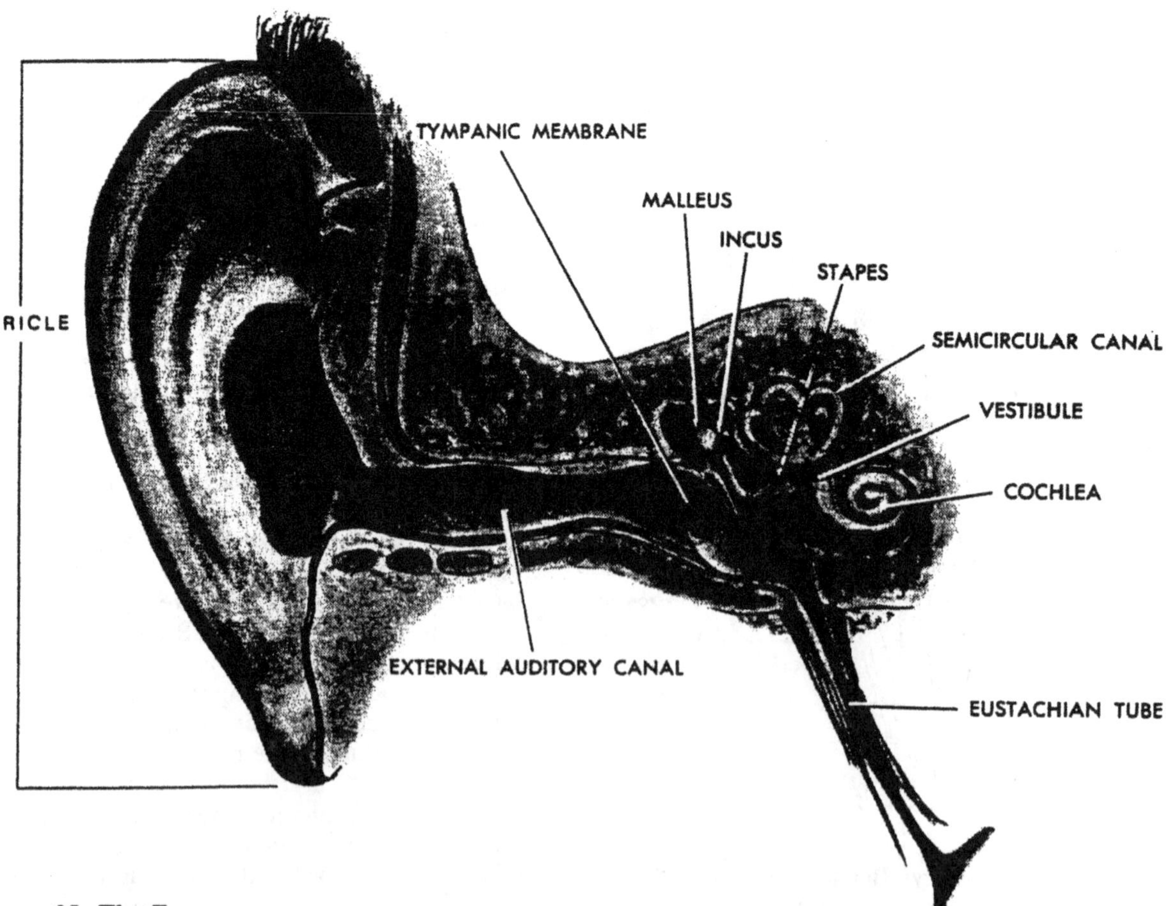

Figure 25. The Ear.

are closely associated. Lymphatic capillaries lie beneath the blood capillaries and collect fluid from the spaces between the cells. When lymph (tissue fluid) enters the lymphatic vessels it carries with it any bacteria that may have invaded these cells. Then, as this lymph proceeds through the lymphatic vessels, these bacteria are filtered out by *lymph nodes* and are destroyed by the action of lymphocytes. The lymph continues on into the main lymph ducts which empty into the neck veins.

SECTION F—THE RESPIRATORY SYSTEM

37. Function of the Respiratory System. The respiratory system includes the structures that are concerned with the exchange of gases (oxygen and carbon dioxide). The exchange of gases is known as respiration or breathing. It involves taking air into the lungs to obtain oxygen in exchange for carbon dioxide which is exhaled. It also involves the exchange of gases at the cellular level. The body requires a constant supply and exchange of these gases to carry on the chemical processes which are vital to life. Figure 30 illustrates the lungs and upper respiratory tract.

38. Anatomy of the Respiratory System. The respiratory system is composed of the nose, pharynx, larynx, trachea, lungs, bronchi, and pleurae. Accessory organs that make breathing possible are the thorax, ribs, diaphragm, and intercostal muscles.

a. *The Nose*. The *nose* is a framework of bone and cartilage with an external covering of skin. The

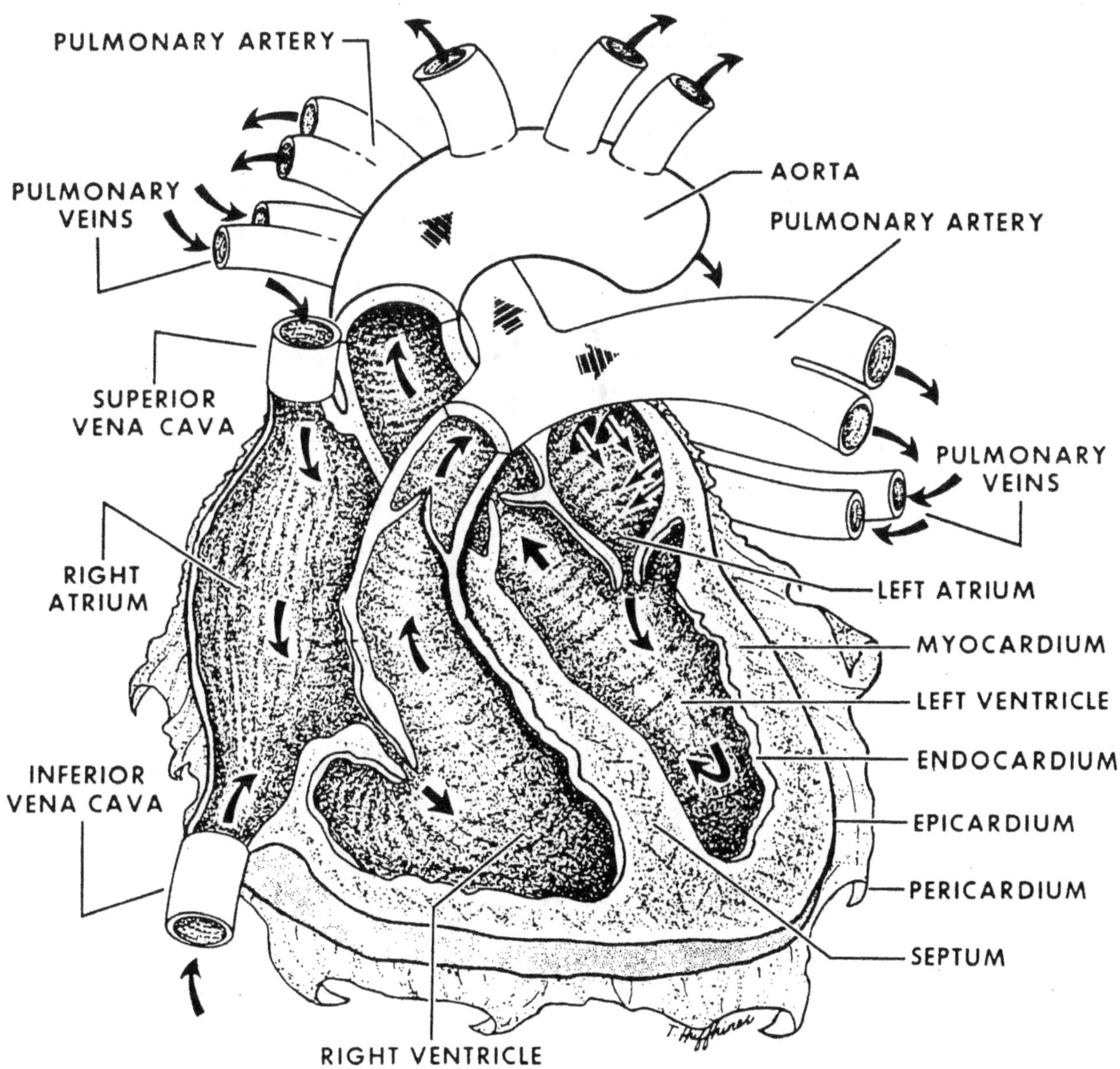

Figure 26. The Heart.

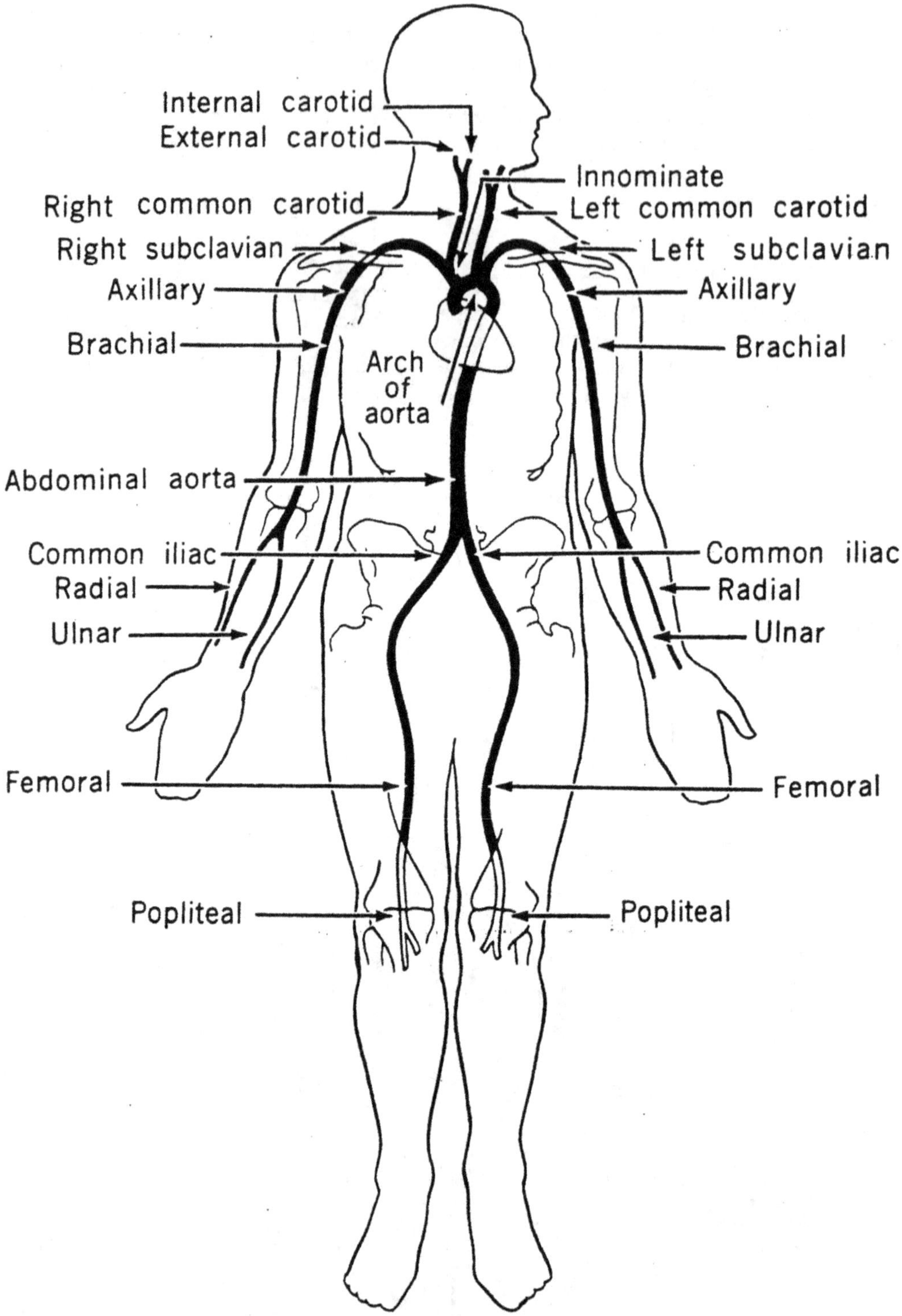

Arteries

Figure 27. Major Arteries.

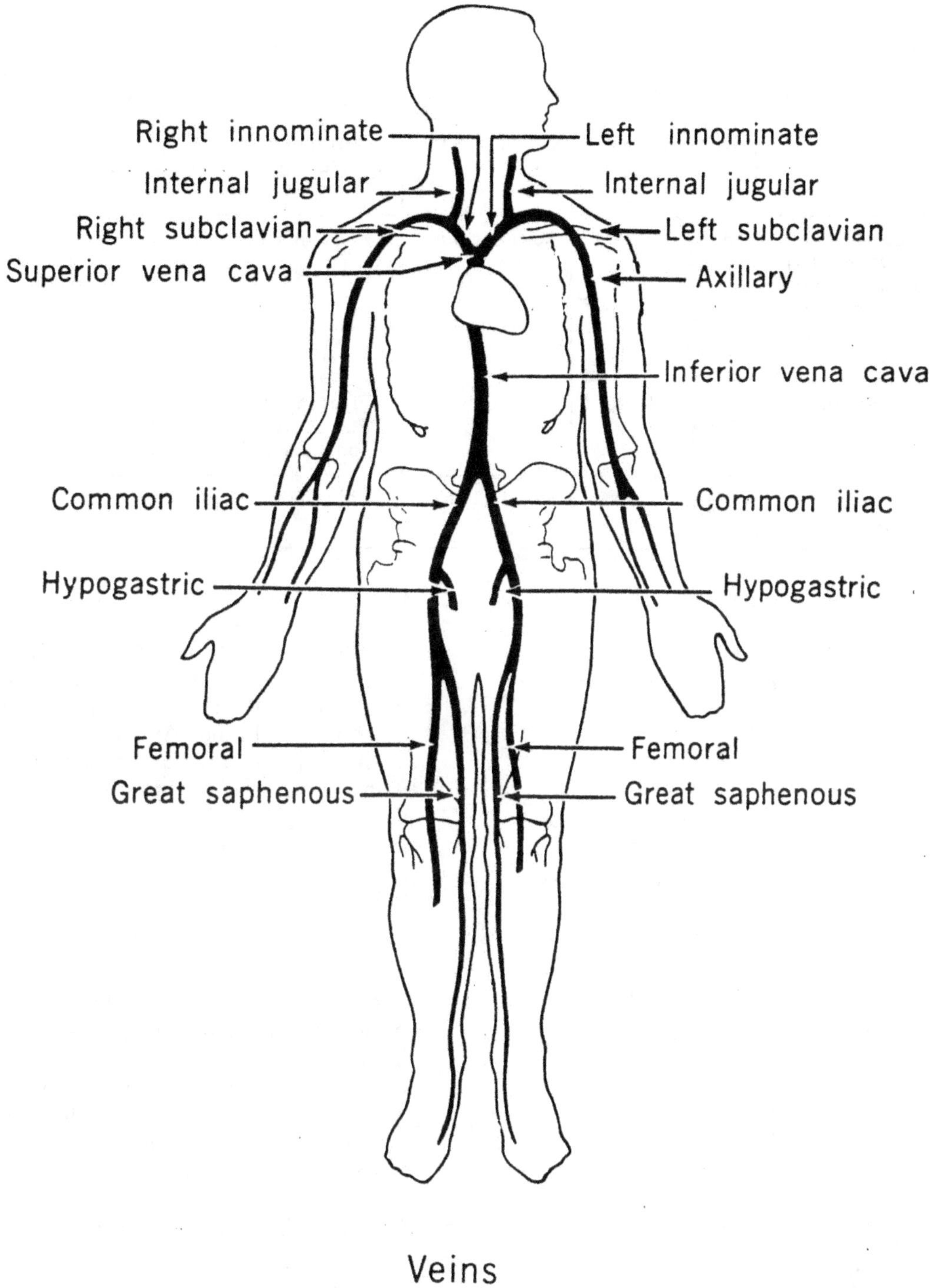

Figure 28. Major Veins.

Table 5. Formed Elements of Blood.

FORMED ELEMENTS OF BLOOD

Element	Source	Area of Destruction	Function
1. Erythrocytes (red cells)	Bone Marrow	Spleen, Liver	Respiration: Hemoglobin portion carries oxygen to cells and carbon dioxide away.
2. Leucocytes (white cells) Granulocytes: Neutrophils Eosinophils Basophils	Bone Marrow	Spleen, Liver	Fight infection
Agranulocytes: Lymphocytes	Lymph Nodes		Fight infection
Monocytes	Unknown		Form scar tissue, Some antibody formation
3. Thrombocytes (platelets)	Bone Marrow	Blood Clots	Coagulation of blood

Table 6. Constituents of Plasma.

CONSTITUENTS OF PLASMA

Substance	Purpose
Water (90% of blood volume)	Regulation of body temperature. Acts as solvent carrying substances to and from cells.
Proteins: Albumin	Buffer; regulates osmotic pressure
Globulin	Immunity
Fibrinogen	Blood clotting
Food: Glucose, Amino acids, Fat	Nourishment of the body
Vitamins Inorganic Salts: *+ions*: sodium, potassium, calcium, magnesium, iron *−ions*: chlorides, carbonates, bicarbonates, sulfates, phosphates, iodides	Metabolism: Acid-base balance, Osmosis, Water distribution throughout body, Irritability in muscles and nerves
Gases: Oxygen, Carbon dioxide, Nitrogen	Respiration
Hormones	Regulation of body functions
Enzymes	Digestion
Antibodies	Immunity to diseases
Waste products	To rid the body of unnecessary products of cell metabolism.

two external openings are called nostrils. They form the nasal cavity, which is divided into two parts by the nasal septum and separated from the mouth by the palate. The roof of the nasal cavity is formed from bones of the skull and face and is lined with mucous membrane. As air passes through the nasal cavity, it is warmed and moistened through contact with the mucous membrane. The air is also filtered; large foreign particles are caught by minute hairlike structures called cilia. The cilia cause wavelike movements of the particles from the anterior part of the nose to the pharynx. From here, these foreign particles are either expelled from the mouth or swallowed.

b. *The Pharynx.* The *pharynx* is the passageway between the nasal chambers, the nose, and the larynx. The *nasopharynx* is the superior portion of the pharynx and contains the two eustachian tubes which communicate with the middle ear. This provides an easy access for throat and nose infections to spread to the middle ear.

c. *The Larynx.* The *larynx*, or "voice box," is a passageway from the pharynx to the trachea. It is a triangular, cartilaginous structure composed of nine cartilages, joined together by ligaments. It lies in the middle of the neck, between the base of the tongue and the trachea. To prevent food from entering the trachea during the act of swallowing, the larynx moves upward and forward, placing it under the base of the tongue. This causes the epiglottis, a cartilaginous flap lying above the larynx, to move back and downward, directing the food into the esophagus. Knowing how this structure works becomes very important when caring for an unconscious or very ill patient. There is a danger that the

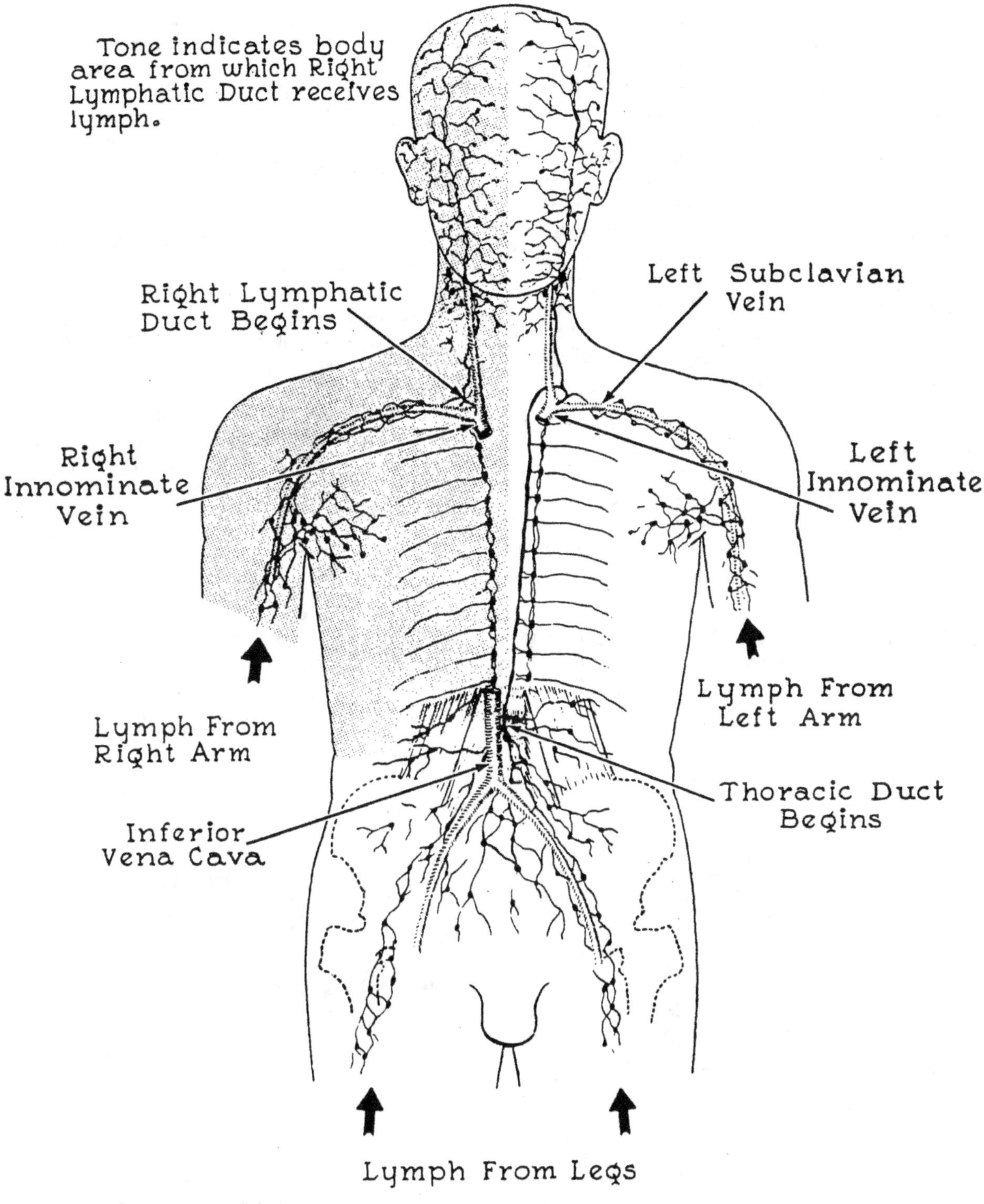

Figure 29. Lymphatic Vessels and Nodes.

tongue and pharyngeal tissues will relax and fall back into the oral pharynx, forcing the epiglottis down over the larynx. This causes obstruction of the airway. It can be relieved by pressing on the lower jaw and pushing it forward, keeping the teeth separated. On some occasions, it may be necessary to grasp the tongue and pull it forward. An artificial airway may be needed as an added precaution.

d. *The Trachea*. The *trachea* extends from the

larynx and terminates when it divides into the right and left bronchi. The trachea is lined with cilia and mucous glands which help entrap dust and foreign matter. The cilia beat upward, moving the particles to the larynx or pharynx, where they can be moved by coughing and expelled from the body.

e. *The Bronchi.* The trachea divides into *two primary bronchi* which convey air from the trachea to the lungs. After entering the lungs, each bronchus divides and sends branches to each lobe of the lungs: three to the right lung and two to the left lung. From here, they further divide into many small branches called bronchioles. These bronchioles go to the alveoli, or air sacs, of the lungs. The alveoli are adapted for easy passage of gases to and from the lung capillaries.

f. *The Lungs.* The *lungs* are the primary organs of respiration. They permit the interchange of gases between the blood and the air. The lungs are contained inside the thoracic cavity and enclosed in the pleurae. The *right lung contains three lobes;* the *left lung contains two lobes.* The lungs are soft and spongy and are constantly changing their form with each respiratory movement.

g. *Diffusion. Diffusion* is the equalization of gases (oxygen and carbon dioxide) between the blood and air. This process takes place in the lungs. Each lung contains thousands of tiny alveoli with blood capillaries in their membrane lining. Here oxygen is theoretically exchanged for carbon dioxide. This exchange also takes place between the capillaries and the tissues of the body. Oxygen cannot be stored by the lung or body tissue, so there is a continuous equalization or exchange of gases. Inhaled air contains about 20 percent oxygen and 0.03 percent carbon dioxide. Exhaled air contains about 16 percent oxygen and 4 percent carbon dioxide.

h. *Pleurae.* The lungs are enclosed in double-walled, serous membranes called the pleurae. Each lung has a separate pleura. The membrane or sac covering the outer surface of the lung is called the visceral layer, and the other layer lining the chest wall is called the parietal layer. The area between these two membranes is called the intrathoracic or pleural space. However, this is only a potential space since the pleural membranes are in very close contact with one another. The only substance separating them is a small amount of pleural fluid, secreted by the membrane. This pleural fluid reduces friction between the two pleural layers during the movements of respiration. Without this fluid a condition known as "dry pleurisy" results, occurring most often in pneumonia. It results in pain because the two pleural membranes rub together (friction fremitus) during each respiration.

i. *The Diaphragm and Intercostal Muscles.* The

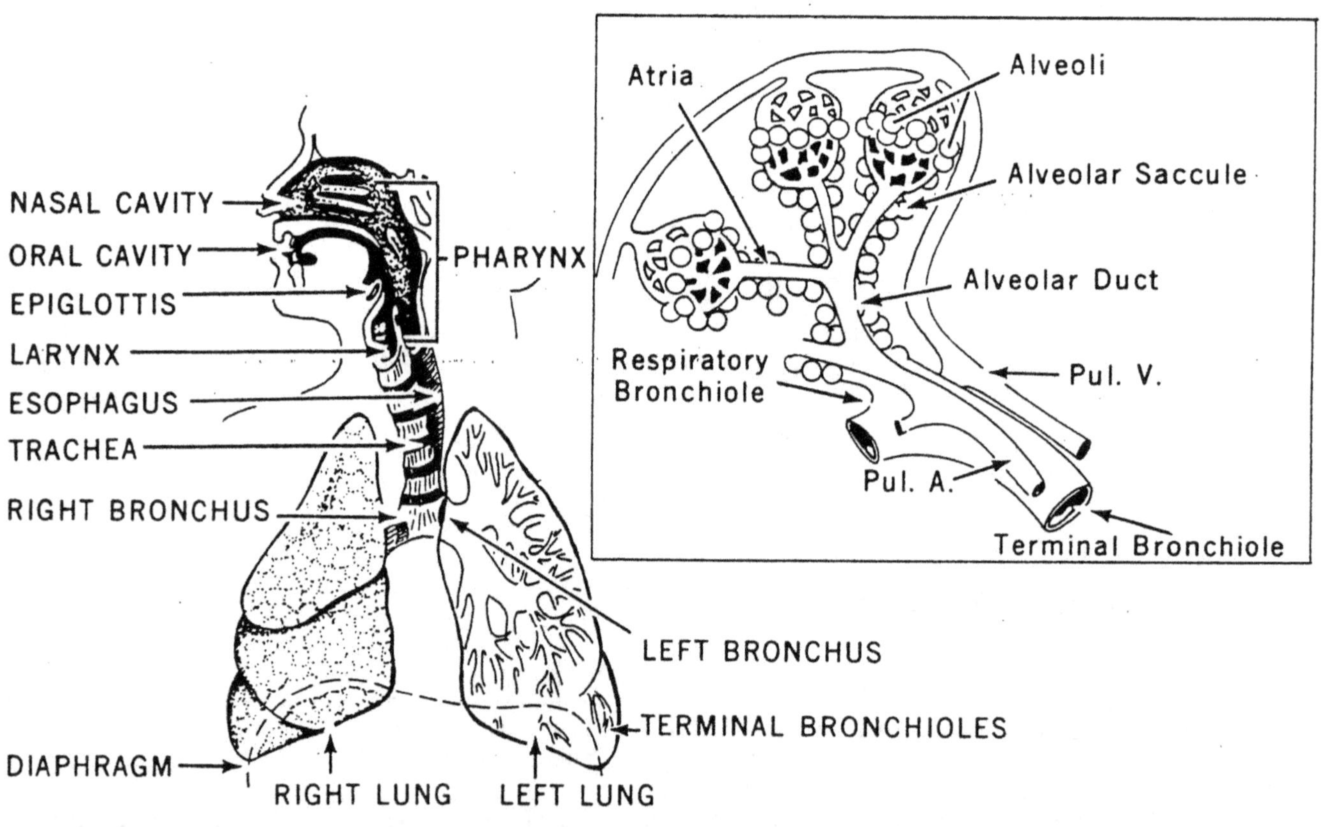

Figure 30. Schematic Drawing of the Lungs and Upper Respiratory Tract.

simple *process of breathing* (inspiration and expiration) is far more complex than it first appears. It is a harmonious interplay of nerve impulses, muscular activity, and mechanical pressure changes, which are all influenced by chemical changes in the blood. The inflation of the lungs occurs because the muscles of respiration contract. These muscles are the *diaphragm* and the *intercostal muscles*.

j. *Inspiration and Expiration.* In the act of *inspiration*, the intercostal muscles contract and help to enlarge the size of the thorax; the ribs move forward and slightly upward, increasing the front-to-back dimensions of the thorax. There is a slight increase in the side-to-side dimensions at the same time. This mechanical change, combined with the downward movement of the diaphragm, enlarges the thorax and produces a pressure decrease in the intrathoracic space—the potential space between the surface of the lungs and the internal lining of the thorax. Since the lungs are inside the thorax, and the interior of the lungs is exposed to the atmospheric pressure outside the body, atmospheric pressure forces air through the conducting passages and into the alveoli. When inspiration is complete, the muscles of inspiration relax, and because of the elasticity of the chest wall and the lungs, expiration occurs.

39. Breathing. Breathing is normally an *involuntary* act controlled by the nervous system. A diffuse group of nerve cells known collectively as the respiratory center is located in the medulla oblongata (brain). The nerve impulses, which cause the muscles of respiration to contract, originate in the cells of the respiratory center. These impulses reach the respiratory muscles by two sets of nerves—the *phrenic nerves* and the *intercostal nerves*. The phrenic nerves pass down into the thorax to the diaphragm. The intercostal nerves leave the spinal cord in the upper region of the back and pass to the intercostal muscles. Nerve impulses from the walls of the alveoli return to the respiratory center through two *vagus nerves* which pass upward through the thorax and neck to the medulla. When the lungs inflate and the walls of the alveoli are stretched to the maximum for the needs of the body at that particular time, nerve impulses return to the respiratory center and stop the impulses to the muscles of inspiration. Passive expiration then follows. This continuing process of inspiration and expiration is primarily involuntary and continues even though a person is asleep or unconscious. *There is a degree of conscious control over breathing*, however. For example, it is possible for a person to hold his or her breath, and it is also possible for the conscious will to control the rate and depth of breathing. This control is from a high voluntary center of the brain in the cerebral cortex. Impulses from these higher centers reach the involuntary respiratory center over specific nerve pathways and temporarily override its automatic function. Nerve impulses from it, then, are in accordance with the desires of the higher center. This control by the higher center is limited by chemical changes in the blood which will occur in time, and the control then reverts back to the involuntary center.

SECTION G—THE DIGESTIVE SYSTEM

40. The Alimentary Canal. The digestive system is divided into two separate divisions—the *alimentary canal* and the *accessory organs of digestion*. The entire system includes all of the organs concerned with the ingestion of food, its absorption, and the nutrition of body cells.

a. *The Mouth.* The mouth contains the *salivary glands*, the *teeth*, and the *tongue*, as illustrated in figure 31. The salivary glands are accessory digestive glands. The teeth aid in the digestive process by masticating food. The tongue is a muscular organ closely associated with the function of taste, mastication, salivation, and swallowing.

b. *The Stomach.* The stomach, shown in figure 32, is a saccular enlargement of the gastrointestinal tract which stores and digests food. It is located in the upper left quadrant of the abdomen just below the diaphragm. Two muscular rings or sphincters guard the entrance to, and the exit from, the stomach. The *cardiac sphincter* at the upper end of the stomach opens and allows food to enter from the esophagus, and the *pyloric sphincter* at the lower end controls the entry of food into the duodenum (the beginning of the small intestine).

(1) Numerous tiny glands in the stomach secrete gastric juice containing enzymes and hydrochloric acid. This gastric juice starts protein digestion. The hydrochloric acid also acts as a disinfectant to destroy any bacteria which may have been taken in with the food. Food remains in the stomach for 3 to 4 hours while peristalsis churns and thoroughly mixes the food with the gastric juices. The result is a semiliquid substance called chyme.

(2) Chyme is released through the pyloric sphincter into the duodenum, where further digestion takes place. Some drugs, a small amount of water, concentrated sugar, and alcohol are absorbed by the stomach, all in small amounts.

c. *The Small Intestine.* The small intestine is a much-coiled muscular tube about 20 feet long. It consists of three parts: the *duodenum*, the *jejunum*, and the *ileum*.

(1) The duodenum is lined with glands which secrete intestinal juices. The bile and pancreatic ducts open into the duodenum, as noted in figure 33.

(2) The jejunum, extending from the duodenum to the ileum, is the middle segment of the small intestine. Minor food absorption takes place here.

(3) The majority of food absorption takes place in the ileum. It is lined with fingerlike processes called villi, which provide a larger absorption area. The villi also contain lymph channels and a network of blood capillaries. After food has been digested, it is absorbed into the capillaries and lymph channels and carried to all parts of the body. Material that cannot be digested and absorbed passes through the ileocecal valve into the large intestine.

d. *The Large Intestine*. The large intestine, often called the colon, consists of the cecum, ascending colon, transverse colon, descending colon, sigmoid colon, and the rectum. The large intestine is about 5 feet in length and about 2 inches in diameter. It absorbs water from the liquid contents it receives.

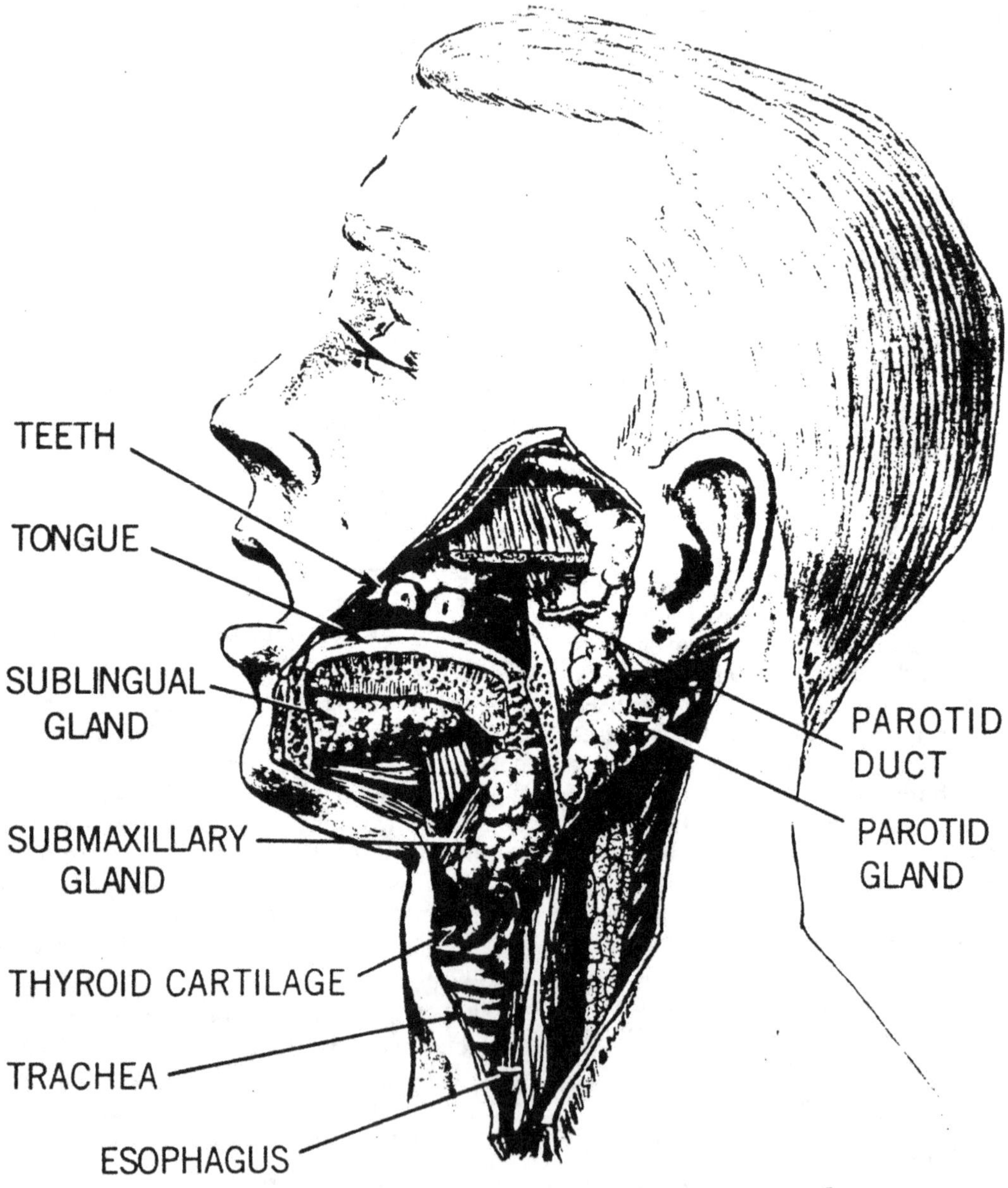

Figure 31. Upper Alimentary Tract.

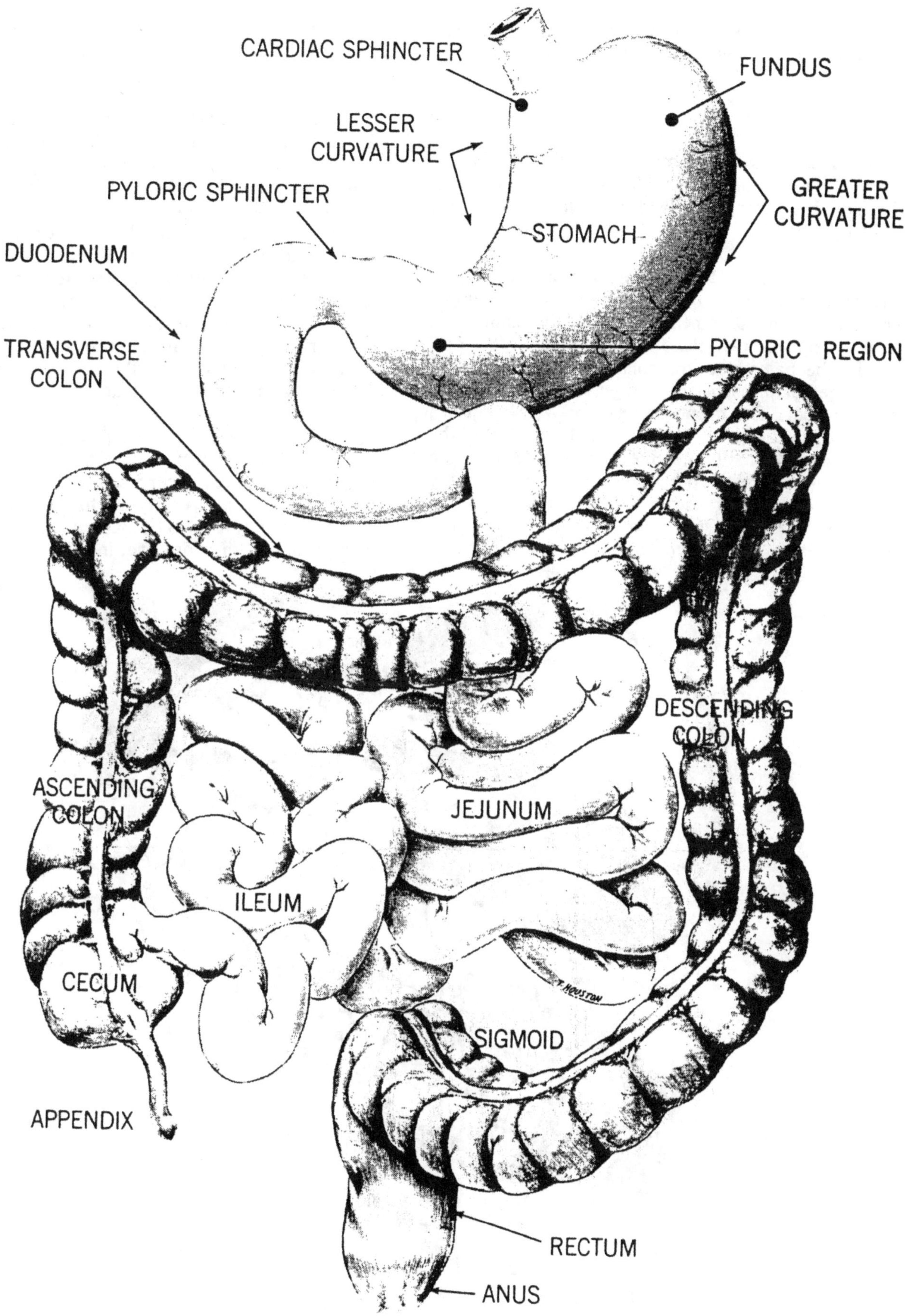

Figure 32. Stomach and Intestines.

Glands in its walls secrete mucus, which mixes with the remaining material and helps form the stool or feces.

41. The Accessory Organs of Digestion. The accessory organs of digestion, illustrated in figure 33, include the liver, gallbladder, pancreas, and the salivary glands.

a. *The Liver.* The liver is one of the largest glands in the body; it is located in the right upper quadrant of the abdomen just below the diaphragm. It is a very vascular gland and is divided into lobes. Each lobe has a duct for collecting bile. The ducts join together in each lobe and leave the liver as the hepatic duct. The hepatic artery and vein furnish a rich supply of blood to the liver. All blood from the stomach and small intestines passes through the liver by means of the portal vein. The liver not only *aids in digestion,* it also *aids in the metabolism of carbohydrates, proteins, and fats; helps maintain the proper level of sugar in the blood; produces heparin and fibrinogen which influence the clotting of blood; and detoxifies substances which might be harmful to the human body.*

b. *The Gallbladder.* The duct system of the liver transports bile from the liver cells to the duodenum or to the gallbladder for storage. The gallbladder is a reservoir for concentrating and storing bile. It is about 3 to 4 inches long and has a capacity of about 50 cm³. It is shaped somewhat like a blackjack and is located in a hollow on the underside of the liver. Its duct, the cystic duct, joins the hepatic duct from the liver to form the common bile duct, which enters the duodenum at the ampulla of Vater. When food arrives in the duodenum, the gallbladder contracts and bile is sent through the cystic duct into the common bile duct and into the duodenum.

c. *The Pancreas.* The pancreas is a long gland with its body or main part lying below the liver and the stomach, and adjacent to the duodenum. Its "tail" extends transversely to the left and terminates near the spleen. The pancreas provides pancreatic juice and the hormone, insulin.

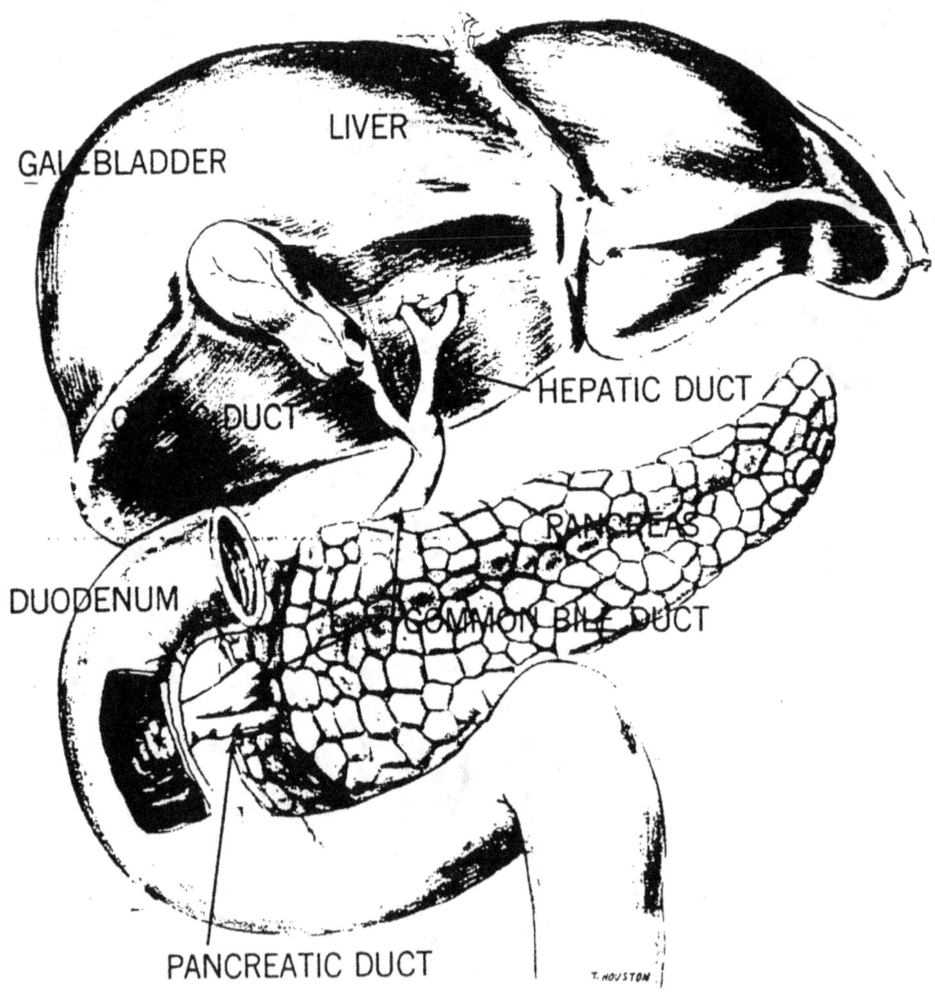

Figure 33. Accessory Organs of Digestion.

d. *The Salivary Glands.* The salivary glands are located in the mouth and are named according to their location.

42. Effect of the Nervous System. The digestive process is also affected by the nervous system. For example, sympathetic impulses that speed up the heart rate and respiratory rate will slow the digestive process. This phenomenon is often evident when a patient has sustained injuries in an accident. Because of the excitement, the digestive processes are delayed, and the stomach may remain filled with undigested food for a long period of time. If the patient is given general anesthetic, the anesthetist must be constantly alert for vomiting as *the anesthetized patient is unable to swallow.* Therefore, any vomitus might be drawn into the trachea and result in suffocation.

SECTION H—THE ENDOCRINE SYSTEM

43. The Glands of Internal Secretion. The endocrine system is composed of the *glands of internal secretion.* They are called ductless and internal glands because they have no ducts to carry away their secretions. Their secretions enter directly into the blood or lymph circulation and eventually reach the organ or organs which they influence or control. Very small quantities of hormones are produced with only a small amount necessary to produce an effect. Some hormones may influence only one part of the body, while others influence the body as a whole. The hormone-producing glands are the pituitary, thyroid, parathyroid, adrenals, pancreas, gonads, intestinal, the pineal body, and the thymus gland. These glands are shown in figure - 34.

a. The pituitary gland is a small gland that has a tremendous influence on the body. It is often referred to as the "master gland," since it has regulatory control over the functions of other glands. It has an *anterior* and a *posterior* lobe and secretes at least nine hormones. Hormones produced by the anterior lobe of the pituitary are growth, thyrotropic, gonadotropic, adrenocorticotropic, and lactogenic. Antidiuretic hormones, vasopressin, and oxytoxin are produced by the posterior lobe of the pituitary gland.

b. The thyroid gland (largest of the endocrine glands) is a butterfly-shaped gland lying in the anterior middle portion of the neck, just below the larynx. It consists of two lateral lobes united by a strip called the isthmus. It has an abundant blood supply furnished by branches of the external carotid and the subclavian arteries. It produces a hormone called thyroxin, which is about 65 percent iodine. Thyroxin performs many functions. It regulates the rate of oxidation and the heat production of the body; it is concerned with growth and differentiation of body organs; it plays a part in mental development; and indirectly affects sexual maturity. It also plays a part in the distribution and the exchange of water, salts, and proteins and has some influence in the production of glucose from amino acids.

c. The adrenal glands are sometimes called the suprarenal glands, since they lie like small caps on the top of each kidney. Each gland has two parts, the medulla and the cortex, and each part produces a different hormone.

(1) The medulla secretes *epinephrine* and norephrine. Epinephrine is one of the most powerful vasopressors known; it increases blood pressure, accelerates the heart muscle, and increases cardiac output. Epinephrine (adrenalin) is used as a cardiac stimulant, a pressor (increases blood pressure) substance, and to relax bronchial smooth muscles.

(2) The cortex secretes several hormones called *cortisones.* The cortex is stimulated by the pituitary hormone. *ACTH* (adrenocorticotropic hormone). Hormones secreted by the cortex help to regulate muscular activity, reproduction, salt metabolism, water electrolyte balance, and kidney function.

d. The pancreas is located behind the stomach and is a double-functioning gland; it produces secretions which are discharged into the duodenum (exocrine or duct gland) and insulin which is discharged into the blood stream (endocrine or ductless gland). *Insulin* is a hormone essential for the use and storage of carbohydrates by the body.

e. The gonads serve a double function in both sexes—the development of reproductive cells (ova and sperm) and the production of hormones.

(1) The principal hormone of the testes is *testosterone.* It regulates the development of secondary sex characteristics, such as hair on the chest and face, deeper voice, and general development of the male stature.

(2) The principal hormones of the female are *estrogen* and *progesterone.* Estrogen is responsible for the secondary sex characteristics, such as body form and development of the mammary glands. Progesterone is responsible for changes in the uterine lining during the second half of the menstrual cycle. It prepares the uterus for the implantation of the fertilized ovum, and for the development of the embryo in the early stages of its growth. It also supplements the action of estrogen on the mammary glands during pregnancy.

f. Other glands which must be considered are the intestinal, the pineal, and the thymus glands. The

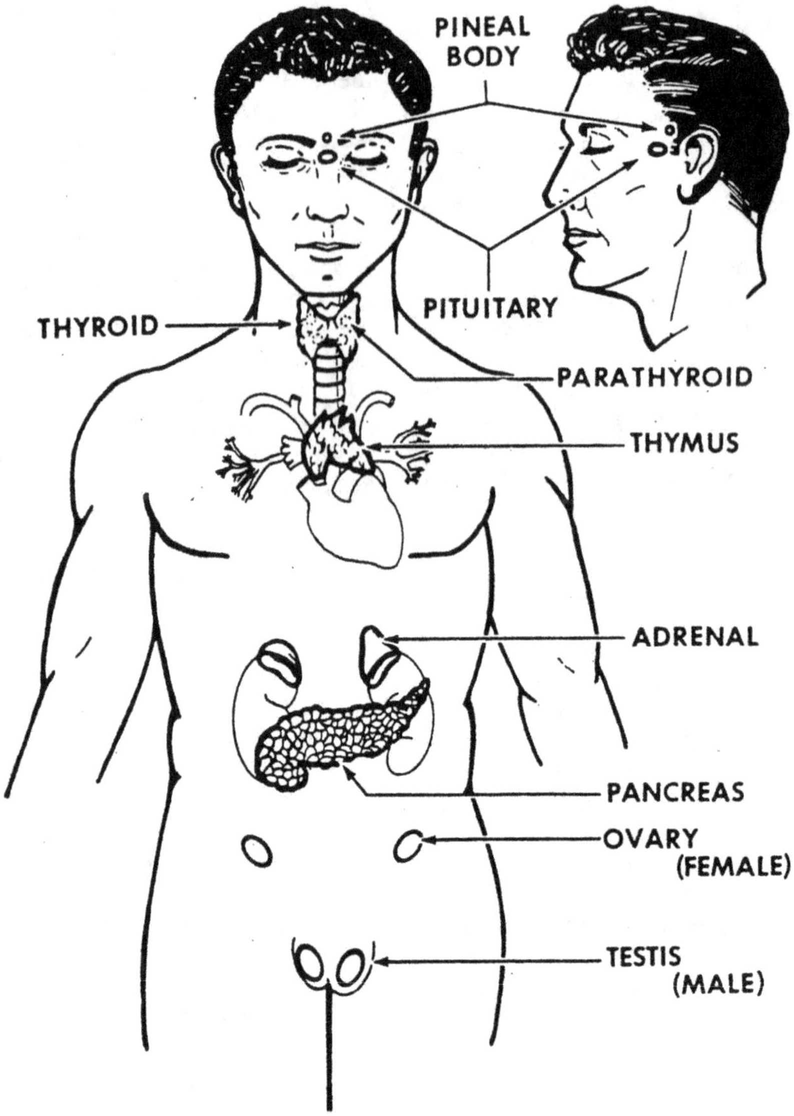

Figure 34. Locations and Approximate Locations of the Endocrine Glands.

intestinal glands secrete a hormone called secretin. Secretin stimulates the secretion of pancreatic juice and bile. The pineal gland is a small gland located within the midpoint of the brain. Its endocrine secretion and function are uncertain. The thymus gland lies within the midline of the chest cavity. Its function is also obscure.

44. The Effect of Endocrine Glands on Surgical Decisions. The functions of the endocrine glands have a decided effect on the decision of the surgeon to remove any one of these glands. If it is deemed necessary to remove the total gland, the doctor must consider the necessity of administering the hormone, originally produced by the gland, by artificial means. For this reason, the surgeon often removes only part of a gland and leaves intact any normal portion which he or she thinks will continue to secrete hormones.

45. Effect of the Endocrine Glands on General Health. Another problem which the surgeon must consider before undertaking procedures that don't actually involve the endocrine organs is that of malfunction of these organs to the extent that ordinary body processes cannot be properly maintained during or after an operative procedure. Treatment of an endocrine malfunction may be necessary before even routine surgery is undertaken.

SECTION I—THE URINARY SYSTEM

46. Anatomy of the Urinary System. The urinary system includes the organs that are concerned with the production and elimination of urine. This system consists of the kidneys, the ureters, the urinary bladder, and the urethra. These structures secrete and eliminate urine, a liquid waste product of cell metabolism. Figure 35 illustrates the structures of the urinary system.

a. *The Kidneys.* The kidneys are paired, bean-shaped organs, located on each side of the vertebral column, posterior to the abdominal cavity, at about the level of the 12th rib. Each is surrounded by fat and connective tissue, and enclosed in a fibrous-type capsule. Each kidney is about 1 inch thick, 2 inches wide, and 4 inches long. It weighs about 6 ounces. The right kidney is slightly lower than the left because of the position of the liver.

(1) The kidney is a highly complex organ with three important functions: to filter the blood, discarding materials no longer needed; to maintain water and electrolyte balance; and to maintain acid-base balance.

(2) Each kidney has two main layers. The outer layer, called the *cortex* and an inner layer called the *medulla*. The medulla contains a number of cone-shaped divisions called pyramids. These pyramids extend into the renal pelvis, which in turn, empties into the ureter.

(3) The artery and vein supplying each kidney are the *renal* artery and the renal vein. The renal artery comes directly from the abdominal aorta, and the renal vein enters the inferior vena cava.

(4) As blood flows through the kidneys, it is filtered and purified by nephron units. Each nephron unit consists of a series of tiny tubules. Each tubule extends from the capsule and joins with other tubules in the medulla region; it descends, loops, ascends, twists, and then terminates into a single collecting tube. The products of filtration pass through the collecting tubules into the funnel-shaped pyramids, to the calyces, and then to the renal pelvis, where they finally enter the ureters. These units are responsible for all the filtering, excreting, and reabsorbing that takes place within the kidneys. A cross section of a kidney is illustrated in figure 36.

b. *Urine.* The end product of kidney filtration is urine. Normally it is amber-colored, free of bacteria, and about 95 percent water. The other 5 percent is made-up of various organic and inorganic compounds. Under normal conditions, an adult excretes from 1500 to 2000 cm^3 of urine in 24 hours. However, this amount can be influenced by such factors as body temperature, humidity, and fluid intake.

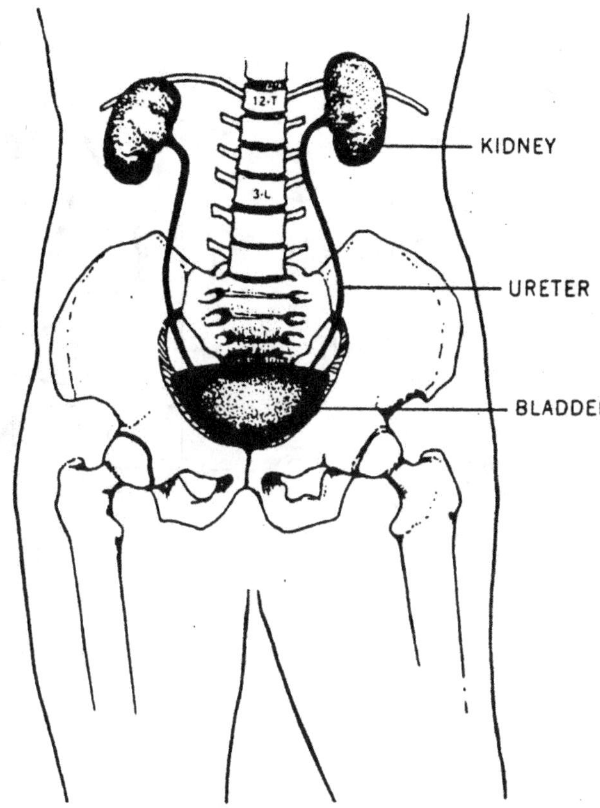

Figure 35. The Urinary System.

SECTION J—THE REPRODUCTIVE SYSTEM

47. Purpose of the Reproductive System. The primary purpose of the reproductive system is to allow for a union of male and female sex cells.

a. *Male Reproductive System.* The male organs of reproduction are the penis, testes, and the associated ducts and glands. The entire system is shown in figure 37.

(1) The *testes* are oval glands suspended by the spermatic cords in a cutaneous pouch, the scrotum. They perform two functions: production of spermatozoa and secretion of the male sex hormone, testosterone. Lying closely adjacent to the superior pole of each testis is the epididymis, a ductal system that collects and transmits sperm cells from the testis. The epididymis runs down the length of the testicle, then turns upward as a straight tube and becomes the vas deferens.

(2) The *scrotum* is part of the male external genitalia. It is a pouchlike sac containing the testes and a part of the spermatic cord. The scrotum, hanging between the legs, exposes the testes to a temperature lower than that of the body, which is

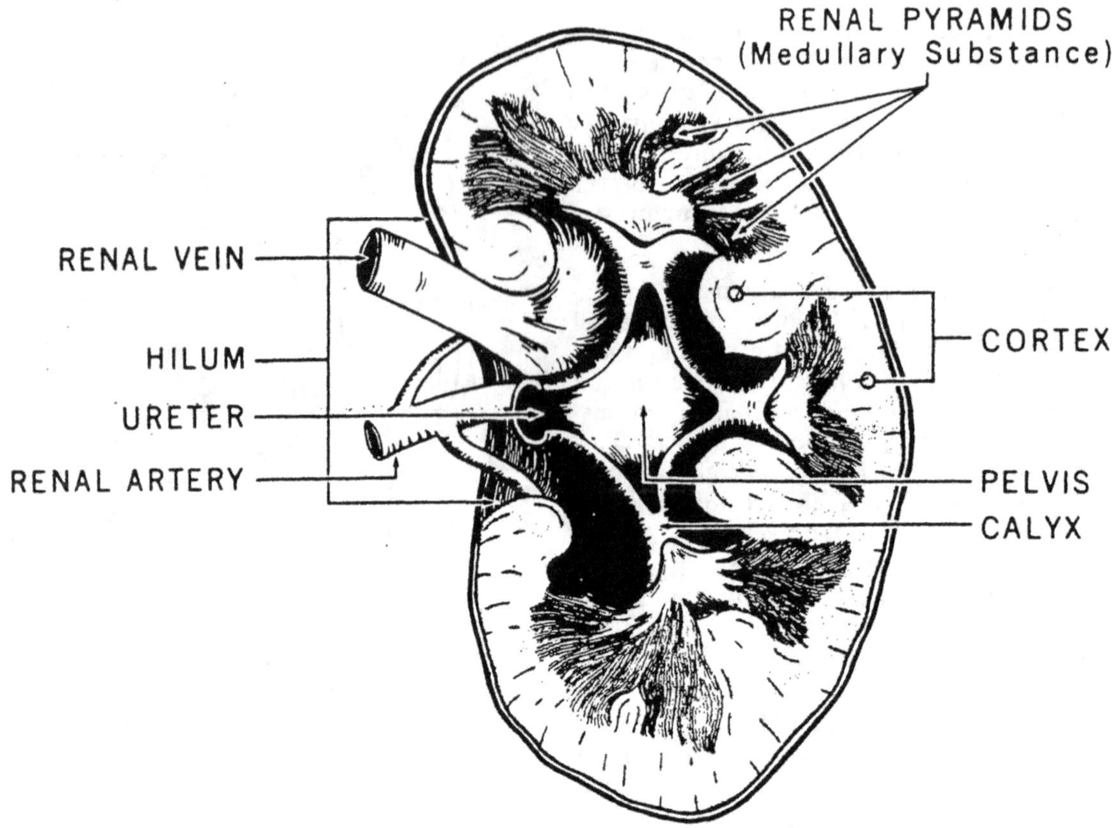

Figure 36. Cross Section of Kidney.

essential for proper development of sperm. Occasionally, a child is born with the testes undescended. This condition, called cryptorchidism, is corrected by surgery.

(3) Two *spermatic cords* each of which suspends and supplies a testis, are formed by the *vas deferens,* spermatic artery, vein, lymphatic vessels, and nerves, and are bound together by connective tissue.

(4) The *vas deferens* (ductus deferens) is a small convoluted tube about 2 feet long that carries sperm cells from the epididymis to the seminal vesicle. There they join and form the ejaculatory duct.

(5) The *seminal vesicles* are two pouches that lie just above the prostate, between the bladder and the rectum. They secrete seminal fluid and serve as a storage place for testicular secretion which is expelled at the time of ejaculation.

(6) The vas deferens and the duct from the seminal vesicles converge and form the ejaculatory duct which leads into the prostatic urethra. Testicular secretion is forced through the ejaculatory duct into the urethra by muscle contraction.

(7) The *prostate gland* is made-up of the smooth muscle and granular tissue that surrounds the proximal portion of the urethra. It resembles a chestnut in size and shape, and secretes an alkaline fluid into the urethra during ejaculation. This fluid keeps the sperm mobile and protects them from the acid secretions of the female vagina. The prostate gland can also be the source of considerable trouble in later life. It has a tendency to enlarge, which may interfere with urination by shutting off the urethra. It also has a tendency to develop cancer and may be surgically removed. Removal is called a prostatectomy. Surgical removal can be accomplished by several different surgical approaches. The physician's choice usually depends upon the age of the patient, the reason for the removal, and the size of the prostate gland.

b. *Female Reproductive System.* The female reproductive system, shown in figure 38, includes the ovaries, fallopian tubes, uterus, vagina, and external genitalia. Although the perineum and the mammary glands are not part of the system, they are clearly associated with its function.

(1) The *ovaries* are two almond-shaped glands that lie on each side of the uterus near the ends of the fallopian tubes. Connecting the ovaries to the uterus are the ovarian ligaments. The ovaries pro-

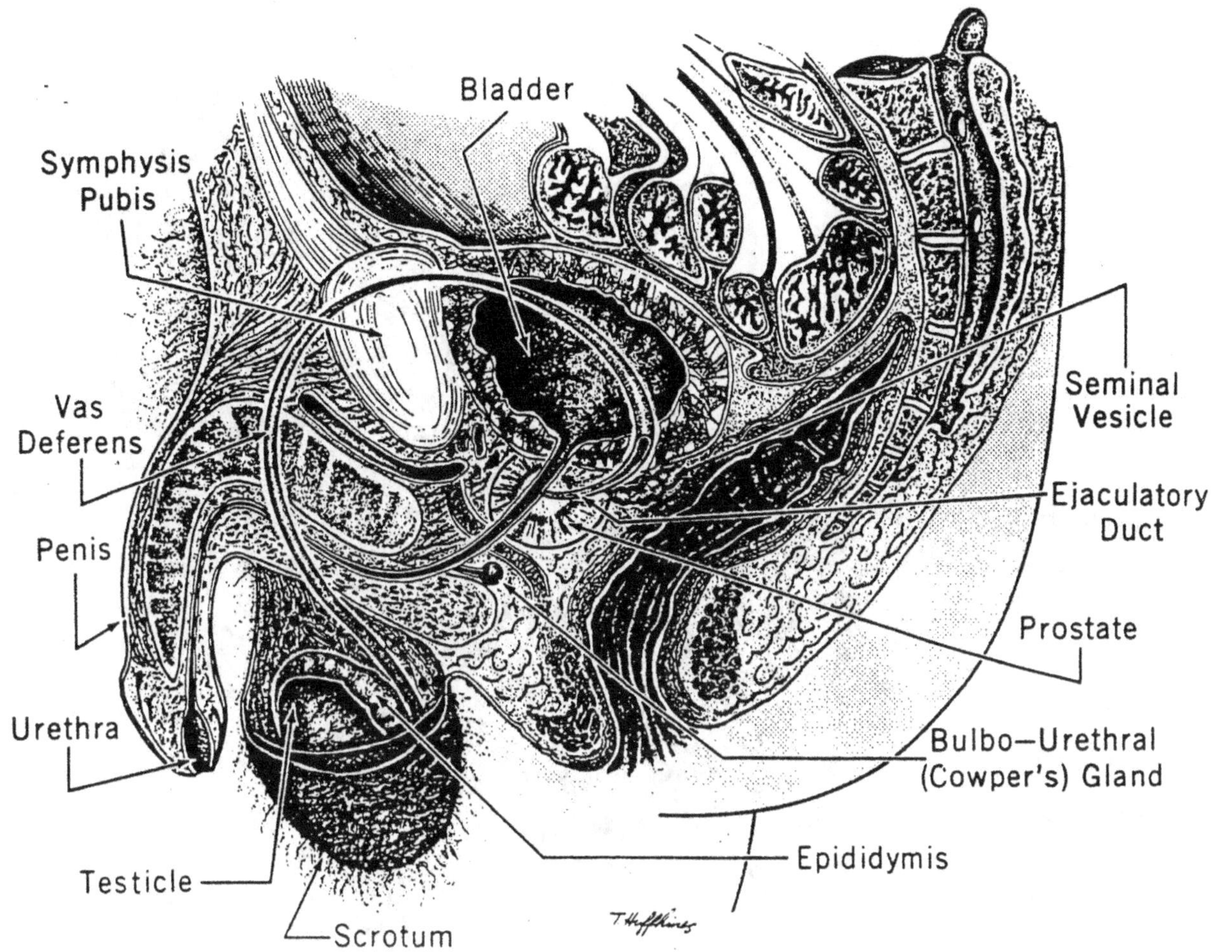

Figure 37. Organs of the Male Reproductive System

duce the female sex cells (ova, or eggs) and the female hormones (estrogen and progesterone). At birth each ovary contains hundreds of potential ova. At puberty, around the age of 12, an ovum matures and is discharged from the ovary. This process is repeated about every 28 days for approximately 30 years. Normally only one ovum matures at a time, with the two ovaries alternating the process at monthly intervals. The discharge of this ovum is called ovulation.

(2) The hormones produced by the ovaries are estrogen and progesterone, which control the sexual development of the female. They are responsible for the form the female body takes, the development of the mammary glands, and the normal functioning of the genital system.

(3) The *fallopian tubes* or, as they are sometimes called, uterine tubes, are two hollow tubes, about 4 inches long, which convey the ovum from an ovary to the uterus.

(4) These tubes lie close to, and partially surround, an ovary, but there is no direct communication between the two. The ovum is actually discharged from an ovary out into the abdominal cavity, where it migrates into the expanded portion of the fallopian tube. The ovum then migrates further into the fallopian tube. If coition has taken place and sperm cells are in the tube, fertilization (union of the male and female sex cells) normally takes place. The "united cell," or the fertilized ovum, then passes through the tube and into the uterus. If no sperm cells are present, the ovum is not fertilized. It fails to develop and disintegrates in its passage to the uterus.

(5) The *uterus* (or womb) is a pear-shaped organ located in the pelvis, between the bladder and the rectum. It is a thick-walled organ measuring about 3 inches in length, 2 inches in width, and 1 inch in thickness in its nonpregnant state. The uterus can be divided into three communicating sections—the fundus, the body, and the cervix. The fundus is the superior portion lying just above the openings for the fallopian tubes. The body is the large, expanded, middle portion. The cervix is the narrow, cylindrical portion just below the uterine body. The cervix is that part of the uterus that protrudes into the vagina. The uterus is held in

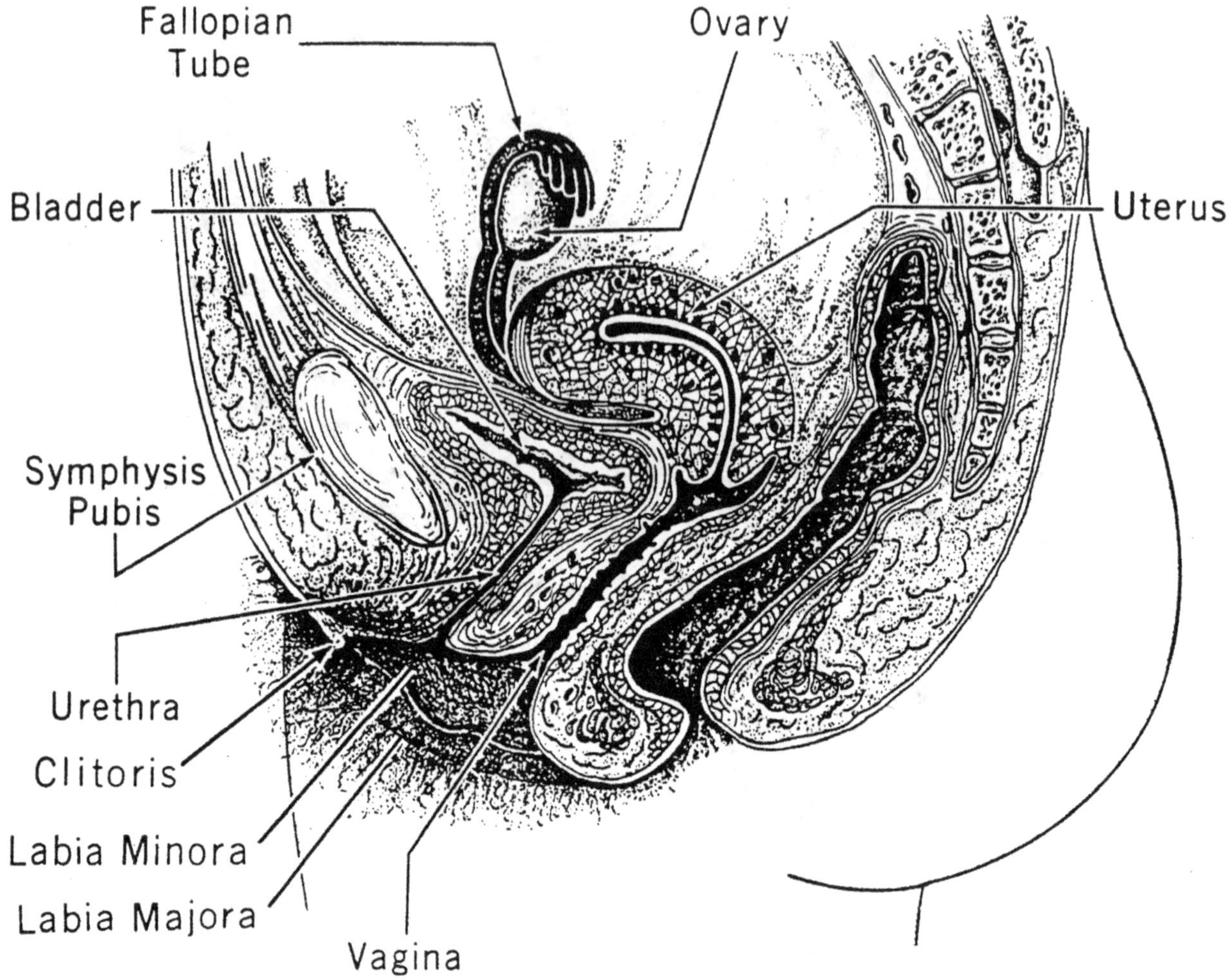

Figure 38. Organs of the Female Reproductive System.

place by several large and strong ligaments. During pregnancy, the uterus increases to several times its normal size, as it houses the unborn child.

(6) The *vagina* is a collapsible musculomembranous canal located between the urethra and the rectum, and behind the urinary bladder. It is about 3 inches in length with its lower opening partially closed by a fold of mucous membrane called the hymen. The hymen covers the vaginal orifice only in the virginal state. The vagina has three essential functions. It serves as an excretory passage for the menstrual flow; it is the female organ of intercourse, receiving the seminal fluid from the male; and it forms the lower part of the birth canal through which the newborn child is delivered. Tissue changes during pregnancy permit the vagina to become greatly distended during the birth of the baby.

(7) The *external genitalia*, collectively referred to as the vulva, include the mons pubis, labia majora, labia minora, clitoris, vestibule, and hymen. Together they serve a secretory and protective function.

(8) The *perineum* is the external surface of the pelvic floor. It includes the area between the anus and the vaginal opening. It is made-up of muscles and fascia which support the pelvic organs. During childbirth this area is often lacerated, or it may be incised to prevent tearing and to facilitate delivery. When a perineal incision is made, the procedure is called an episiotomy.

(9) Anatomically, the breasts, or *mammary glands*, are large, modified skin glands, and belong to the integumentary system. However, their development and function are related to the reproductive system, because their growth and development are regulated by hormones from the ovaries and pituitary glands. The mammary glands undergo noticeable change in the female at puberty, during pregnancy, during and after lactation, and at menopause. Their purpose is milk production for the newborn infant. On occasion, cystic masses occur in breast

tissue, and these, as well as several types of malignant and nonmalignant tumors, are the cause of surgical procedures which range from minor biopsies to radical mastectomies.

(10) *Menstruation* is the periodic sloughing off of the endometrial lining of the uterus. Each month the uterine lining becomes thicker, the blood supply is increased, and hormones are secreted to prepare the uterus for a fertilized ovum. This lining is not needed if the ovum has not been fertilized, and it is expelled through the vagina in the form of a bloody discharge. When an ovum is fertilized and the woman becomes pregnant, the menstrual periods cease until the infant is born.

(11) Pregnancy is that period of time between fertilization and birth, during which the fetus is developing within the uterus. A pregnancy that terminates from premature expulsion of a nonviable fetus is called abortion. Occasionally, the ovum develops outside the uterus, resulting in an ectopic pregnancy. The most common site of an ectopic pregnancy is the fallopian tube. Abortion may necessitate surgical intervention and ectopic pregnancy must be surgically terminated.

c. *Considerations Prior to Surgery*. The surgeon must consider both the hormonal and sex cell functions of the gonads when procedures involving the reproductive organs are being performed.

SECTION K—THE INTEGUMENTARY SYSTEM

48. The Skin. Skin is composed of epidermis and dermis. The epidermis is made-up of epithelial tissue. Below this, as can be seen in figure 3–39, is the dermis, which is composed of connective tissue. Located throughout are the various sweat glands and ducts; hair roots and follicles; sebaceous glands; capillaries, and nerve endings for pain, heat, cold, touch, and pressure. The ceruminous glands that secrete earwax, the mammary glands, and the nails are also considered derivatives of the skin.

49. Functions of the Skin. The skin excretes waste in sweat, secretes exocrine glandular materials, cools or warms the blood through the dilatation and constriction of capillaries, receives sensory nerve stimulation, and acts as a protective shield against the entrance of infectious agents.

50. The Healing Process. Since the majority of surgical procedures require an incision, it is well to

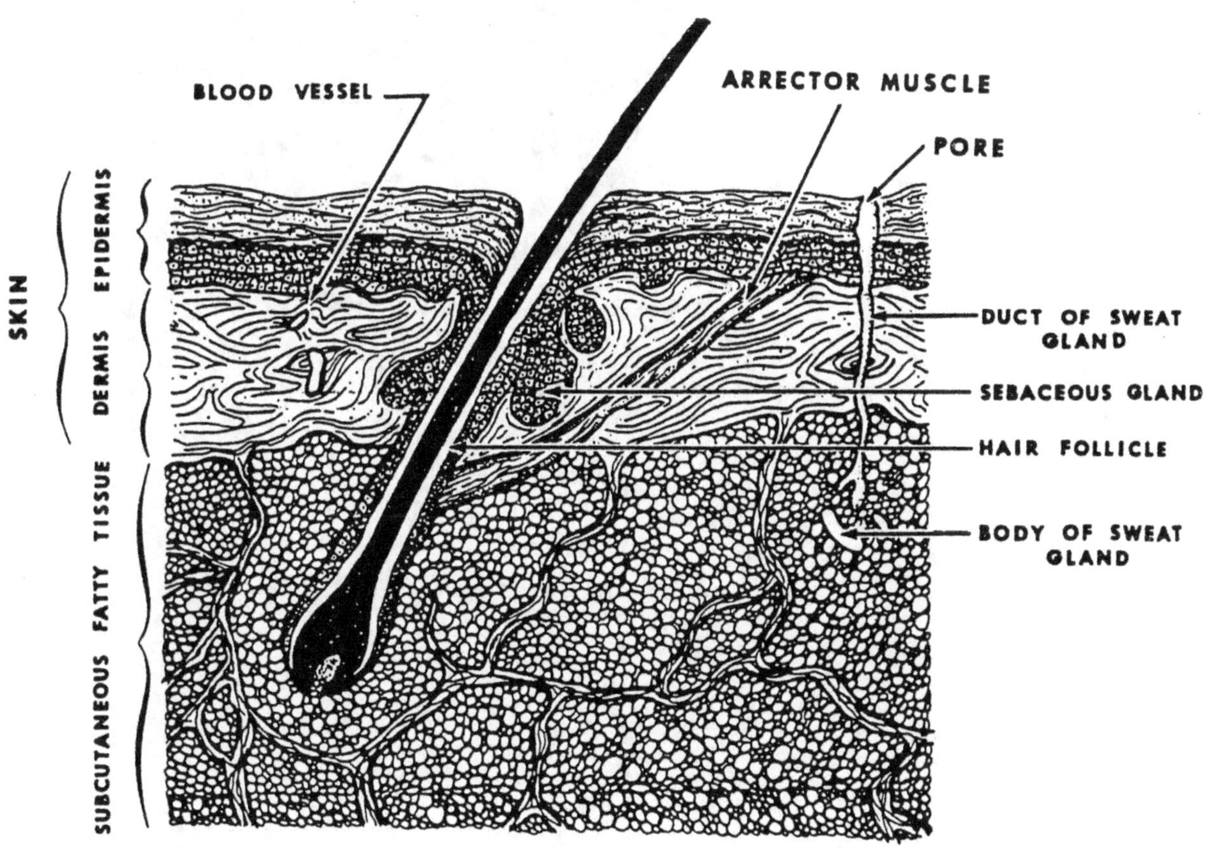

Figure 39. Cross Section of Skin.

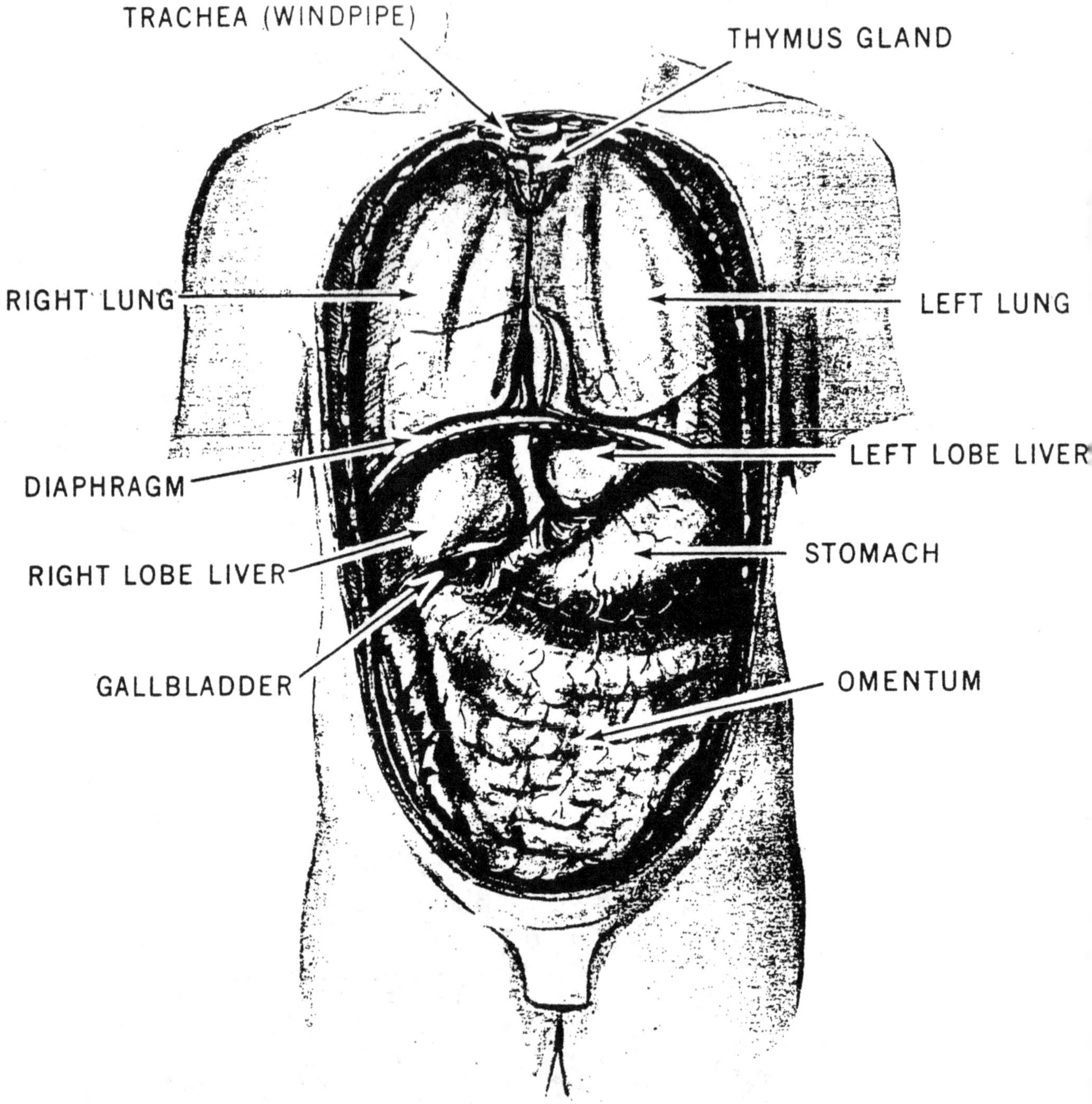

Figure 40. Organs as They Occupy the Thoracic and Abdominal Cavities.

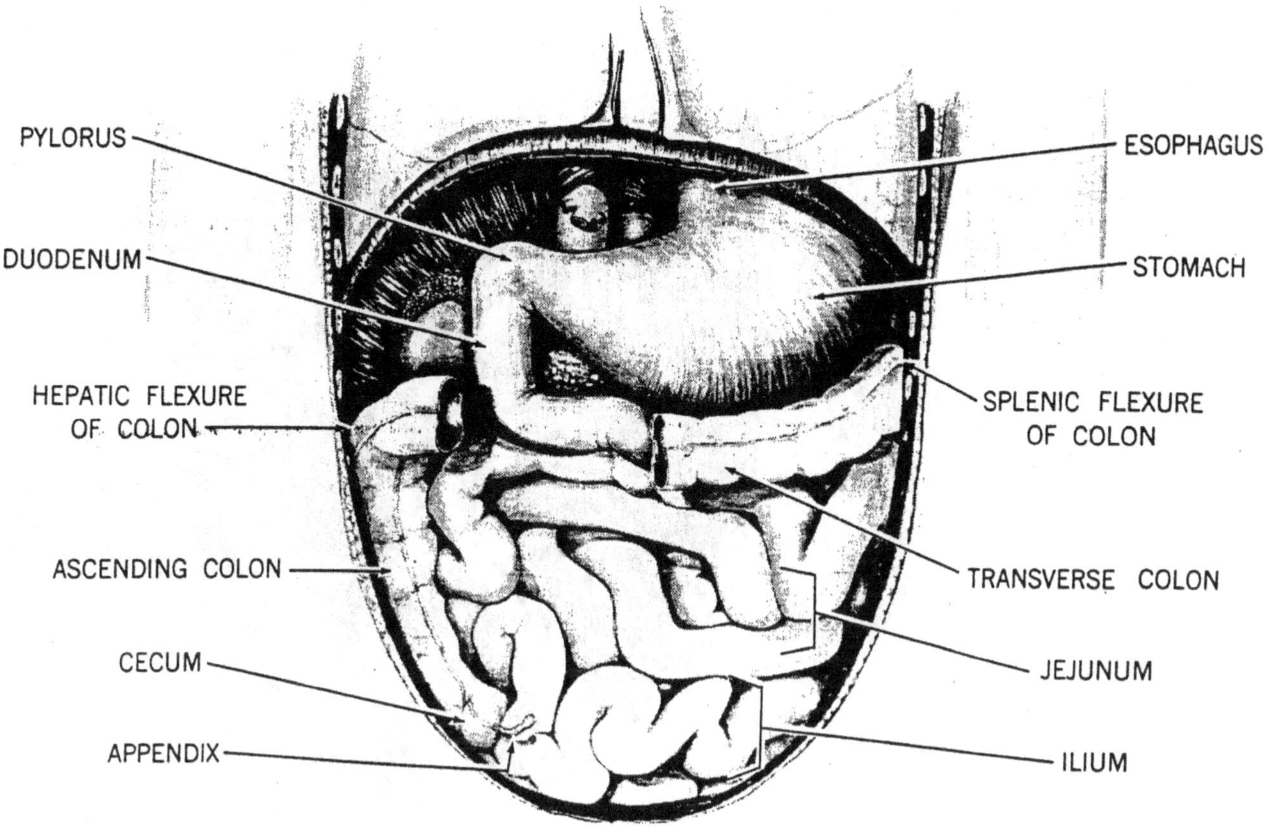

Figure ³ 40. Continued.

know the role of the integumentary system in the healing process and in the formation of scar tissue. The minute bleeding into cut edges and the intact living cells on either side of the incision go through a process whereby new cells are formed. These new cells stretch across the wound and gradually close it. This is called healing by "first intention" or without scar formation. Healing by "second intention" is more common among wounds that have been made by a surgical incision. This involves the filling of the area between the wound edges with granulation tissue formed by the blood and connective tissue cells. This process tends to start in the deeper areas of the wound and work its way toward the surface. This process results in tough, pinkish-gray tissue known as a scar.

SECTION L—THE ORGANS AS THEY OCCUPY THE THORACIC AND ABDOMINAL CAVITIES

51. Interrelationship and Interdependence of the Body Systems. The various systems of the body are interrelated and interdependent. Although each is studied separately, it is necessary to understand how they are situated within the body in relationship to each other. See figure · 40 which shows the organs as they occupy the thoracic and abdominal cavities and how each structure would be exposed through a thoraco-abdominal incision. The nervous system, the circulatory system, and the numerous layers of connective tissue have been eliminated to provide a clear picture of the internal structures.

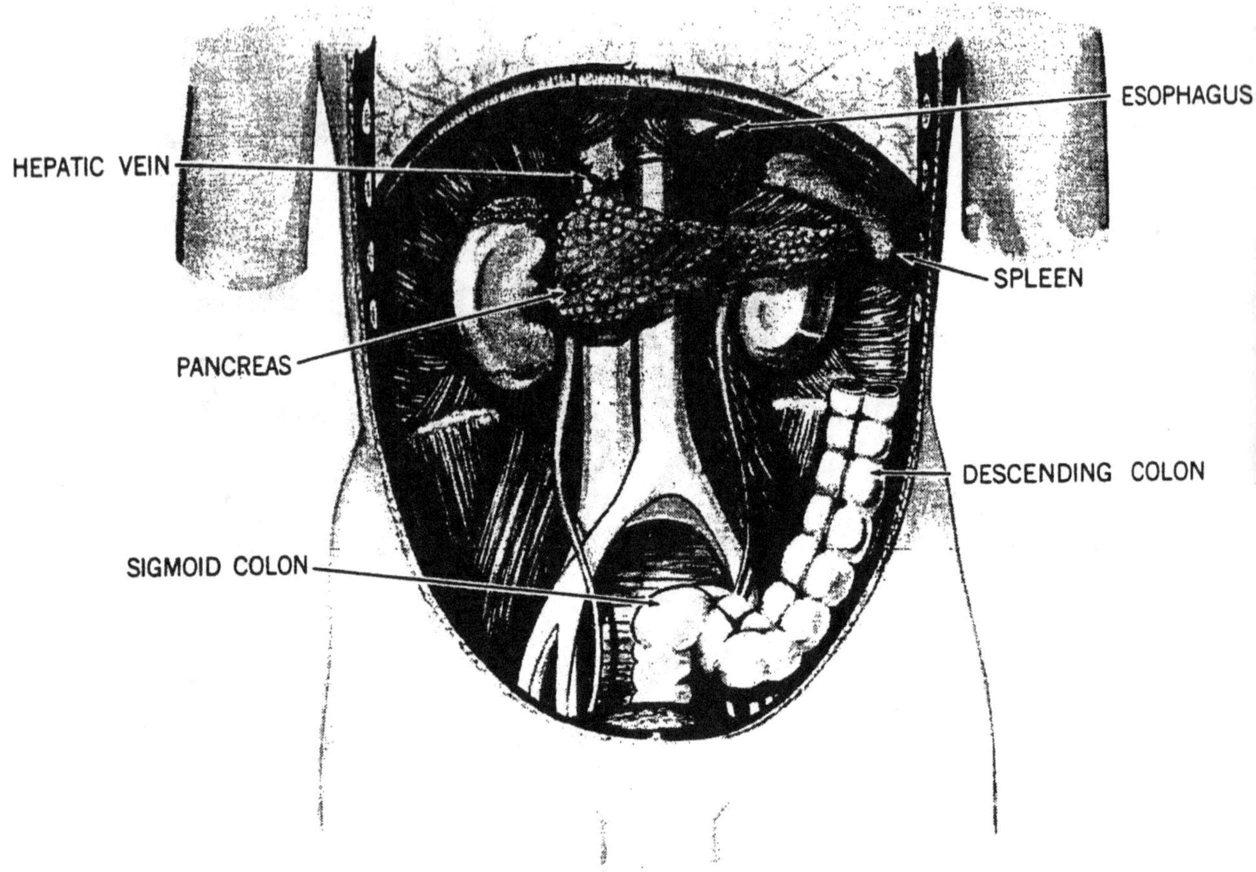

Figure 40. Continued.

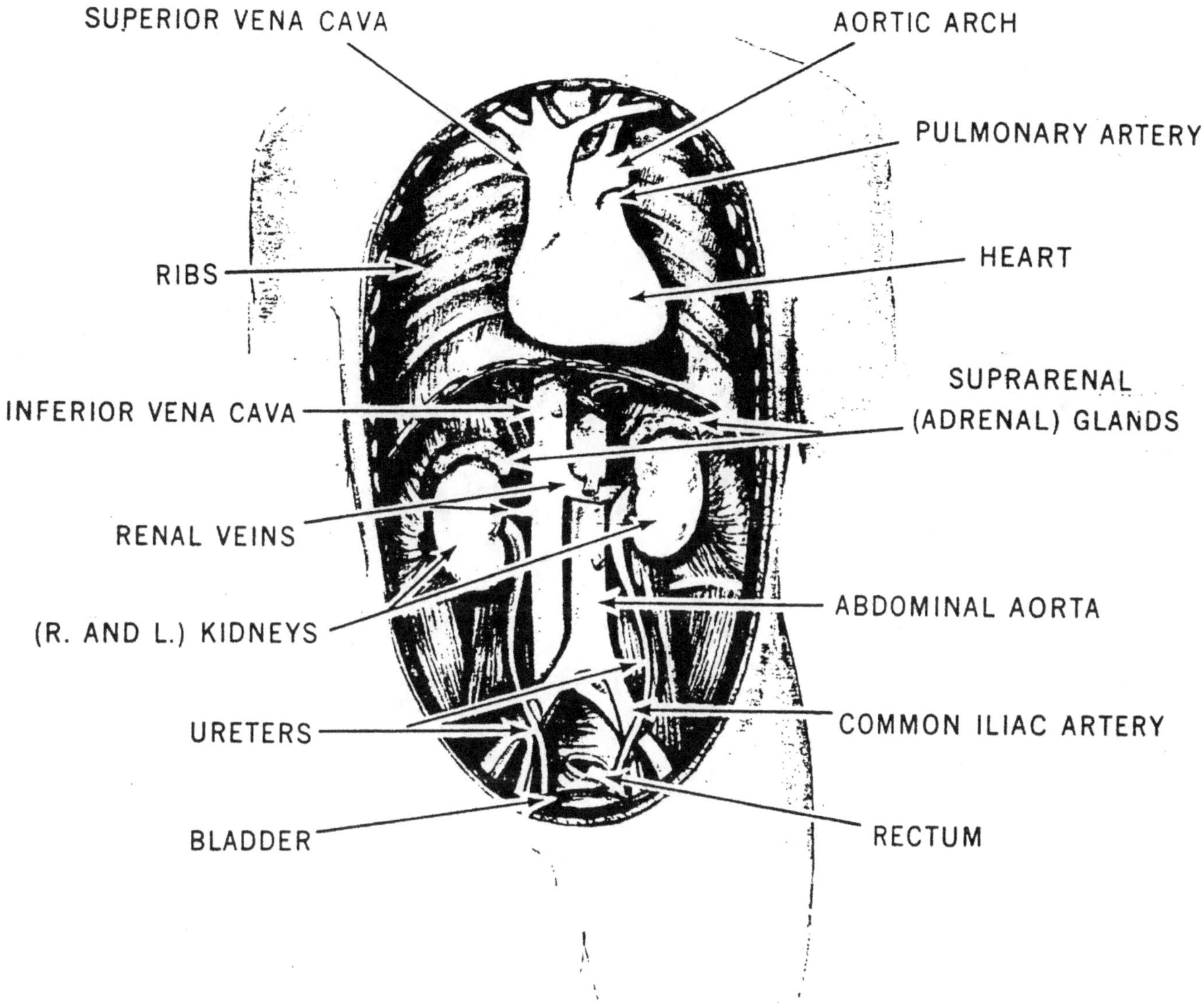

Figure 40. Continued.

www.ingramcontent.com/pod-product-compliance
Lightning Source LLC
LaVergne TN
LVHW080022210926
848481LV00011B/3089

* 9 7 8 1 7 9 9 3 5 8 0 4 6 *